Medical-
Surgical
Nursing

LIPPINCOTT
MANUAL *of*
NURSING
PRACTICE
POCKET
GUIDES

Medical-Surgical Nursing

Lippincott Williams & Wilkins
a Wolters Kluwer business
Philadelphia · Baltimore · New York · London
Buenos Aires · Hong Kong · Sydney · Tokyo

The clinical treatments described and recommended in this publication are based on research and consultation with nursing, medical, and legal authorities. To the best of our knowledge, these procedures reflect currently accepted practice. Nevertheless, they can't be considered absolute and universal recommendations. For individual applications, all recommendations must be considered in light of the patient's clinical condition and, before administration of new or infrequently used drugs, in light of the latest package-insert information. The authors and publisher disclaim any responsibility for any adverse effects resulting from the suggested procedures, from any undetected errors, or from the reader's misunderstanding of the text.

Library of Congress
Cataloging-in-Publication Data

Medical-surgical nursing.
    p. ; cm.—(Lippincott manual of nursing practice pocket guides)
   Includes bibliographical references and index.
   1. Operating room nursing—Handbooks, manuals, etc. I. Lippincott Williams & Wilkins. II. Title. III. Series.
   [DNLM: 1. Perioperative Nursing—Handbooks. WY 49 M4892 2007]
RD32.3.M42 2007
617'.0231--dc22
ISBN 1-58255-897-3 (alk. paper) 2006002039

Contents

Contributors
and consultants

Katrina Davis Allen, RN, MSN, CCRN
Nursing Faculty (ADN) Program
Faulkner State Community College
Bay Minette, Ala.

Mary Ann Boucher, RN, APRN,BC, ND
Consultant
Livingston, Tex.

Joanna E. Cain, RN, BSN, BA
President
Auctorial Pursuits Inc.
Wilmington, N.C.

Kim Cooper, RN, MSN
Nursing Department Program Chair
Ivy Tech Community College
Terre Haute, Ind.

Colleen Davenport, RN, MSN
Staff Nurse
Wrangell (Alaska) Medical Center

Rebecca Crews Gruener, RN, MS
Associate Professor of Nursing
Louisiana State University at Alexandria

Sharon L.G. Lee, APRN, MS, CCRN
Emergency RN/Family Nurse
    Practitioner/Instructor
BryanLGH Medical Center/BryanLGH College
    of Health Sciences
Lincoln, Neb.

Shelly Luger, RN, BA, BSN
Instructor Community Health Nursing
Mount Marty College
Yankton, S. Dak.

Susan Sample, MSN, CRNP
Program Manager – Cardiothoracic Surgery
Lancaster (Pa.) General Hospital

Donna Scemons, RN, MSN, CNS, CWOCN, FNP-C
President
Healthcare Systems
Castaic, Calif.

Catherine Shields, RN
Instructor of Practical Nursing
Ocean County Vocational-Technical School
Lakehurst, N.J.

Allison J. Terry, RN, PhD
Director of Community Certification
Alabama Department of Mental Health,
    Mental Retardation Division
Montgomery

Part one

Disorders

Acceleration-deceleration injuries

DESCRIPTION

- Injury resulting from sharp hyperextension and flexion of the neck that damages muscles, ligaments, disks, and nerve tissue
- Excellent prognosis; symptoms usually subside with symptomatic treatment
- Also called *whiplash*

PATHOPHYSIOLOGY

- Unexpected force causes the head to jerk back and then forward.
- The neck bones snap out of position, causing injury.
- Irritated nerves can interfere with blood flow and transmission of nerve impulses.
- Pinched nerves can affect certain body part functions.

CAUSES

- Fall
- Motor vehicle accident (absence of head restraint)
- Sports accident

ASSESSMENT FINDINGS

- Back or shoulder pain, initially minimal but increasing 12 to 72 hours after accident
- Dizziness
- Headache
- Vision disturbances
- Tinnitus
- Neck muscle asymmetry
- Gait disturbances
- Arm rigidity or numbness
- Tenderness at exact location of injury
- Decreased active and passive range of motion of neck and affected extremities

TEST RESULTS

- Full cervical spine X-ray shows cervical fracture.

TREATMENT

- Soft cervical collar (see *Applying a cervical collar*)

APPLYING A CERVICAL COLLAR

Cervical collars are used to support an injured or weakened cervical spine and to maintain alignment during healing. The soft cervical collar, made of spongy foam, provides gentler support and reminds the patient to avoid cervical spine motion.

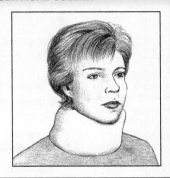

- Ice packs
- Physical therapy
- Limited activity during the first 72 hours after the injury
- Limited neck movement
- Limited strenuous activities, such as lifting and contact sports, until full recovery has been established (which may take more than 2 years)
- Oral analgesics (acetaminophen, nonsteroidal anti-inflammatory drugs, opioids)
- Muscle relaxants
- Corticosteroids
- Surgical stabilization (may be necessary in severe cervical acceleration-deceleration injuries)

KEY PATIENT OUTCOMES

The patient will:
- identify factors that intensify pain
- modify behavior to limit movement and avoid extended injury
- develop effective coping mechanisms
- attain the highest degree of mobility possible
- state feelings and fears about the injury.

NURSING INTERVENTIONS

- Protect the spine during all care.
- Give prescribed medication and evaluate effectiveness.

- Apply a soft cervical collar.
- Evaluate pain control.
- Monitor for complications.
- Reassess neurologic status regularly.

PATIENT TEACHING

Be sure to cover:
- activity restrictions
- proper application of a soft cervical collar
- medication administration, dosage, and possible adverse effects
- instructions about driving and the use of alcohol while taking opioids.

Acute pyelonephritis

DESCRIPTION

- Inflammation of the kidney occurring mainly in the interstitial tissue and renal pelvis and occasionally in the renal tubules
- Affecting one or both kidneys
- Good prognosis; extensive permanent damage rare
- Also called *acute infective tubulointerstitial nephritis*

PATHOPHYSIOLOGY

- Infection spreads from the bladder to the ureters to the kidneys, commonly through vesicoureteral reflux.
- Vesicoureteral reflux may result from congenital weakness at the junction of the ureter and bladder.
- Bacteria refluxed to intrarenal tissues may create colonies of infection within 24 to 48 hours.
- Female anatomy allows for higher incidence of infection.

CAUSES

- Bacterial infection of the kidneys

ASSESSMENT FINDINGS

- History of urinary urgency and frequency
- Burning during urination
- Dysuria, nocturia, hematuria
- Anorexia, vomiting, diarrhea
- Fatigue
- Symptoms that develop rapidly over a few hours or a few days

- Pain on flank palpation
- Cloudy urine
- Ammonia-like or fishy odor to urine
- Fever of 102° F (38.9° C) or higher, shaking chills

TEST RESULTS

- Urinalysis and culture and sensitivity testing reveal pyuria, significant bacteriuria, low specific gravity and osmolality, slightly alkaline urine pH, or proteinuria, glycosuria, and ketonuria (less frequent).
- White blood cell count, neutrophil count, and erythrocyte sedimentation rate are elevated.
- Kidney-ureter-bladder radiography reveals calculi, tumors, or cysts in the kidneys or urinary tract.
- Excretory urography reveals asymmetrical kidneys, possibly indicating a high frequency of infection.

TREATMENT

- Identification and correction of predisposing factors to infection, such as obstruction or calculi
- Short courses of therapy for uncomplicated infections
- Increased fluid intake
- Antibiotics
- Urinary analgesics such as phenazopyridine (Prodium)

KEY PATIENT OUTCOMES

The patient will:
- maintain fluid balance
- maintain urine specific gravity within the designated limits
- identify risk factors that exacerbate decreased tissue perfusion and modify lifestyle appropriately
- report increased comfort.

NURSING INTERVENTIONS

- Give prescribed medication.
- Check vital signs, intake and output, and daily weight.
- Monitor characteristics of urine and the pattern of urination.
- Monitor renal function studies.

PATIENT TEACHING

Be sure to cover:

- the disorder, diagnosis, and treatment
- avoidance of bacterial contamination by following hygienic toileting practices (wiping the perineum from front to back after bowel movements for women)
- proper technique for collecting a clean-catch urine specimen
- medication administration, dosage, and possible adverse effects
- routine checkup with a history of urinary tract infections
- signs and symptoms of recurrent infection.

Acute tubular necrosis

DESCRIPTION

- Injury to the nephron's tubular segment resulting from ischemic or nephrotoxic injury and causing renal failure and uremic syndrome
- Also known as *acute tubulointerstitial nephritis*

PATHOPHYSIOLOGY

- Ischemic injury, circulatory collapse, severe hypotension, trauma, hemorrhage, dehydration, cardiogenic or septic shock, surgery, anesthetics, and reactions to transfusions may cause disruption of blood flow to the kidneys.
- Nephrotoxic injury may follow ingestion of certain chemical agents, such as contrast medium or antibiotics, or result from a hypersensitive reaction of the kidneys.

CAUSES

- Diseased tubular epithelium
- Ischemic injury to glomerular epithelial cells or vascular endothelium
- Obstructed urine flow

ASSESSMENT FINDINGS

- Diagnosis usually delayed until condition has progressed to an advanced stage
- History of ischemic or nephrotoxic injury
- Low urine output (less than 400 ml/24 hours)
- Evidence of bleeding abnormalities, such as petechiae and ecchymosis
- Dry, pruritic skin

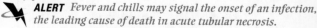

ALERT *Fever and chills may signal the onset of an infection, the leading cause of death in acute tubular necrosis.*

- Dry mucous membranes
- Uremic breath
- Cardiac arrhythmia, if hyperkalemic
- Muscle weakness

TEST RESULTS

- Urinary sediment testing reveals red blood cells (RBCs) and casts.
- Urine specific gravity is 1.010.
- Urine osmolality is less than 400 mOsm/kg.
- Urine sodium level is 40 to 60 mEq/L.
- Blood urea nitrogen and serum creatinine levels are elevated.
- Anemia is evident.
- Platelet adherence is defective.
- Metabolic acidosis is revealed.
- Hyperkalemia is shown.
- Electrocardiogram may show arrhythmias and, with hyperkalemia, a widening QRS complex, disappearing P waves, and tall, peaked T waves.

TREATMENT

Acute phase
- Vigorous supportive measures until normal kidney function resumes

Long-term management
- Daily replacement of projected and calculated fluid loss (including insensible loss)
- Peritoneal dialysis or hemodialysis if the patient is catabolic or if hyperkalemia and fluid volume overload aren't controlled by other measures
- Fluid restriction
- Low-sodium, low-potassium diet
- Rest periods when fatigued
- Diuretics
- Transfusion of packed RBCs
- Epoetin alfa
- Antibiotics
- Emergency I.V. administration of 50% glucose, regular insulin, and sodium bicarbonate (for hyperkalemia)
- Sodium polystyrene sulfonate (Kayexalate) with sorbitol by mouth or enema (for hyperkalemia)

KEY PATIENT OUTCOMES

The patient will:
- maintain fluid balance
- maintain hemodynamic stability
- maintain urine specific gravity within the designated limits
- have improved kidney function.

NURSING INTERVENTIONS

- Give prescribed medication and blood products.
- Restrict food containing high sodium and potassium levels.
- Use aseptic technique, particularly when handling catheters.
- Perform passive range-of-motion exercises.
- Provide good skin care.
- Check vital signs and intake and output.
- Monitor laboratory studies.
- Monitor for complications.

PATIENT TEACHING

Be sure to cover:
- the disorder, diagnosis, and treatment
- signs of infection and when to report them to the physician
- dietary restrictions
- how to set goals that are realistic for the patient's prognosis
- appropriate supportive services or social service.

Adrenal hypofunction

DESCRIPTION

- Primary adrenal hypofunction or insufficiency (Addison's disease) originating within the adrenal gland and characterized by the decreased secretion of mineralocorticoids, glucocorticoids, and androgens
- Secondary adrenal hypofunction due to a disorder outside the gland such as impaired pituitary secretion of corticotropin; characterized by decreased glucocorticoid secretion
- Adrenal crisis (addisonian crisis), a critical deficiency of mineralocorticoids and glucocorticoids generally following acute stress, sepsis, trauma, surgery, or the omission of steroid therapy in patients who have chronic adrenal insufficiency

 ALERT *Adrenal crisis is a medical emergency that needs immediate, vigorous treatment.*

PATHOPHYSIOLOGY

- The disorder results from the partial or complete destruction of the adrenal cortex.
- The disorder is a clinical syndrome in which the symptoms are associated with deficient production of the adrenocortical hormones cortisol, aldosterone, and androgen.
- Corticotropin and corticotropin-releasing hormone levels are high.
- Addison's disease involves all zones of the cortex, causing deficiencies of the adrenocortical secretions, glucocorticoids, androgens, and mineralocorticoids.
- Cortisol deficiency causes decreased liver gluconeogenesis (the formation of glucose from molecules that aren't carbohydrates), resulting in low blood glucose levels that can become dangerously low in patients who take insulin routinely.
- Aldosterone deficiency causes increased renal sodium loss and enhances potassium reabsorption.
- Hypotension develops from sodium excretion.
- Increased production of angiotensin II results from low plasma volume and arteriolar pressure.
- Androgen deficiency may decrease hair growth in axillary and pubic areas (less noticeable in men) as well as on the extremities of women.

CAUSES

Primary hypofunction

- Autoimmune process in which circulating antibodies react specifically against the adrenal tissue
- Bilateral adrenalectomy
- Family history of autoimmune disease (may predispose the patient to Addison's disease and other endocrinopathies)
- Hemorrhage into the adrenal gland
- Infections (histoplasmosis, cytomegalovirus)
- Neoplasms
- Tuberculosis (the chief cause in the past; now responsible for less than 20% of adult cases)

Secondary hypofunction

- Abrupt withdrawal of long-term corticosteroid therapy
- Hypopituitarism
- Removal of a corticotropin-secreting tumor

Adrenal crisis
- Exhausted body stores of glucocorticoids in a patient with adrenal hypofunction after trauma, surgery, or other physiologic stress

ASSESSMENT FINDINGS
- History of synthetic steroid use, adrenal surgery, or recent infection
- Muscle weakness, poor coordination
- Fatigue
- Weight loss, dehydration
- Craving for salty food
- Decreased tolerance for stress
- GI disturbances
- Amenorrhea (in women)
- Impotence (in men)
- Decreased axillary and pubic hair (in women)
- Bronze coloration of the skin, darkening of scars
- Areas of vitiligo
- Increased pigmentation of mucous membranes
- Weak, irregular pulse
- Hypotension

TEST RESULTS
- In the rapid corticotropin stimulation test, a low corticotropin level indicates a secondary disorder; an elevated level indicates a primary disorder.
- Plasma cortisol level declines (less than 10 mcg/dl in the morning; lower in the evening).
- Serum sodium and fasting blood glucose levels decline.
- Serum potassium, calcium, and blood urea nitrogen levels increase.
- Hematocrit and lymphocyte and eosinophil counts increase.
- Chest X-ray shows a small heart in severe disease.
- Computed tomography scan of the abdomen shows adrenal calcification if the cause is infectious.

TREATMENT
- I.V. fluids
- Periods of rest
- Small, frequent, high-protein meals
- Lifelong corticosteroid replacement, usually with cortisone (Cortone Acetate) or hydrocortisone (Cortef)
- Oral fludrocortisone (Florinef Acetate)
- I.V. saline and glucose solutions (for adrenal crisis)

KEY PATIENT OUTCOMES

The patient will:
- maintain stable vital signs
- maintain an adequate fluid balance
- remain free from signs and symptoms of infection
- develop adequate coping skills.

NURSING INTERVENTIONS

- Until onset of mineralocorticoid effect, encourage fluids to replace excessive fluid loss.
- Arrange for a diet that maintains sodium and potassium balances; if the patient is anorexic, suggest six small meals per day to increase caloric intake.
- Observe for cushingoid signs such as fluid retention around the eyes and face.
- Check for petechiae.
- If the patient receives glucocorticoids alone, observe for orthostatic hypotension or electrolyte abnormalities.
- Check vital signs, intake and output, and daily weight.
- Watch for signs of shock (decreased level of consciousness and urine output).
- Observe for hyperkalemia before treatment and hypokalemia after treatment.
- Monitor cardiac rhythm.
- Check blood glucose levels.
- Refer the patient to the National Adrenal Diseases Foundation for support and information.

PATIENT TEACHING

Be sure to cover:
- life-long steroid therapy requirement
- symptoms of steroid overdose (swelling, weight gain) and steroid underdose (lethargy, weakness)
- that dosage may need to be increased during times of stress or illness (when the patient has a cold, for example)
- that infection, injury, or profuse sweating in hot weather may precipitate adrenal crisis
- importance of carrying a medical identification card that states the patient is on steroid therapy (name of the medication and its dosage should be included on the card)
- how to give a hydrocortisone injection and the need to keep an emer-

gency kit containing hydrocortisone in a prepared syringe available for
use in times of stress
- stress management techniques.

Alzheimer's disease

DESCRIPTION
- Degenerative disorder of the cerebral cortex (especially the frontal lobe),
  characterized by progressive dementia
- Accounts for more than 50% of all cases of dementia
- Poor prognosis
- No cure or definitive treatment
- Gradual loss of recent and remote memory

PATHOPHYSIOLOGY
- Chromosome 21 shows a genetic abnormality.
- Brain damage is caused by a genetic substance, amyloid.
- Three distinguishing features of brain tissue are neurofibrillary tangles,
  neuritic plaques, and granulovacuolar degeneration.

CAUSES
- Unknown

ASSESSMENT FINDINGS
- History obtained from a family member or caregiver
- Insidious onset
- Initial changes almost imperceptible
- Forgetfulness and subtle memory loss
- Recent memory loss
- Difficulty learning and remembering new information
- General deterioration in personal hygiene
- Inability to concentrate
- Tendency to perform repetitive actions and to be restless
- Negative personality changes (irritability, depression, paranoia, hostility)
- Nocturnal awakening
- Disorientation
- Suspicious and fearful of imaginary people and situations
- Misperceives own environment
- Misidentifies objects and people
- Complains of stolen or misplaced objects

- Emotions may be described as labile
- Mood swings, sudden angry outbursts, and sleep disturbances
- Impaired sense of smell (usually an early symptom)
- Impaired stereognosis
- Gait disorders
- Tremors
- Loss of recent memory
- Positive snout reflex
- Organic brain disease in adults
- Urinary or fecal incontinence
- Seizures

TEST RESULTS

- Diagnosis is made by exclusion.
- Positive diagnosis is made on autopsy.
- Positron emission tomography reveals metabolic activity of the cerebral cortex.
- Computed tomography scan reveals excessive and progressive brain atrophy.
- Magnetic resonance imaging rules out intracranial lesions.
- Cerebral blood flow studies reveals abnormalities in blood flow to the brain.
- Cerebrospinal fluid analysis reveals chronic neurologic infection.
- EEG shows slowing of the brain waves in late stages of the disease.
- Neuropsychologic test results show impaired cognitive ability and reasoning.

TREATMENT

▶ *COLLABORATION Consult with a neuropsychiatrist, psychologist, social worker, dietitian, and occupational therapist to evaluate the patient's strengths and weaknesses and teach the patient and his family behavioral strategies to improve quality of life.*
- Well-balanced diet (may need to be monitored)
- Safe activities as tolerated (may need to be monitored)
- Cerebral vasodilators
- Psychostimulators
- Antidepressants
- Anxiolytics
- Neurolytics
- Anticonvulsants (experimental)
- Anti-inflammatories (experimental)

- Anticholinesterase agents
- Vitamin E

KEY PATIENT OUTCOMES

The patient (or family) will:
- perform activities of daily living to maximum ability
- maintain daily calorie requirements
- remain free from signs and symptoms of infection
- perform self-care needs to maximum ability
- use support systems and develop adequate coping behaviors.

NURSING INTERVENTIONS

- Provide an effective communication system.
- Use soft tones and a slow, calm manner when speaking to the patient.
- Allow the patient sufficient time to answer questions.
- Protect the patient from injury.
- Provide rest periods.
- Provide an exercise program.
- Encourage independence.
- Offer frequent toileting.
- Assist with hygiene and dressing.
- Give prescribed medication.
- Provide familiar objects to help with orientation and behavior control.
- Evaluate response to medications.
- Monitor fluid intake and nutrition status.
- Adjust environment for safety.
- Refer the patient (and his family or caregivers) to social services for additional support.

PATIENT TEACHING

Be sure to cover (with the patient and his caregivers):
- the disease process
- exercise regimen
- importance of cutting food and providing finger foods, if indicated
- use of plates with rim guards, built-up utensils, and cups with lids
- independence
- how to access the Alzheimer's Association
- location of a local support group.

Amyotrophic lateral sclerosis

DESCRIPTION
- Most common motor neuron disease of muscular atrophy
- Chronic, progressive, and debilitating disease that's invariably fatal
- Also known as *Lou Gehrig disease*

PATHOPHYSIOLOGY
- An excitatory neurotransmitter accumulates to toxic levels.
- Motor units no longer innervate.
- Progressive degeneration of axons cause loss of myelin.
- Upper and lower motor neurons progressively degenerate.
- Motor nuclei in the cerebral cortex and corticospinal tracts progressively degenerate.

CAUSES
- Exact cause unknown
- Immune complexes such as those formed in autoimmune disorders
- Inherited as an autosomal dominant trait in 10% of patients
- Virus that creates metabolic disturbances in motor neurons

ASSESSMENT FINDINGS
- Mental function intact
- Family history of amyotrophic lateral sclerosis (ALS)
- Asymmetrical weakness first noticed in one limb
- Easy fatigue and easy cramping in the affected muscles
- Fasciculations in the affected muscles
- Progressive weakness in muscles of the arms, legs, and trunk
- Brisk and overactive stretch reflexes
- Difficulty talking, chewing, swallowing, and breathing
- Shortness of breath and occasional drooling

TEST RESULTS
- Cerebrospinal fluid has increased protein.
- Computed tomography scan and EEG rule out other disorders.
- Muscle biopsy discloses atrophic fibers.
- Electromyography shows the electrical abnormalities of involved muscles.
- Nerve conduction studies appear normal.

TREATMENT

- Rehabilitative measures
- May need tube feedings
- Activity as tolerated
- Dantrolene (Dantrium) or baclofen (Lioresal) for muscle spasticity
- I.V. or intrathecal administration of thyrotropin-releasing hormone
- Riluzole (Rilutek) to delay progression of disease

KEY PATIENT OUTCOMES

The patient will:
- maintain a patent airway and adequate ventilation
- maintain joint mobility and range of motion (ROM)
- maintain daily calorie requirements
- seek support systems and exhibit adequate coping behaviors
- remain free from infection.

NURSING INTERVENTIONS

- Provide emotional and psychological support.

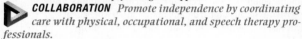 **COLLABORATION** *Promote independence by coordinating care with physical, occupational, and speech therapy professionals.*

- Turn and reposition the patient frequently.
- Give prescribed medication.
- Provide airway and respiratory management.
- Promote nutrition.
- Maintain aspiration precautions.
- Monitor muscle weakness, respiratory status, speech, and swallowing ability.
- Maintain skin integrity.
- Evaluate nutritional status.
- Adjust the patient's environment for safety.
- Evaluate response to treatment.
- Assess for complications, signs, and symptoms of infection.
- Establish an alternative communication plan for when the patient is unable to speak or write.

PATIENT TEACHING

Be sure to cover:
- the disorder, diagnosis, and treatment
- swallowing therapy regimen
- medications and adverse effects

MODIFYING THE HOME FOR A PATIENT WITH ALS

To help the patient with amyotrophic lateral sclerosis (ALS) live safely at home, follow these guidelines:

- Explain basic safety precautions, such as keeping stairs and pathways free from clutter; using nonskid mats in the bathroom and in place of loose throw rugs; keeping stairs well lit; installing handrails in stairwells and the shower, tub, and toilet areas; and removing electrical and telephone cords from traffic areas.
- Discuss the need for rearranging the furniture, moving items in or out of the patient's care area, and obtaining a hospital bed, a commode, or oxygen equipment.
- Recommend devices to ease the patient's and caregiver's work, such as extra pillows or a wedge pillow to help the patient sit up, a draw sheet to help him move up in bed, a lap tray for eating, or a bell for calling the caregiver.
- Help the patient adjust to changes in the environment. Encourage independence.
- Advise the patient to keep a suction machine handy to reduce the fear of choking due to secretion accumulation and dysphagia. Teach him how to suction himself when necessary.

- skin care
- ROM exercises
- deep-breathing and coughing exercises
- safety in the home (see *Modifying the home for a patient with ALS*)
- how to access a local ALS support group.

 Life-threatening disorder

Anaphylaxis

DESCRIPTION

- Dramatic, acute atopic reaction to an allergen
- Marked by sudden onset of rapidly progressive urticaria and respiratory distress
- More severe the sooner signs and symptoms appear after exposure to the antigen
- Severe reactions possibly initiating vascular collapse, leading to systemic shock and, possibly, death

PATHOPHYSIOLOGY

- After initial exposure to an antigen, the immune system produces specific immunoglobulin (Ig) antibodies in the lymph nodes. Helper T cells enhance the process.
- The antibodies (IgE) then bind to membrane receptors located on mast cells and basophils.
- After the body re-encounters the antigen, the IgE antibodies, or cross-linked IgE receptors, recognize the antigen as foreign; this activates the release of powerful chemical mediators.
- IgG or IgM enters into the reaction and activates the release of complement factors.

CAUSES

- Systemic exposure to sensitizing drugs, foods, insect venom, or other specific antigens

ASSESSMENT FINDINGS

- Immediately after exposure, complaints of a feeling of impending doom or fright and exhibiting apprehension, restlessness, cyanosis, cool and clammy skin, erythema, edema, tachypnea, weakness, sweating, sneezing, dyspnea, nasal pruritus, and urticaria
- A "lump" in the patient's throat caused by angioedema
- Complaints of chest tightness
- Hoarseness or stridor and wheezing
- Severe abdominal cramps, nausea, and diarrhea
- Urinary urgency and incontinence
- Dizziness, drowsiness, headache, and seizures
- Hypotension and shock; sometimes, angina and cardiac arrhythmias

TEST RESULTS

- No tests are required to identify anaphylaxis because the patient's history and signs and symptoms establish the diagnosis.
- Skin testing may help to identify a specific allergen.

TREATMENT

- Establishing and maintaining a patent airway
- Cardiopulmonary resuscitation, if cardiac arrest occurs
- Nothing by mouth, until stable
- Bed rest, until stable

- Immediate injection of epinephrine 1:1,000 aqueous solution, subQ, or I.V.
- Corticosteroids to reduce inflammatory reaction
- Diphenhydramine (Benadryl) I.V.
- Volume expander infusions as needed
- Vasopressors to support blood pressure
- Norepinephrine (Levophed) to restore blood pressure, if needed
- Dopamine (Dobutrex) to support blood pressure
- Aminophylline (Truphylline) I.V. to dilate bronchi
- Antihistamines to counteract histamine reaction

KEY PATIENT OUTCOMES

The patient will:
- maintain a patent airway
- maintain adequate ventilation
- express feelings of increased comfort and decreased pain
- maintain normal cardiac output and normal heart rate
- identify causative allergen.

NURSING INTERVENTIONS

- Provide supplemental oxygen and prepare to assist with insertion of an endotracheal tube, if needed.
- Insert a peripheral I.V. line.
- Continually reassure the patient, and explain all tests and treatments.
- If the patient undergoes skin or scratch testing, monitor for signs of a serious allergic response. Keep emergency resuscitation equipment readily available.

ALERT If a patient must receive a medication to which he's allergic, prevent a severe reaction by making sure he receives careful desensitization with gradually increasing doses of the antigen or with advance administration of corticosteroids. Closely monitor the patient during testing, and have resuscitation equipment and epinephrine readily available.

- Check vital signs.
- Observe for adverse reactions from radiographic contrast media.
- Monitor respiratory and neurologic status and the degree of edema.
- Observe for serious allergic response after skin or scratch testing.
- Evaluate response to treatment.
- Assess for complications.

PATIENT TEACHING

Be sure to cover:
- risk for delayed symptoms and importance of reporting them immediately
- avoidance of exposure to known allergens
- importance of carrying and becoming familiar with an anaphylaxis kit and learning to use it before the need arises
- need for medical identification jewelry to identify allergy.

Anemia, aplastic

DESCRIPTION

- Potentially fatal marrow failure syndrome resulting from injury to or destruction of stem cells in bone marrow or the bone marrow matrix
- Causes pancytopenia (anemia, leukopenia, thrombocytopenia) and bone marrow hypoplasia

PATHOPHYSIOLOGY

- The disorder usually develops when damaged or destroyed stem cells inhibit red blood cell (RBC) production.
- The disorder less commonly develops when damaged bone marrow microvasculature creates an unfavorable environment for cell growth and maturation

CAUSES

- Congenital hypoplastic anemia, also known as *Blackfan-Diamond anemia*, which develops between ages 2 and 3 months, and Fanconi's syndrome, developing between birth and age 10
- Immunologic factors; severe disease, especially hepatitis; viral infection, especially in children; and preleukemic and neoplastic infiltration of bone marrow
- May be idiopathic
- Result of adverse drug reaction

ASSESSMENT FINDINGS

- Weight loss
- Dizziness
- Syncope
- Bruising

- Nosebleeds
- Shortness of breath
- Pallor, ecchymosis, petechiae, or retinal hemorrhage
- Alterations in level of consciousness
- Weakness, fatigue
- Bibasilar crackles, tachycardia, and a gallop murmur
- Fever
- Oral and rectal ulcers and sore throat
- Nausea
- Decreased hair and skin quality

TEST RESULTS

- RBC count is 1 million/mm^3 or less, usually with normochromic and normocytic cells; absolute reticulocyte count is very low.
- Serum iron levels are elevated (unless bleeding occurs), but total iron-binding capacity is normal or slightly reduced.
- Serum platelet and white blood cell counts are decreased.
- Bone marrow biopsies performed at several sites may reveal a dry tap or showing severely hypocellular or aplastic marrow, with a varying amount of fat, fibrous tissue, or gelatinous replacement; absence of tagged iron and megakaryocytes; and depression of erythroid elements.

TREATMENT

- Treatment of underlying cause
- Vigorous supportive measures, such as packed RBCs, platelets, and experimental histocompatibility antigen-matched leukocyte transfusions
- Respiratory support with oxygen
- Prevention of infection ranging from frequent hand washing to filtered airflow
- Well-balanced diet
- Neutropenic precautions, if appropriate
- Antibiotics
- Corticosteroids
- Marrow-stimulating agents, such as androgens, antilymphocyte globulin (experimental), and immunosuppressants
- Granulocyte colony-stimulating factor, granulocyte-macrophage colony-stimulating factor, and erythropoietic-stimulating factor
- Bone marrow transplantation (for severe aplasia and patients who need constant RBC transfusions)

KEY PATIENT OUTCOMES

The patient will:
- state the need to increase activity level gradually
- maintain vital signs within prescribed limits during activity
- maintain normal cardiac output
- exhibit adequate ventilation
- express feelings of increased comfort and decreased pain.

NURSING INTERVENTIONS

- Help the patient to prevent or manage hemorrhage, infection, adverse effects of medication therapy, and blood transfusion reaction.
- If the patient's platelet count is low (less than 20,000/mm^3), prevent hemorrhage by avoiding I.M. injections and by suggesting the use of an electric razor and a soft toothbrush. Apply pressure to venipuncture sites until bleeding stops.
- Follow neutropenic precautions.
- Make sure throat, urine, nasal, stool, and blood cultures are done regularly and correctly to check for infection.
- Schedule frequent rest periods.
- Administer oxygen therapy.
- Ensure a comfortable environmental temperature.
- If blood transfusions are necessary, administer according to facility policy and assess for transfusion reactions.
- Monitor blood studies with patients receiving anemia-inducing drugs.

PATIENT TEACHING

Be sure to cover:
- avoidance of contact with potential sources of infection, such as crowds, soil, and standing water that can harbor organisms
- disorder and its treatment
- prescribed medication and possible adverse reactions and when to report them
- normal lifestyle with appropriate restrictions until remission occurs (for the patient who doesn't require hospitalization)
- how to access the Aplastic Anemia Foundation of America for additional information, assistance, and support.

Anemia, iron deficiency

DESCRIPTION

- Decreased total iron body content diminishing erythropoiesis
- Produces smaller (microcytic) cells with less color on staining (hypochromia)

PATHOPHYSIOLOGY

- Body stores of iron, including plasma iron, decrease.
- Transferrin, which binds with and transports iron, also decreases.
- Insufficient body stores of iron lead to a depleted red blood cell (RBC) mass and to a decreased hemoglobin concentration.
- The result is decreased oxygen-carrying capacity of the blood. (See *Iron absorption and storage.*)

CAUSES

- Blood loss secondary to drug-induced GI bleeding or due to heavy menses, hemorrhage from trauma, GI ulcers, malignant tumors, and varices
- Can be related to lead poisoning in children
- Inadequate dietary intake of iron
- Intravascular hemolysis-induced hemoglobinuria or paroxysmal nocturnal hemoglobinuria
- Iron malabsorption

FOCUS IN
IRON ABSORPTION AND STORAGE

Found in abundance throughout the body, iron is needed for erythropoiesis. Two-thirds of total-body iron is found in hemoglobin; the other third, mostly in the reticuloendothelial system (liver, spleen, and bone marrow), with small amounts in muscle, serum, and body cells.

Adequate iron in the diet and recirculation of iron released from disintegrating red blood cells maintain iron supplies. The duodenum and upper part of the small intestine absorb dietary iron. Such absorption depends on gastric acid content, the amount of reducing substances (ascorbic acid, for example) present in the alimentary canal, and amount of iron intake. If iron intake is deficient, the body gradually depletes its iron stores, causing decreased hemoglobin levels and, eventually, signs and symptoms of iron deficiency anemia.

- Mechanical erythrocyte trauma caused by a prosthetic heart valve or vena cava filter
- Pregnancy

ASSESSMENT FINDINGS

- Can persist for years without signs and symptoms
- Fatigue
- Inability to concentrate
- Headache, shortness of breath (especially on exertion)
- Increased frequency of infections
- Pica, an uncontrollable urge to eat strange things, such as clay, starch, ice and, in children, lead
- Menorrhagia
- Dysphagia
- Vasomotor disturbances
- Numbness and tingling of the extremities
- Neuralgic pain
- Red, swollen, smooth, shiny, and tender tongue (glossitis)
- Corners of the mouth may be eroded, tender, and swollen (angular stomatitis)
- Spoon-shaped, brittle nails
- Tachycardia

TEST RESULTS

- Serum hemoglobin level decreases (males, less than 12 g/dl; females, less than 10 g/dl) or mean corpuscular hemoglobin level decreases in severe anemia.
- Serum hematocrit decreases (males, less than 47 ml/dl; females, less than 42 ml/dl).
- Level of serum iron with high binding capacity decreases.
- Serum ferritin level decreases.
- Serum RBC count decreases (in early stages, RBC count may be normal, except in infants and children) with increased microcytic and hypochromic cells.
- Bone marrow studies reveal depleted or absent iron stores (done by staining) as well as normoblastic hyperplasia.
- GI studies, such as guaiac stool tests, barium swallow and enema, endoscopy, and sigmoidoscopy, rule out or confirm the diagnosis of bleeding causing the deficiency.

TREATMENT

- Underlying cause determined
- Nutritious, nonirritating foods
- Planned rest periods during activity
- Oral preparation of iron or a combination of iron and ascorbic acid
- I.M. iron in rare cases
- Total-dose I.V. infusions of supplemental iron for pregnant and elderly patients with severe disease

KEY PATIENT OUTCOMES

The patient will:
- maintain weight without further loss
- maintain vital signs within prescribed limits during activity
- express feelings of increased energy
- express feelings of increased comfort and decreased pain.

NURSING INTERVENTIONS

- Note the patient's signs or symptoms of decreased perfusion to vital organs.
- Provide oxygen therapy as needed.
- Assess the family's dietary habits for iron intake, noting the influence of childhood eating patterns, cultural food preferences, and family income on adequate nutrition.
- Ask the dietitian to give the patient nonirritating foods.
- Give prescribed analgesics for headache and other discomfort.
- Evaluate the patient's drug history. Certain drugs, such as pancreatic enzymes and vitamin E, can interfere with iron metabolism and absorption; aspirin, steroids, and other drugs can cause GI bleeding.
- Provide frequent rest periods.
- If the patient receives iron I.V., monitor the infusion rate carefully and observe for an allergic reaction.
- Use the Z-track injection method when administering iron I.M. to prevent skin discoloration, scarring, and irritating iron deposits in the skin.
- Provide good nutrition and meticulous care of I.V. sites.
- Check vital signs.
- Monitor compliance with prescribed iron supplement therapy.
- Assess for iron replacement overdose. (See *Recognizing iron overdose*, page 26.)

RECOGNIZING IRON OVERDOSE

Excessive iron replacement may produce such signs and symptoms as diarrhea, fever, severe stomach pain, nausea, and vomiting.

When these signs and symptoms occur, notify the physician and give prescribed treatment, which may include chelation therapy, vigorous I.V. fluid replacement, gastric lavage, whole-bowel irrigation, and supplemental oxygen.

PATIENT TEACHING

Be sure to cover:
- the disorder, diagnosis, and treatment
- dangers of lead poisoning, especially if the patient reports pica
- importance of continuing therapy, even after the patient begins to feel better
- absorption interference of iron supplementation with milk or antacid
- increased absorption with vitamin C
- avoidance of staining teeth by drinking liquid supplemental iron through a straw
- when to report adverse effects of iron therapy
- basics of a nutritionally balanced diet
- importance of avoiding infection and when to report signs of infection
- need for regular checkups
- compliance with prescribed treatment.

Anemia, sickle cell

DESCRIPTION

- Congenital hemolytic disease that results from a defective hemoglobin (Hb) molecule (HbS) that causes red blood cells (RBCs) to become sickle shaped
- Sickle-shaped cells impairing circulation, resulting in chronic ill health (fatigue, dyspnea on exertion, swollen joints), periodic crises, long-term complications, and premature death
- Forms of crisis including painful crisis (most common crisis and the hallmark of the disease; usually appears periodically after age 5), aplastic crisis, acute sequestration crisis (occurs in infants 8 months to 2 years), and hemolytic crisis
- No cure

PATHOPHYSIOLOGY

- The abnormal HbS found in the patient's RBCs becomes insoluble whenever hypoxia occurs.
- RBCs become rigid, rough, and elongated, forming a crescent or sickle shape.
- Sickling can produce hemolysis (cell destruction).
- The altered cells accumulate in capillaries and smaller blood vessels, making the blood more viscous.
- Normal circulation is impaired, causing pain, tissue infarctions, and swelling.

CAUSES

- Homozygous inheritance of the HbS-producing gene (defective Hb gene from each parent)

ASSESSMENT FINDINGS

- Signs and symptoms usually absent before age 6 months
- Chronic fatigue
- Unexplained dyspnea, or dyspnea on exertion
- Joint swelling; aching bones
- Chest pain
- Ischemic leg ulcers
- Increased susceptibility to infection
- Pulmonary infarctions and cardiomegaly
- Jaundice or pallor
- May appear small in stature for age
- Delayed growth and puberty
- Spiderlike body build (narrow shoulders and hips, long extremities, curved spine, and barrel chest) in adult
- Tachycardia
- Hepatomegaly and, in children, splenomegaly
- Systolic and diastolic murmurs
- Sleepiness with difficulty awakening
- Hematuria
- Pale lips, tongue, palms, and nail beds
- Body temperature over 104° F (40° C) or a temperature of 100° F (37.8° C) that persists for 2 or more days

In painful crisis

- Severe abdominal, thoracic, muscle, or bone pain
- Increased jaundice

- Dark urine
- Low-grade fever

In aplastic crisis
- Pallor
- Lethargy
- Sleepiness
- Dyspnea
- Possible coma
- Markedly decreased bone marrow activity
- RBC hemolysis

In acute sequestration crisis
- Lethargy
- Pallor
- Progression to hypovolemic shock and death, if untreated

In hemolytic crisis
- Liver congestion
- Hepatomegaly

TEST RESULTS
- Stained blood smear shows sickle cells, and hemoglobin electrophoresis shows HbS. (Electrophoresis should be done on umbilical cord blood samples at birth to provide sickle cell disease screening for all neonates at risk.)
- RBC count and erythrocyte sedimentation rate decrease, white blood cell and platelet counts and serum iron level increase.
- RBC survival and reticulocytosis decrease; hemoglobin level is normal or low.
- Ophthalmoscopic examination reveals corkscrew- or comma-shaped vessels in the conjunctivae.
- A lateral chest X-ray reveals the characteristic "Lincoln log" deformity. (This spinal abnormality develops in many adults and some adolescents with sickle cell anemia, leaving the vertebrae resembling logs that form the corner of a cabin.)

TREATMENT
- Avoidance of extreme temperatures
- Avoidance of stress
- Well-balanced diet

- Adequate amounts of folic acid–rich foods
- Adequate fluid intake
- Bed rest with crises
- Activity, as tolerated
- Vaccines, such as polyvalent pneumococcal vaccine and *Haemophilus influenzae* B vaccine
- Anti-infectives
- Analgesics
- Iron supplements
- Transfusion of packed RBCs, if Hb level decreases suddenly or if condition deteriorates rapidly
- Sedation and administration of analgesics, blood transfusion, oxygen therapy, and large amounts of oral or I.V. fluids, in an acute sequestration crisis

KEY PATIENT OUTCOMES

The patient will:
- demonstrate age-appropriate skills and behaviors to the extent possible
- exhibit adequate ventilation
- maintain collateral circulation
- maintain balanced fluid volume where input will equal output
- express feelings of increased comfort and decreased pain
- maintain normal peripheral pulses
- maintain normal skin color and temperature.

NURSING INTERVENTIONS

 COLLABORATION *Promote optimum care by coordinating with dietitian, respiratory therapist, and psychologist.*
- Encourage the patient to talk about his fears and concerns.
- If a male patient develops sudden, painful priapism, reassure him that such episodes are common and have no permanent harmful effects.
- Ensure that the patient receives adequate amounts of folic acid–rich foods such as green, leafy vegetables.
- Encourage adequate fluid intake.
- Apply warm compresses, warmed thermal blankets, and warming pads or mattresses to painful areas of the patient's body, unless he has neuropathy.
- Administer analgesics and antipyretics, as needed.
- When cultures demonstrate the presence of infection, give prescribed antibiotics.

- Give prescribed prophylactic antibiotics.
- Use strict sterile technique when performing treatments.
- Encourage bed rest with the head of the bed elevated to decrease tissue oxygen demand.
- Administer oxygen as needed.
- Administer blood transfusions.
- If the patient requires general anesthesia for surgery, help ensure that he receives adequate ventilation to prevent hypoxic crisis.
- Check vital signs and intake and output.
- Monitor complete blood count and other laboratory test results.
- Refer parents of children with sickle cell anemia for genetic counseling to answer their questions about the risk to future offspring.
- Refer other family members for genetic counseling to determine whether they're heterozygote carriers.
- If necessary, refer the patient for psychological counseling to help him cope.
- Refer women with sickle cell anemia for birth control counseling.

PATIENT TEACHING

Be sure to cover:
- avoidance of tight clothing that restricts circulation
- conditions that provoke hypoxia, such as strenuous exercise, vasoconstricting medications, cold temperatures, unpressurized aircraft, and high altitude
- importance of normal childhood immunizations, meticulous wound care, good oral hygiene, regular dental checkups, and a balanced diet as safeguards against infection
- need for prompt treatment of infection
- need to increase fluid intake to prevent dehydration, which can cause increased blood viscosity
- symptoms of vaso-occlusive crisis
- need for hospitalization in a vaso-occlusive crisis in which I.V. fluids, parenteral analgesics, oxygen therapy, and blood transfusions may be necessary
- need to inform all health care providers that the patient has this disease before undergoing any treatment, especially major surgery
- pregnancy and the disease; birth control options and resources
- balanced diet, including folic acid supplements during pregnancy.

Aneurysm, abdominal aortic

DESCRIPTION

■ Abnormal dilation in the arterial wall of the aorta, commonly between the renal arteries and iliac branches
■ Can be fusiform (spindle-shaped), saccular (pouchlike), or dissecting

PATHOPHYSIOLOGY

■ Focal weakness in the tunica media layer of the aorta caused by degenerative changes allows the tunica intima and tunica adventitia layers to stretch outward.
■ Blood pressure within the aorta progressively weakens vessel walls and enlarges the aneurysm.

CAUSES

■ Arteriosclerosis or atherosclerosis (95% of causes)
■ Syphilis; other infections
■ Trauma

ASSESSMENT FINDINGS

■ Asymptomatic until the aneurysm enlarges and compresses surrounding tissue
■ Syncope when the aneurysm ruptures
■ When clot forms and bleeding stops, may again be asymptomatic or have abdominal pain because of bleeding into the peritoneum

Intact aneurysm

■ Gnawing, generalized, steady abdominal pain
■ Lower back pain unaffected by movement
■ Gastric or abdominal fullness
■ Sudden onset of severe abdominal pain or lumbar pain with radiation to flank and groin

> **ALERT** *Watch for possible pulsating masses in the peri-umbilical area. Don't palpate this mass because doing so may lead to rupture of the aneurysm.*

Ruptured aneurysm

■ Into the peritoneal cavity: severe, persistent abdominal and back pain
■ Into the duodenum: GI bleeding with massive hematemesis and melena
■ Mottled skin; poor distal perfusion

- Absent peripheral pulses distally
- Decreased level of consciousness
- Diaphoresis
- Hypotension
- Tachycardia
- Oliguria
- Distended abdomen
- Ecchymosis or hematoma in the abdominal, flank, or groin area
- Paraplegia if aneurysm rupture reduces blood flow to the spine
- Systolic bruit over the aorta
- Tenderness over affected area

TEST RESULTS

- Abdominal ultrasonography or echocardiography reveals size, shape, and location of the aneurysm.
- Anteroposterior and lateral abdominal X-rays reveal aortic calcification, which outlines the mass, at least 75% of the time.
- Computed tomography scan visualizes the aneurysm's effect on nearby organs.
- Aortography reveals the condition of vessels proximal and distal to the aneurysm, as well as the extent of the aneurysm. The aneurysm diameter may be underestimated because it shows only the flow channel and not the surrounding clot.

TREATMENT

- Surgery (may be delayed if aneurysm is small and asymptomatic)
- Careful control of hypertension
- Fluid and blood replacement
- Weight reduction, if appropriate
- Low-fat diet
- Activity as tolerated
- Beta-adrenergic blockers
- Antihypertensives
- Analgesics
- Antibiotics
- Endovascular grafting or resection of large aneurysms or those that produce symptoms (see *Endovascular grafting for repair of AAA*)
- Bypass procedures for poor perfusion distal to aneurysm
- Repair of ruptured aneurysm with a graft replacement

ENDOVASCULAR GRAFTING FOR REPAIR OF AAA

Endovascular grafting is a minimally invasive procedure for the patient who requires repair of an abdominal aortic aneurysm (AAA). Endovascular grafting reinforces the walls of the aorta to prevent rupture and prevents expansion of the size of the aneurysm.

The procedure is performed with fluoroscopic guidance, whereby a delivery catheter with an attached compressed graft is inserted through a small incision into the femoral or iliac artery over a guidewire. The delivery catheter is advanced into the aorta, where it's positioned across the aneurysm. A balloon on the catheter expands the graft and affixes it to the vessel wall. The procedure usually takes 2 to 3 hours to perform. Patients are instructed to walk the first day after surgery and are discharged from the hospital in 1 to 3 days.

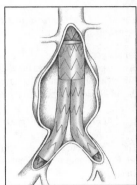

KEY PATIENT OUTCOMES

The patient will:
- maintain adequate cardiac output
- maintain hemodynamic stability
- maintain palpable pulses distal to the aneurysm site
- maintain adequate urine output (output equivalent to intake)
- express feelings of increased comfort and decreased pain.

NURSING INTERVENTIONS

In a nonacute situation
- Allow the patient to express his fears and concerns, and identify effective coping strategies.
- Offer the patient and his family psychological support.
- Before elective surgery, weigh the patient, insert an indwelling urinary catheter and an I.V. line, and assist with insertion of the arterial line and pulmonary artery catheter to monitor hemodynamic balance.
- Give prescribed preventive antibiotics.

In an acute situation

- Insert an I.V. line with at least a 14G needle to facilitate blood replacement.
- Obtain blood samples for laboratory tests, as ordered.
- Give prescribed medication.

 ALERT *Be alert for signs of rupture, which may be immediately fatal. If rupture does occur, surgery needs to be immediate. Medical antishock trousers may be used while transporting the patient to surgery.*

After surgery

- Assess peripheral pulses for graft failure or occlusion.
- Watch for signs of bleeding retroperitoneally from the graft site.
- Maintain blood pressure in the prescribed range with fluids and medications.

 ALERT *Assess the patient for severe back pain, which can indicate that the graft is tearing.*

- Have the patient cough, or suction the endotracheal tube, as needed.
- Provide frequent turning, and assist with ambulation as soon as the patient is able.
- Monitor cardiac rhythm and hemodynamics.
- Assess vital signs, intake and output hourly, neurologic status, and pulse oximetry.
- Check respirations and breath sounds at least every hour.
- Monitor arterial blood gas values as ordered.
- Monitor the patient's fluid status and daily weight.
- Check the patient's nasogastric intubation for patency and amount and type of drainage.
- Monitor laboratory studies as ordered.
- Check the patient's abdominal dressings frequently, and monitor the wound site for infection.

PATIENT TEACHING

Be sure to cover:

- surgical procedure and the expected postoperative care
- importance of taking all medications as prescribed and carrying a list of medications at all times, in case of an emergency
- activity restrictions
- need for regular examination and ultrasound checks to monitor progression of the aneurysm, if surgery wasn't performed.

Aortic insufficiency

DESCRIPTION

- A heart condition in which blood flows back into the left ventricle, causing excess fluid volume
- Also called *aortic regurgitation*

PATHOPHYSIOLOGY

- Blood flowing back into the left ventricle during diastole causes increased left ventricular diastolic pressure.
- Aortic insufficiency results in volume overload, dilation, and, eventually, hypertrophy of the left ventricle.
- Excess fluid volume also eventually results in increased left atrial pressure and increased pulmonary vascular pressure.

CAUSES

- Aortic aneurysm
- Aortic dissection
- Connective tissue diseases
- Hypertension
- Idiopathic valve calcification
- Infective endocarditis
- Primary disease of either the wall or the aortic root
- Rheumatic fever
- Trauma

ASSESSMENT FINDINGS

- Exertional dyspnea
- Orthopnea
- Paroxysmal nocturnal dyspnea
- Sensation of a forceful heartbeat, especially in supine position
- Angina, especially nocturnal
- Fatigue
- Palpitations, pounding head
- Wide pulse pressure
- Diffuse, hyperdynamic apical impulse, displaced laterally and inferiorly
- Systolic thrill at base or suprasternal notch
- S_3 gallop with increased left ventricular end-diastolic pressure
- High frequency, blowing, early-peaking, diastolic decrescendo murmur

IDENTIFYING THE MURMUR OF AORTIC INSUFFICIENCY

A high-pitched, blowing decrescendo murmur that radiates from the aortic valve
area to the left sternal border characterizes aortic insufficiency.

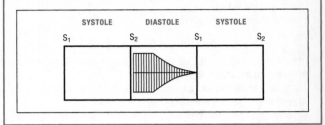

best heard with the patient sitting leaning forward and in deep fixed expi-
ration (see *Identifying the murmur of aortic insufficiency*)
- Head bobbing with each heartbeat
- Tachycardia, peripheral vasoconstriction, and pulmonary edema, if severe
  aortic insufficiency
- Corrigan's sign (hard full pulse followed by a sudden collapse in pulse)
- Bisferious pulse (pulse with palpable peaks)
- Pulsating nail beds (Quincke's sign)
- Symptoms of heart failure (in late stages)

TEST RESULTS

- Chest X-rays may show left ventricular enlargement and pulmonary vein
  congestion.
- Echocardiography may show left ventricular enlargement, increased motion of the septum and posterior wall, thickening of valve cusps, prolapse
  of the valve, flail leaflet, vegetations, or dilation of the aortic root.
- Electrocardiography shows sinus tachycardia, left axis deviation, left ventricular hypertrophy, and left atrial hypertrophy in severe disease.
- Cardiac catheterization shows presence and degree of aortic insufficiency,
  left ventricular dilation and function, and coexisting coronary artery disease.

TREATMENT

- Periodic noninvasive monitoring of aortic insufficiency and left ventricular function with echocardiogram
- Medical control of hypertension

- Low-sodium diet
- Planned periodic rest periods to avoid fatigue
- Cardiac glycosides
- Diuretics
- Vasodilators
- Antihypertensives
- Antiarrhythmics
- Infective endocarditis prophylaxis

> ⚡ **ALERT** *Avoid using beta-adrenergic blockers because of their negative inotropic effects.*

- Valve replacement, if severe

KEY PATIENT OUTCOMES

The patient will:
- carry out activities of daily living without excess fatigue or decreased energy
- maintain cardiac output, demonstrate hemodynamic stability, and not develop arrhythmias
- maintain adequate fluid balance
- maintain adequate ventilation.

NURSING INTERVENTIONS

- Give prescribed medication.
- If the patient needs bed rest, stress its importance; provide a bedside commode.
- Alternate periods of activity and rest.
- Allow the patient to express his concerns about the effects of activity restrictions on his responsibilities and routines.
- Keep the patient's legs elevated while he sits in a chair.
- Place the patient in an upright position, if necessary, and administer oxygen.

> ▶ **COLLABORATION** *Keep the patient on a low-sodium diet. Consult a dietitian to help in the construction of a suitable meal plan.*

- Monitor for signs and symptoms of heart failure or pulmonary edema.
- Check for adverse reactions to drug therapy.
- Observe for complications.

After surgery
- Monitor vital signs and cardiac rhythm frequently.
- Watch for hypotension, arrhythmias, and thrombus formation.

- Assess heart sounds.
- Observe chest tube drainage for amount and color.
- Monitor neurologic status.
- Record intake and output; daily weight.
- Monitor blood chemistry studies, prothrombin time, and International Normalized Ratio values and arterial blood gas levels.
- Monitor chest X-ray results.
- Assess pulmonary artery catheter pressures.
- Refer the patient to an outpatient cardiac rehabilitation program, if indicated.
- Refer the patient to a smoking-cessation program, if indicated.
- Refer the patient to a weight-reduction program, if indicated.

PATIENT TEACHING

Be sure to cover:
- the disorder, diagnosis, and treatment
- medications and potential adverse reactions
- when to notify the physician
- periodic rest periods in the patient's daily routine
- leg elevation whenever the patient sits
- dietary restrictions
- signs and symptoms of heart failure
- importance of consistent follow-up care
- monitoring of pulse rate and rhythm
- blood pressure control.

Aortic stenosis

DESCRIPTION

- Narrowing of the aortic valve that affects blood flow in the heart
- Classified as either *acquired* or *rheumatic*

PATHOPHYSIOLOGY

- Stenosis of the aortic valve results in impedance to forward blood flow.
- The left ventricle requires greater pressure to open the aortic valve.
- Added workload increases myocardial oxygen demands.
- Diminished cardiac output reduces coronary artery blood flow.
- Left ventricular hypertrophy and failure result.

CAUSES

- Atherosclerosis
- Congenital aortic bicuspid valve
- Idiopathic fibrosis and calcification
- Rheumatic fever

ASSESSMENT FINDINGS

- Possibly asymptomatic
- Dyspnea on exertion
- Angina
- Exertional syncope
- Fatigue
- Palpitations
- Paroxysmal nocturnal dyspnea
- Small, sustained arterial pulses that rise slowly
- Distinct lag between carotid artery pulse and apical pulse
- Orthopnea
- Prominent jugular vein waves
- Peripheral edema
- Diminished carotid pulses with delayed upstroke
- Apex of the heart possibly displaced inferiorly and laterally
- Suprasternal thrill
- Split S_2 develops as stenosis becomes more severe
- Prominent S_4
- Harsh, rasping, mid- to late-peaking systolic murmur that's best heard at the base and commonly radiates to carotids and apex (see *Identifying the murmur of aortic stenosis*, page 40)
- An early systolic ejection murmur may be present in children and adolescents who have noncalcified valves. The murmur is low-pitched, rough, and rasping and is loudest at the base in the second intercostal space.

TEST RESULTS

- Chest X-ray shows valvular calcification, left ventricular enlargement, pulmonary vein congestion and, in later stages, left atrial, pulmonary artery, right atrial, and right ventricular enlargement.
- Echocardiography shows decreased valve area, increased gradient, and increased left ventricular wall thickness.
- Cardiac catheterization shows increased pressure gradient across the aortic valve, increased left ventricular pressures, and presence of coronary artery disease.

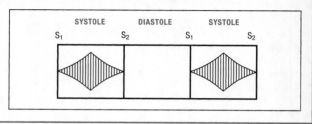

IDENTIFYING THE MURMUR OF AORTIC STENOSIS

A low-pitched, harsh crescendo-decrescendo murmur that radiates from the aortic valve area to the carotid artery characterizes aortic stenosis.

- Electrocardiography may show left ventricular hypertrophy, atrial fibrillation, or other arrhythmia.

TREATMENT

- Periodic noninvasive evaluation of the severity of valve narrowing
- Lifelong treatment and management of congenital aortic stenosis
- Low-sodium, low-fat, low-cholesterol diet
- Planned rest periods
- Cardiac glycosides
- Antibiotic infective endocarditis prophylaxis

> **ALERT** *The use of diuretics and vasodilators may lead to hypotension and inadequate stroke volume.*

- In adults, valve replacement after becoming symptomatic with hemodynamic evidence of severe obstruction
- Percutaneous balloon aortic valvuloplasty
- In children without calcified valves, simple commissurotomy under direct visualization
- Ross procedure in patients younger than age 5

KEY PATIENT OUTCOMES

The patient will:
- perform activities of daily living without excess fatigue or exhaustion
- avoid complications
- maintain cardiac output
- demonstrate hemodynamic stability
- maintain balanced fluid status

- maintain joint mobility and range of motion
- develop and demonstrate adequate coping skills.

NURSING INTERVENTIONS

- Give prescribed medication.

> **COLLABORATION** *Maintain the patient on a low-sodium, low-fat, low-cholesterol diet. Consult with a dietitian when constructing a meal plan.*

- If the patient requires bed rest, stress its importance. Provide a bedside commode.
- Alternate periods of activity and rest.
- Allow the patient to voice concerns about the effects of activity restrictions.
- Keep the patient's legs elevated while he sits in a chair.
- Place the patient in an upright position and administer oxygen, as needed.
- Allow the patient to express his fears and concerns.
- Check vital signs, intake and output, and hemodynamics.
- Assess for signs and symptoms of heart failure, progressive aortic stenosis, and thrombus formation.
- Obtain daily weight.
- Monitor for arrhythmias.
- Observe respiratory status and arterial blood gas results.
- Monitor blood chemistry and chest X-ray results.
- Refer the patient to a weight-reduction program, if indicated.
- Refer the patient to a smoking-cessation program, if indicated.

PATIENT TEACHING

Be sure to cover:
- the disorder, diagnosis, and treatment
- medications and potential adverse reactions
- when to notify the physician
- periodic rest in the patient's daily routine
- leg elevation whenever the patient sits
- dietary and fluid restrictions
- importance of consistent follow-up care
- signs and symptoms of heart failure
- infective endocarditis prophylaxis
- pulse rate and rhythm
- monitoring for atrial fibrillation and other arrhythmias.

Arterial occlusive disease

DESCRIPTION

- An obstruction or narrowing of the lumen of the aorta and its major branches
- May affect arteries, including the carotid, vertebral, innominate, subclavian, femoral, iliac, renal, mesenteric, and celiac
- Prognosis dependent on location of the occlusion and development of collateral circulation that counteracts reduced blood flow

PATHOPHYSIOLOGY

- Narrowing of vessel leads to interrupted blood flow, usually to the legs and feet.
- During times of increased activity or exercise, blood flow to surrounding muscles is unable to meet the metabolic demand.
- The condition results in pain in the affected areas.

CAUSES

- Atheromatous debris (plaques)
- Atherosclerosis
- Direct blunt or penetrating trauma
- Embolism
- Fibromuscular disease
- Immune arteritis
- Indwelling arterial catheter
- Raynaud's disease
- Thromboangiitis obliterans
- Thrombosis

ASSESSMENT FINDINGS

- One or more risk factors: smoking, hypertension, dyslipidemia, diabetes mellitus, and advanced age
- Family history of vascular disease
- Intermittent claudication
- Pain at rest
- Poorly healing wounds or ulcers
- Impotence
- Dizziness or near syncope
- Transient ischemic attack symptoms
- Trophic changes of involved arm or leg

- Diminished or absent pulses in arm or leg
- Presence of ischemic ulcers
- Pallor with elevation of arm or leg
- Dependent rubor
- Arterial bruit
- Hypertension
- Pulselessness distal to the occlusion
- Paralysis and paresthesia occurring in the affected arm or leg
- Poikilothermy (temperature of affected part varying with environmental factors)

TEST RESULTS

- Arteriography shows type, location, and degree of obstruction, and the establishment of collateral circulation.
- Ultrasonography and plethysmography show decreased blood flow distal to the occlusion.
- Doppler ultrasonography shows a relatively low-pitched sound and a monophasic waveform.
- EEG and computed tomography scan may show the presence of brain lesions.
- Segmental limb pressures and pulse volume measurements show the location and extent of the occlusion.
- Ophthalmodynamometry shows the degree of obstruction in the internal carotid artery.
- Electrocardiogram may show the presence of cardiovascular disease.

TREATMENT

- Smoking cessation
- Hypertension, diabetes, and dyslipidemia control
- Foot and leg care
- Weight control
- Low-fat, low-cholesterol, high-fiber diet
- Regular walking program
- Antiplatelets
- Lipid-lowering agents
- Hypoglycemic agents
- Antihypertensives
- Thrombolytics
- Anticoagulation
- Niacin or vitamin B complex
- Embolectomy

- Endarterectomy
- Atherectomy
- Laser angioplasty
- Endovascular stent placement
- Percutaneous transluminal angioplasty
- Laser surgery
- Patch grafting
- Bypass graft
- Lumbar sympathectomy
- Amputation
- Bowel resection

KEY PATIENT OUTCOMES

The patient will:
- report increased comfort and decreased pain
- maintain palpable pulses and collateral circulation
- maintain skin integrity
- maintain joint mobility and range of motion
- develop no signs or symptoms of infection.

NURSING INTERVENTIONS

 COLLABORATION *Consult with an endocrinologist to assist with glucose control if the patient has diabetes.*

Chronic arterial occlusive disease

- Use preventive measures, such as minimal pressure mattresses, heel protectors, a foot cradle, or a footboard.
- Avoid using restrictive clothing such as antiembolism stockings.
- Give prescribed drugs.
- Allow the patient to express fears and concerns.

Preoperative care during an acute episode

- Assess the patient's circulatory status.
- Give prescribed analgesics.
- Give prescribed heparin (Heparin Sodium Injection) or thrombolytics.
- Wrap the patient's affected foot in soft cotton batting, and reposition it frequently to prevent pressure on any one area.
- Strictly avoid elevating or applying heat to the affected leg.

Postoperative care

- Watch the patient closely for signs of hemorrhage.
- In mesenteric artery occlusion, connect a nasogastric tube to low intermittent suction.

- Give prescribed analgesics.
- Assist with early ambulation, but don't allow the patient to sit for an extended period.
- If amputation has occurred, check the residual limb carefully for drainage and note and record its color and amount and the time.
- Elevate the residual limb as ordered.
- Monitor for signs and symptoms of fluid or electrolyte imbalance, renal failure, or stroke.
- Check vital signs, intake and output, distal pulses, neurologic status, and bowel sounds.
- Refer the patient to a physical and occupational therapist, if indicated.

PATIENT TEACHING

Be sure to cover:
- the disorder, diagnosis, and treatment
- medications and potential adverse reactions
- when to notify the physician
- dietary restrictions
- regular exercise program
- foot care
- signs and symptoms of graft occlusion
- signs and symptoms of arterial insufficiency and occlusion
- avoidance of constrictive clothing, or crossing legs
- risk factor modification
- avoidance of temperature extremes
- referral to a podiatrist for foot care as needed
- how to access a smoking-cessation program as indicated.

Asthma

DESCRIPTION

- A chronic reactive airway disorder involving episodic, reversible airway obstruction resulting from bronchospasms, increased mucus secretions, and mucosal edema
- May begin dramatically, with simultaneous onset of severe, multiple symptoms, or insidiously, with gradually increasing respiratory distress
- Signs and symptoms that range from mild wheezing and dyspnea to life-threatening respiratory failure
- Signs and symptoms of bronchial airway obstruction that may persist between acute episodes

PATHOPHYSIOLOGY

- Tracheal and bronchial linings overreact to various stimuli, causing episodic smooth-muscle spasms that severely constrict the airways.
- Mucosal edema and thickened secretions further block the airways.
- Immunoglobulin (Ig) E antibodies, attached to histamine-containing mast cells and receptors on cell membranes, initiate intrinsic asthma attacks.
- When exposed to an antigen such as pollen, the IgE antibody combines with the antigen. On subsequent exposure to the antigen, mast cells degranulate and release mediators.
- The mediators cause the bronchoconstriction and edema of an asthma attack.
- During an asthma attack, expiratory airflow decreases, trapping gas in the airways and causing alveolar hyperinflation.
- Atelectasis may develop in some lung regions.
- The increased airway resistance initiates labored breathing.

CAUSES

- Animal dander
- Bronchoconstriction
- Cold air
- Drugs, such as aspirin, beta-adrenergic blockers, and nonsteroidal anti-inflammatory drugs
- Emotional stress
- Exercise
- Food additives containing sulfites and any other sensitizing substance
- Genetic factors
- Hereditary predisposition
- House dust mites or mold
- Kapok or feather pillows
- Pollen
- Psychological stress
- Sensitivity to allergens or irritants such as pollutants (extrinsic or atopic asthma)
- Internal, nonallergenic factors (intrinsic or nonatopic asthma)
- Tartrazine dye, a common coloring agent in some foods and drugs
- Viral infections

ASSESSMENT FINDINGS

- Intrinsic asthma typically preceded by severe respiratory tract infections, especially in adults; may be aggravated by irritants, emotional stress, fatigue, endocrine changes and temperature and humidity variations

- Exposure to a particular allergen followed by sudden onset of dyspnea and wheezing and by tightness in the chest accompanied by a cough that produces thick, clear, or yellow sputum
- Visibly dyspneic
- Ability to speak only a few words before pausing for breath
- Use of accessory respiratory muscles
- Diaphoresis
- Increased anteroposterior thoracic diameter (if severe)
- Hyperresonance
- Tachycardia; tachypnea; mild systolic hypertension
- Inspiratory and expiratory wheezes
- Prolonged expiratory phase of respiration
- Diminished breath sounds
- Cyanosis, confusion, and lethargy indicating the onset of life-threatening status asthmaticus and respiratory failure

TEST RESULTS

- Arterial blood gas (ABG) analysis reveals hypoxemia.
- Serum IgE level is increased from an allergic reaction.
- Complete blood count with differential shows increased eosinophil count.
- Chest X-rays may show hyperinflation with areas of focal atelectasis.
- Pulmonary function studies show decreased peak flows and forced expiratory volume in 1 second, low-normal or decreased vital capacity, and increased total lung and residual capacities.
- Skin testing identifies specific allergens.
- Bronchial challenge testing shows the clinical significance of allergens identified by skin testing.
- Pulse oximetry measurements show decreased oxygen saturation.

TREATMENT

- Identification and avoidance of precipitating factors
- Desensitization to specific antigens
- Establishment and maintenance of a patent airway
- Fluid replacement
- Activity as tolerated
- Bronchodilators
- Corticosteroids
- Histamine antagonists
- Leukotriene antagonists
- Anticholinergic bronchodilators

- Low-flow oxygen
- Antibiotics
- Heliox trial (before intubation)
- I.V. magnesium sulfate (controversial because of potential for causing respiratory depression)

> **ALERT** *The patient with increasingly severe asthma who doesn't respond to drug therapy is usually admitted for treatment with corticosteroids, epinephrine, and sympathomimetic aerosol sprays. He may require endotracheal intubation and mechanical ventilation.*

KEY PATIENT OUTCOMES

The patient will:
- maintain adequate ventilation
- maintain a patent airway
- use effective coping strategies
- report feelings of comfort
- maintain skin integrity.

NURSING INTERVENTIONS

- Give prescribed drugs.
- Place the patient in high Fowler's position.
- Encourage pursed-lip and diaphragmatic breathing.
- Administer prescribed humidified oxygen.
- Monitor ABG results, pulmonary function test results, and pulse oximetry.
- Adjust oxygen according to the patient's vital signs and ABG values.
- Assist with intubation and mechanical ventilation, if appropriate.
- Perform postural drainage and chest percussion, if tolerated.
- Suction an intubated patient as needed.
- Treat the patient's dehydration with I.V. or oral fluids as tolerated.
- Anticipate bronchoscopy or bronchial lavage.
- Keep the room temperature comfortable.
- Use an air conditioner or a fan in hot, humid weather.
- Check vital signs and intake and output.
- Monitor response to treatment.
- Watch for signs and symptoms of theophylline toxicity and complications of corticosteroids.
- Auscultate breath sounds.
- Assess level of anxiety.

- Refer the patient to a local asthma support group through the American Lung Association or Asthma and Allergy Foundation of America.

PATIENT TEACHING

Be sure to cover:
- the disorder, diagnosis, and treatment
- medications and potential adverse reactions
- when to notify the physician
- avoidance of known allergens and irritants
- metered-dose inhaler or dry powder inhaler use
- pursed-lip and diaphragmatic breathing
- use of peak flow meter
- effective coughing techniques
- maintaining adequate hydration.

Atrial fibrillation

DESCRIPTION

- Rhythm disturbance of the atria
- Characterized by an irregularly irregular cardiac rate and rhythm (see *Recognizing atrial fibrillation*, page 50)

PATHOPHYSIOLOGY

- Rapid discharges from numerous ectopic foci in the atria lead to erratic and uncoordinated atrial rhythm.

CAUSES

- Atrial fibrosis
- Cardiomyopathy
- Cardiothoracic surgery
- Heart failure
- Hypersympathetic state associated with acute alcohol ingestion
- Hypertension
- Hyperthyroidism
- Myocardial infarction (MI)
- Pericarditis
- Pulmonary embolism
- Valvular disease

RECOGNIZING ATRIAL FIBRILLATION

The following rhythm strip shows atrial fibrillation.

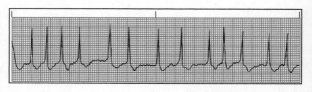

- Rhythm: irregular
- Rate: atrial — indiscernible; ventricular — 130 beats/minute
- P wave: absent; replaced by fine fibrillatory waves
- PR interval: indiscernible
- QRS complex: 0.08 second
- T wave: indiscernible
- QT interval: unmeasurable
- Other: none

ASSESSMENT FINDINGS

- Palpitations
- Fatigue
- Dyspnea
- Chest pain
- Syncope
- Irregular pulse; possible tachycardia
- Hypotension
- Signs of heart failure

TEST RESULTS

- Cardiac enzymes show myocardial damage (with MI).
- Thyroid function studies reveal hyperthyroidism.
- Complete blood count shows decreased hemoglobin level and hematocrit, if blood loss has occurred.
- Chest X-ray may reveal pulmonary edema.
- Echocardiogram or transesophageal echocardiography may reveal valvular disease, left ventricular dysfunction, or atrial clots.
- Electrocardiogram may reveal irregular rhythm.
- Holter monitoring may reveal paroxysmal atrial fibrillation.

TREATMENT

- Possible electrical cardioversion
- Atrial fibrillation suppression pacemaker
- Ablation
- Low-fat, low-sodium diet
- Fluid restriction, if indicated
- Planned rest periods as needed
- Calcium channel blockers
- Beta-adrenergic blockers
- Other antiarrhythmics
- Cardiac glycosides
- Anticoagulants

KEY PATIENT OUTCOMES

The patient will:
- report ways to reduce activity intolerance
- identify effective coping mechanisms to manage anxiety
- discuss the causes of fatigue
- verbalize understanding of medication regimen.

NURSING INTERVENTIONS

- Give prescribed drugs.
- Encourage the patient and his family to talk about feelings and concerns.
- Plan rest periods.
- Check vital signs at rest and after physical activity, intake and output, and daily weight.
- Monitor for signs and symptoms of embolism and abnormal bleeding.
- Refer the patient to programs such as "Coumadin Clinic" where available, or instruct him to contact his physician within 3 days to arrange follow-up testing to monitor anticoagulant therapy.

PATIENT TEACHING

Be sure to cover:
- the disorder, diagnosis, and treatment
- medications and potential adverse reactions
- when to notify the physician
- instructions on how to monitor pulse
- anticoagulation precautions and the need for regular blood testing
- abnormal bleeding
- signs and symptoms of embolic events.

Benign prostatic hyperplasia

DESCRIPTION

- Prostate gland enlarges sufficiently to compress the urethra, causing overt urinary obstruction
- May be treated surgically or symptomatically, depending on the size of prostate, age and health of patient, and extent of obstruction
- Referred to as *BPH*

PATHOPHYSIOLOGY

- Changes occur in periurethral glandular tissue.
- Prostate enlarges and may extend into the bladder.
- Compression or distortion of the prostatic urethra obstructs urine outflow.
- BPH may cause a diverticulum musculature, retaining urine.

CAUSES

- Unknown
- Recent evidence suggests a link with hormonal activity

ASSESSMENT FINDINGS

- Decreased urine stream caliber and force
- Interrupted urinary stream
- Urinary hesitancy and frequency
- Difficulty initiating urination
- Nocturia, hematuria
- Dribbling, incontinence
- Urine retention
- Visible midline mass above the symphysis pubis
- Distended bladder
- Enlarged prostate on digital rectal examination

TEST RESULTS

- Elevated blood urea nitrogen and serum creatinine levels suggest impaired renal function.
- Bacterial count over $100,000/mm^3$ reveals hematuria, pyuria, and urinary tract infection (UTI).
- Excretory urography may indicate urinary tract obstruction, hydronephrosis, calculi or tumors, and bladder filling and emptying defects.

- Cystourethroscopy reveals prostate enlargement, bladder wall changes, calculi, and raised bladder (also determines best surgical intervention).
- International Prostate Symptom Score classifies the disorder's severity.

TREATMENT

- Short-term fluid restriction (prevents bladder distention)
- No sexual intercourse for several weeks after surgery; regular sexual intercourse if surgery not indicated
- Antibiotics, if infection present
- Alpha$_1$-adrenergic blockers such as terazosin (Hytrin)
- Transurethral Microwave Thermotherapy
- 5-alpha-reductase inhibitors such as finasteride (Proscar)
- Surgery for relief of acute urine retention, hydronephrosis, severe hematuria, and recurrent UTI or for palliative relief of intolerable symptoms
- Suprapubic (transvesical) prostatectomy
- Perineal prostatectomy
- Retropubic (extravesical) prostatectomy
- Transurethral resection
- Balloon dilatation, ultrasound needle ablation, and use of stents

KEY PATIENT OUTCOMES

The patient will:
- express feelings of increased comfort
- express understanding of disorder and treatment
- demonstrate skill in managing urinary elimination
- express feelings about potential or actual changes in sexual activity.

NURSING INTERVENTIONS

- Give prescribed medication.

　　ALERT *Avoid giving tranquilizers, alcohol, antidepressants, or anticholinergics, which can worsen the obstruction.*

- Provide I.V. therapy as ordered.
- Check vital signs, intake and output, and daily weight.

　　ALERT *Watch for signs of postobstructive diuresis, characterized by polyuria exceeding 2 qt (2 L) in 8 hours and excessive electrolyte losses. Although usually self-limiting, it can result in vascular collapse and death if not promptly treated.*

- Ensure pain control after surgery.
- Monitor catheter function and drainage.
- Watch for signs of infection.

PATIENT TEACHING

Be sure to cover:
- the disorder, diagnosis, and treatment
- signs of UTI that should be reported
- avoidance of lifting, performing strenuous exercises, and taking long automobile rides for at least 1 month after surgery
- when to seek medical care (fever, unable to void, or passing bloody urine).

Bladder cancer

DESCRIPTION

- Malignant tumor that develops on the bladder wall surface or grows within the wall and quickly invades underlying muscles
- Less common bladder tumors include adenocarcinomas, epidermoid carcinomas, squamous cell carcinomas, sarcomas, tumors in bladder diverticula, and carcinoma in situ
- Most common cancer of the urinary tract

PATHOPHYSIOLOGY

- About 90% of bladder cancers are transitional cell carcinomas, arising from the transitional epithelium of mucous membranes. (They may result from malignant transformation of benign papillomas.)

CAUSES

- Exact cause unknown
- Associated with chronic bladder irritation and infection in people with renal calculi, indwelling urinary catheters, chemical cystitis caused by cyclophosphamide, or pelvic irradiation

ASSESSMENT FINDINGS

- Gross, painless, intermittent hematuria, usually with clots
- Suprapubic pain after voiding, which suggests invasive lesions
- Bladder irritability, urinary frequency, nocturia, and dribbling
- Flank pain and tenderness that may indicate an obstructed ureter

TEST RESULTS

- Complete blood count may reveal anemia.
- Urinalysis detects blood and malignant cells in the urine.
- Excretory urography may identify a large, early-stage tumor or an infil-

trating tumor; delineates functional problems in the upper urinary tract; and shows hydronephrosis and rigid deformity of the bladder wall.
- Retrograde cystography evaluates bladder structure and integrity for functional or anatomical abnormalities; it also helps confirm bladder cancer diagnosis.
- Bone scan may reveal metastasis.
- Computed tomography scan reveals thickness of the involved bladder wall and enlarged retroperitoneal lymph nodes.
- Ultrasonography reveals metastases in tissues beyond the bladder and distinguishes a bladder cyst from a bladder tumor.
- Cystoscopy and biopsy confirm bladder cancer diagnosis. (If the test results show cancer cells, further studies determine the cancer stage and treatment.)
- Bimanual examination (during a cystoscopy, if the patient has received an anesthetic) helps to determine whether the bladder is fixed to the pelvic wall.

TREATMENT

- Influenced by cancer's stage and patient's lifestyle, other health problems, and mental outlook
- Initially postoperatively, avoid heavy lifting and contact sports; after recovery, no activity restrictions
- Intravesical chemotherapy, such as thiotepa (Thioplex), doxorubicin (Adriamycin), and mitomycin (Mutamycin)
- Attenuated bacille Calmette-Guérin vaccine live
- Transurethral resection (cystoscopic approach) and fulguration (electrically)
- Segmental bladder resection
- Radical cystectomy
- Ureterostomy, nephrostomy, continent vesicostomy (Kock pouch), ileal bladder, and ureterosigmoidostomy

KEY PATIENT OUTCOMES

The patient will:
- maintain adequate fluid balance
- express feelings of increased comfort and decreased pain
- exhibit adequate coping mechanisms
- express feelings about potential or actual changes in sexual activity.

NURSING INTERVENTIONS

- Provide support and encourage verbalization.
- Give prescribed drugs.
- Provide preoperative teaching; discuss procedure and postoperative course.
- Inspect wound site.
- Monitor for postoperative complications.
- Check vital signs and intake and output.
- Ensure pain control.
- While the patient is hospitalized, refer him to an enterostomal therapist for training and to other resource and support services such as the American Cancer Society.
- Before discharge, arrange for follow-up home nursing care.

PATIENT TEACHING

Be sure to cover:
- the disorder, diagnosis, and treatment
- stoma care
- skin care and evaluation
- avoidance of heavy lifting and contact sports (postoperatively with a urinary stoma)
- encouragement of participation in usual athletic and physical activities.

 Life-threatening disorder

Blood transfusion reaction

DESCRIPTION

- A hemolytic reaction following the transfusion of mismatched blood
- Accompanies or follows I.V. administration of blood components
- Mediated by immune or nonimmune factors
- Severity varying from mild to severe

PATHOPHYSIOLOGY

- Recipient's antibodies, immunoglobulin (Ig) G or IgM, attach to donor red blood cells (RBCs), leading to widespread clumping and destruction of recipient's RBCs.
- Transfusion with Rh-incompatible blood triggers a less serious reaction, known as Rh isoimmunization, within several days to 2 weeks. (See *Understanding the Rh system*.)

FOCUS IN
UNDERSTANDING THE Rh SYSTEM

The Rh system contains more than 30 antibodies and antigens. Of the world's population, about 85% are Rh positive, which means that their red blood cells carry the D or Rh antigen. The rest of the population are Rh negative and don't have this antigen.

Effects of sensitization
When an Rh-negative person receives Rh-positive blood for the first time, he becomes sensitized to the D antigen but shows no immediate reaction to it. If he receives Rh-positive blood a second time, he experiences a massive hemolytic reaction.

For example, an Rh-negative mother who delivers an Rh-positive baby is sensitized by the baby's Rh-positive blood. During her next Rh-positive pregnancy, her sensitized blood will cause a hemolytic reaction in the fetal circulation.

Preventing sensitization
To prevent the formation of antibodies against Rh-positive blood, an Rh-negative mother should receive $Rh_o(D)$ immune globulin (human) (RhoGAM) I.M. within 72 hours after delivering an Rh-positive baby.

- A febrile nonhemolytic reaction — the most common type of reaction — develops when cytotoxic or agglutinating antibodies in the recipient's plasma attack antigens on transfused lymphocytes, granulocytes, or plasma cells.

CAUSES
- Transfusion with incompatible blood

ASSESSMENT FINDINGS
- Chills
- Nausea
- Vomiting
- Chest tightness
- Chest and back pain
- Mild to severe fever within the first 15 minutes of transfusion or within 2 hours after its completion
- Tachycardia and hypotension

- Dyspnea and apprehension
- Urticaria and angioedema
- Wheezing
- In a surgical patient, blood oozing from mucous membranes or the incision site
- In a hemolytic reaction, fever, an unexpected decrease in serum hemoglobin level, frank blood in urine, and jaundice

TEST RESULTS

- Serum hemoglobin level decreases.
- Serum bilirubin and indirect bilirubin levels increase.
- Urinalysis reveals hemoglobinuria.
- Result of indirect Coombs' test or serum antibody screen is positive for serum anti-A or anti-B antibodies.
- Prothrombin time increases and fibrinogen level decreases.
- Blood urea nitrogen and serum creatinine levels increase.

TREATMENT

- Immediate halt of transfusion
- Dialysis (may be necessary if acute tubular necrosis occurs)
- Diet as tolerated
- Bed rest
- Osmotic or loop diuretics
- I.V. normal saline solution
- I.V. vasopressors
- Epinephrine
- Diphenhydramine
- Corticosteroids
- Antipyretics

KEY PATIENT OUTCOMES

The patient will:
- maintain hemodynamic stability
- show no signs of active bleeding
- maintain adequate ventilation
- express understanding of disorder.

NURSING INTERVENTIONS

- Stop the blood transfusion.
- Maintain a patent I.V. line with normal saline solution.
- Insert an indwelling urinary catheter.

- Report early signs of complications.
- Cover the patient with blankets to ease chills.
- Administer supplemental oxygen as needed.
- Document the transfusion reaction on the patient's chart, noting the duration of the transfusion and the amount of blood absorbed.
- Follow your facility's blood transfusion policy and procedures.

> *ALERT Double-check the patient's name, identification number, blood type, and Rh status before administering blood. If you find any discrepancy, don't administer the blood. Notify the blood bank immediately and return the unopened unit.*

- Check vital signs throughout the transfusion.
- Monitor intake and output.
- Watch for signs of shock.
- Monitor laboratory results.

PATIENT TEACHING

Be sure to cover:
- signs and symptoms of transfusion reaction
- type of transfusion after recovery.

Life-threatening disorder

Botulism

DESCRIPTION

- Life-threatening paralytic illness
- Results from an exotoxin produced by the gram-positive, anaerobic bacillus *Clostridium botulinum*
- Occurs as botulism food poisoning, wound botulism, and infant botulism (see *Infant botulism*, page 60)
- Mortality about 25%, with death most commonly caused by respiratory failure during the first week of illness
- Onset within 24 hours a signal of a critical and potentially fatal illness

> *ALERT Immediately report all cases of botulism to the local board of health.*

PATHOPHYSIOLOGY

- Endotoxin acts at the neuromuscular junction of skeletal muscle, preventing acetylcholine release and blocking neural transmission, eventually resulting in paralysis.

INFANT BOTULISM

Infant botulism, which usually afflicts neonates and infants between 3 and 20 weeks old, is typically caused by ingesting the spores of *botulinum* bacteria, which then grow in the intestines and release toxin. This disorder can produce floppy infant syndrome, characterized by constipation, a feeble cry, a depressed gag reflex, and an inability to suck. The infant also exhibits a flaccid facial expression, ptosis, and ophthalmoplegia—the result of cranial nerve deficits.

As the disease progresses, the infant develops generalized weakness, hypotonia, areflexia, and sometimes a striking loss of head control. Nearly 50% of affected infants develop respiratory arrest.

Intensive supportive care allows most infants to recover completely. Antitoxin therapy isn't recommended because of the risk of anaphylaxis.

CAUSES

- *C. botulinum* bacteria from eating improperly preserved foods, use of injectable street drugs, and possible terrorist attack

ASSESSMENT FINDINGS

- History revealing consumption of home-canned food 18 to 30 hours before onset of symptoms or heroin use
- Vertigo
- Sore throat
- Weakness
- Nausea and vomiting
- Constipation or diarrhea
- Diplopia, blurred vision
- Dysphagia
- Dyspnea
- Ptosis and dilated, nonreactive pupils
- Appearance of dry, red, and crusted oral mucous membranes
- Abdominal distention with absent bowel sounds
- Descending weakness or paralysis of muscles in the extremities or trunk
- Deep tendon reflexes intact, diminished, or absent
- Unexplained postural hypotension
- Urinary retention
- Photophobia
- Slurred speech

TEST RESULTS

- Mouse bioassay detects toxin found in the patient's serum, stool, or gastric contents.
- Electromyogram shows diminished muscle action potential after a single supramaximal nerve stimulus.

TREATMENT

- Supportive measures
- Early tracheotomy and ventilatory assistance in respiratory failure
- Nasogastric suctioning
- Total parenteral nutrition
- Bed rest
- I.V. or I.M. *botulinum* antitoxin
- Debridement of wounds to remove source of toxin-producing bacteria

KEY PATIENT OUTCOMES

The patient will:
- maintain tissue perfusion and cellular oxygenation
- maintain adequate ventilation
- maintain stable neurologic status.

NURSING INTERVENTIONS

- Obtain history of food intake for the past several days.
- Obtain family history of similar symptoms and food intake.
- Administer I.V. fluids as ordered.
- Administer oxygen as needed.
- Perform nasogastric suctioning as needed.
- Monitor neurologic status and cardiac and respiratory function.
- Assess cough and gag reflexes.
- Check vital signs and input and output.
- Review arterial blood gas levels.

PATIENT TEACHING

Be sure to cover:
- the disorder, diagnosis, and treatment
- proper techniques in processing and preserving foods
- never tasting food from a bulging can or one with a peculiar odor
- sterilizing utensils by boiling what came in contact with suspected contaminated food
- not feeding honey to infants (can be fatal if contaminated).

Brain tumor, malignant

DESCRIPTION

- Abnormal growth among cells within the intracranial space
- May affect brain tissue, meninges, pituitary gland, and blood vessels
- Gliomas and meningiomas most common tumor types in adults; usually occur above the covering of the cerebellum or as supratentorial tumors
- Astrocytomas, medulloblastomas, ependymomas, and brain stem gliomas most common tumor types in children

PATHOPHYSIOLOGY

- Classification is based on histology or grade of cell malignancy.
- Central nervous system changes are caused by cancer cells invading and destroying tissues and by secondary effect — mainly compression of the brain, cranial nerves, and cerebral vessels; cerebral edema; and increased intracranial pressure (ICP).

CAUSES

- Unknown

ASSESSMENT FINDINGS

- Insidious onset of headaches
- Nausea and vomiting
- Vision disturbances
- Weakness, paralysis
- Aphasia, dysphagia
- Ataxia, incoordination
- Seizure

TEST RESULTS

- Skull X-rays confirm presence of tumor.
- Brain scan confirms presence of tumor.
- Computed tomography scan confirms presence of tumor.
- Magnetic resonance imaging confirms presence of tumor.
- Cerebral angiography confirms presence of tumor.
- Positron emission tomography confirms presence of tumor.
- Tissue biopsy confirms type of tumor.
- Lumbar puncture reveals increased cerebrospinal fluid (CSF) pressure, which reflects ICP, increased protein levels, decreased glucose levels and, occasionally, tumor cells in CSF.

TREATMENT

- Varies depending on the tumor's histologic type, radiosensitivity, and location
- No dietary restrictions unless swallowing impaired
- Possibly, altered physical restrictions based on neurologic status
- Chemotherapy
- Steroids
- Antacids and histamine-receptor antagonists
- Anticonvulsants

For glioma

- Resection by craniotomy, followed by radiation therapy and chemotherapy

For low-grade cystic cerebellar astrocytoma

- Surgical resection

For astrocytoma

- Repeated surgeries, radiation therapy, and shunting of fluid from obstructed CSF pathways

For oligodendroglioma and ependymoma

- Surgical resection and radiation therapy

For medulloblastoma

- Surgical resection
- Possibly, intrathecal infusion of methotrexate (Rheumatrex) or another antineoplastic drug

For meningioma

- Surgical resection, including dura mater and bone

For schwannoma

- Microsurgical technique

KEY PATIENT OUTCOMES

The patient will:

- recognize limitations imposed by illness and express feelings about them
- continue to function in usual roles as much as possible
- enlist support from available sources
- express feelings of increased comfort.

NURSING INTERVENTIONS

- Maintain a patent airway.
- Take steps to protect the patient's safety.
- Give prescribed drugs.
- After supratentorial craniotomy, elevate the head of the bed about 30 degrees.
- After infratentorial craniotomy, keep the patient flat for 48 hours.
- As appropriate, instruct the patient to avoid Valsalva's maneuver and isometric muscle contractions when moving or sitting up in bed.

> ▶ **COLLABORATION** *Consult with occupational, speech, and physical therapists to maintain patient safety and independence in activities of daily living and to develop a postdischarge care plan.*

- Refer the patient to resource and support services.
- Provide emotional support.
- Monitor neurologic status.
- Check vital signs.
- Observe wound site for infection and bleeding.
- Assess for postoperative complications.

PATIENT TEACHING

Be sure to cover:
- the disease process, diagnosis, and treatment
- signs of infection or bleeding that may result from chemotherapy
- adverse effects of chemotherapy and other treatments and actions that may alleviate them
- early signs of tumor recurrence.

Breast cancer

DESCRIPTION

- Malignant proliferation of epithelial cells lining the ducts or lobules of the breast
- Early detection and treatment influencing prognosis considerably

> ⚡ **ALERT** *The most reliable detection method of breast cancer is regular breast self-examination, followed by an immediate professional evaluation of any abnormality. (Theoretically, slow-growing breast cancer may take up to 8 years to become palpable at 1 cm.)*

PATHOPHYSIOLOGY

■ Breast cancer spreads by way of the lymphatic system and the blood-stream through the right side of the heart to the lungs and to the other breast, chest wall, liver, bone, and brain.

Classification

■ Adenocarcinoma (ductal) — arising from the epithelium
■ Intraductal — developing within the ducts (includes Paget's disease)
■ Infiltrating — occurring in the breast's parenchymal tissue
■ Inflammatory (rare) — growing rapidly and causing overlying skin to become edematous, inflamed, and indurated
■ Lobular carcinoma in situ — involving the lobes of glandular tissue
■ Medullary or circumscribed — enlarging tumor with rapid growth rate

CAUSES

■ No known cause
■ Risk factors: family history of breast cancer, early onset of menses, late menopause, high-fat diet, estrogen therapy, endometrial or ovarian cancer, and use of alcohol or tobacco

ASSESSMENT FINDINGS

■ Detection of a painless lump or mass in the breast (see *Breast tumor sources and sites*, page 66)
■ Change in breast tissue
■ History of risk factors
■ Clear, milky, or bloody nipple discharge, nipple retraction, scaly skin around the nipple, and skin changes, such as dimpling or inflammation
■ Arm edema
■ Hard lump, mass, or thickening of breast tissue
■ Lymphadenopathy

TEST RESULTS

■ Alkaline phosphatase level and liver function test results reveal distant metastasis.
■ Hormonal receptor assay determines whether the tumor is estrogen- or progesterone-dependent; it also guides decisions to use therapy that blocks the action of the estrogen hormone that supports tumor growth.
■ Mammography may show a tumor that's too small to palpate.
■ Ultrasonography distinguishes between a fluid-filled cyst and a solid mass.

BREAST TUMOR SOURCES AND SITES

About 90% of all breast tumors arise from the epithelial cells lining the ducts. About half of all breast cancers develop in the breast's upper outer quadrant— the section containing the most glandular tissue.

The second most common cancer site is the nipple, where all the breast ducts converge.

The next most common site is the upper inner quadrant, followed by the lower outer quadrant and, finally, the lower inner quadrant.

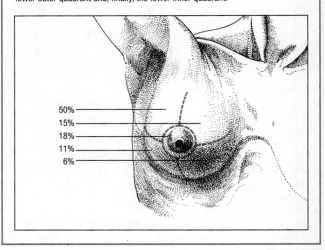

- Chest X-rays pinpoint metastases in the chest.
- Scans of the bone, brain, liver, and other organs detect distant metastasis.

TREATMENT

- The choice of treatment usually depends on the stage and type of disease, the woman's age and menopausal status, and any disfiguring effects of surgery. With adjunctive therapy, 70% to 75% of women with negative nodes survive 10 years or more, compared to 20% to 25% of women with positive nodes.
- Primary radiation therapy
- Preoperative breast irradiation

- Chemotherapy such as a combination of drugs including cyclophosphamide (Cytoxan), fluorouracil (Efudex), methotrexate, doxorubicin (Adriamycin), vincristine (Oncovin), paclitaxel (Taxol), and prednisone (Deltasone)
- Regimen of cyclophosphamide, methotrexate, and fluorouracil
- Antiestrogen therapy such as tamoxifen (Nolvadex)
- Hormonal therapy, including estrogen, progesterone, androgen, or anti-androgen aminoglutethimide therapy
- Lumpectomy
- Partial, total, or modified radical mastectomy

KEY PATIENT OUTCOMES

The patient will:
- recognize limitations imposed by illness and express feelings about these limitations
- express positive feelings about self
- report feelings of comfort
- express increased sense of well-being
- use situational supports to reduce fear.

NURSING INTERVENTIONS

- Provide information about the disease process, diagnostic tests, and treatment.
- Give prescribed drugs.
- Provide emotional support and monitor psychological status.
- Observe wound site for infection or bleeding, and change dressings.
- Monitor for postoperative complications.
- Check vital signs and intake and output.
- Track white blood cell count.
- Help maintain pain control.

PATIENT TEACHING

Be sure to cover:
- procedures and treatments
- activities or exercises that promote healing
- breast self-examination
- risks and signs and symptoms of recurrence
- avoidance of venipuncture or blood pressure monitoring on the affected arm
- how to access local and national support groups.

Burns

DESCRIPTION

- Heat or chemical injury to tissue
- May be permanently disfiguring and incapacitating
- May be partial thickness or full thickness

PATHOPHYSIOLOGY

First-degree burns (superficial, partial thickness)

- The epidermis sustains a localized injury.
- These burns aren't life-threatening.

Second-degree burns (deep, partial thickness)

- Epidermis and some dermis are destroyed.
- Thin-walled, fluid-filled blisters develop.
- Nerve endings are exposed to air as blisters break.
- Pain develops when blisters are exposed to air.
- The barrier function of the skin is lost.

Third-degree burns (full thickness)

- These burns affect every body system and organ.
- Burn extends into the subcutaneous tissue layer.
- Muscle, bone, and interstitial tissues are damaged.
- Interstitial fluids result in edema.
- Immediate immunologic response occurs.
- Wound sepsis is a threat.
- These burns are painless initially due to destruction of nerves.

CAUSES

- Chewing electric cords
- Child or elder abuse
- Contact with faulty electrical wiring
- Contact with high-voltage power lines
- Contact, ingestion, inhalation, or injection of acids, alkali, or vesicants
- Friction or abrasion
- Improper handling of firecrackers
- Improper use or handling of matches
- Improperly stored gasoline
- Motor vehicle accidents
- Residential fires
- Scalding accidents

- Space heater or electrical malfunctions
- Sun exposure

ASSESSMENT FINDINGS

- *Major burns* — more than 10% of a patient's body surface area (BSA); more than 20% of a child's BSA
- *Moderate burns* — 3% to 10% of a patient's BSA; 10% to 20% of a child's BSA
- *Minor burns* — less than 3% of a patient's BSA; less than 10% of a child's BSA
- Respiratory distress and cyanosis
- Edema
- Alteration in pulse rate, strength, and regularity
- Stridor, wheezing, crackles, and rhonchi
- S_3 or S_4
- Hypotension
- Singed nasal hair
- Sores in mouth or nose
- Voice changes
- Coughing, wheezing
- Darkened sputum
- Localized pain and erythema, usually without blisters in the first 24 hours (first-degree burn)
- Chills, headache, localized edema, and nausea and vomiting (more severe first-degree burns)
- Thin-walled, fluid-filled blisters appearing within minutes of the injury, with mild-to-moderate edema and pain (second-degree superficial partial-thickness burn)
- White waxy appearance to damaged area (second-degree deep partial-thickness burn)
- White, brown, or black leathery and visible thrombosed vessels, without blisters (third-degree burn)
- Silver raised or charred area, usually at the site of contact (electrical burn)

TEST RESULTS

- Arterial blood gas levels show evidence of smoke inhalation and may show decreased alveolar function and hypoxia.
- Complete blood count shows decreased hemoglobin level and hematocrit, if blood loss occurs.
- Electrolyte levels are abnormal because of fluid losses and shifts.
- Blood urea nitrogen level is increased if fluid loss occurs.

- Glucose level is decreased in children because of limited glycogen storage.
- Urinalysis shows myoglobinuria and hemoglobinuria.
- Carboxyhemoglobin level is increased.
- Electrocardiogram may show myocardial ischemia, injury, or arrhythmias, especially in electrical burns.
- Fiber-optic bronchoscopy may show edema of the airways.

TREATMENT

ALERT *In an emergency situation, immediately stop the burn source, secure the patient's airway, and take measures to prevent hypoxia.*

COLLABORATION *Obtain collaboration among physical, occupational, and respiratory therapists, dietitians, and social services for optimal pain management and rehabilitation of burn patients.*

- I.V. fluids through a large-bore I.V. line (see *Fluid replacement after a burn*)
  – Adult: maintaining urine output of 30 to 50 ml/hour
  – Child weighing less than 66 lb (29.9 kg): maintaining urine output of 1 ml/kg/hour
- Nasogastric tube and urinary catheter insertion
- Wound care
- Nothing by mouth until severity of burn is established, then high-protein, high-calorie diet as ordered
- Increase hydration with high-calorie, high-protein drinks, not free water
- Total parenteral nutrition, if unable to take food by mouth
- Activity limitation based on extent and location of burn
- Physical therapy
- Booster of tetanus toxoid
- Analgesics
- Antibiotics
- Antianxiety agents
- Loose tissue and blister debridement (optional)
- Escharotomy (optional)
- Skin grafting (optional)

KEY PATIENT OUTCOMES

The patient will:
- maintain a patent airway
- maintain fluid balance within the acceptable range
- report increased comfort and decreased pain

FLUID REPLACEMENT AFTER A BURN

To replace fluid in an adult with a burn, use one of the following formulas.

First 24 hours
Evans
- 1 ml × patient's weight in kg × % total body surface area (TBSA) burn (0.9% normal saline solution)
- 1 ml × patient's weight in kg × % TBSA burn (colloid solution)

Brooke
- 1.5 ml × patient's weight in kg × % TBSA burn (lactated Ringer's solution)
- 0.5 ml × patient's weight in kg × % TBSA burn (colloid solution)

Parkland
- 4 ml × patient's weight in kg × % TBSA burn (lactated Ringer's solution) (Give one-half of volume in first 8 minutes; then infuse remainder over 16 minutes.)

Second 24 hours
Evans
- 50% of first 24-hour replacement (0.9% normal saline solution)
- 2,000 ml (dextrose 5% in water [D_5W])

Brooke
- 50% to 75% of first 24-hour replacement (lactated Ringer's solution)
- 2,000 ml (D_5W)

Parkland
- 30% to 60% of calculated plasma volume (25% albumin)
- Volume to maintain desired urine output (D_5W)

- attain the highest degree of mobility
- demonstrate effective coping techniques.

NURSING INTERVENTIONS

- Apply immediate, aggressive burn treatment.
- Use strict sterile technique.
- Remove clothing that's still smoldering.
- Remove constricting items.
- Perform appropriate wound care.

- Provide adequate hydration.
- Weigh the patient daily.
- Encourage verbalization and provide support.
- Check vital signs and intake and output.
- Monitor respiratory status.
- Observe for signs of infection.
- Maintain hydration and nutritional status.
- Refer the patient to rehabilitation, if appropriate.
- Refer the patient to psychological counseling, if needed.
- Refer the patient to resource and support services.

PATIENT TEACHING

Be sure to cover:
- the injury, diagnosis, and treatment
- appropriate wound care
- medication administration, dosage, and possible adverse effects
- developing a dietary plan
- signs and symptoms of complications.

Cellulitis

DESCRIPTION

- Acute infection of the dermis and subcutaneous tissue causing inflammation of the cells
- May follow damage to the skin, such as a bite or wound
- Prognosis usually good with timely treatment
- With other comorbidities, such as diabetes, increased risk of developing or spreading cellulitis

PATHOPHYSIOLOGY

- A break in skin integrity almost always precedes infection.
- As the offending organism invades the compromised area, it overwhelms the defensive cells, including the neutrophils, eosinophils, basophils, and mast cells, that normally contain and localize the inflammation.
- As cellulitis progresses, the organism invades tissue around the initial wound site.

CAUSES

- Bacterial infections, usually by *Staphylococcus aureus* and *group A beta-hemolytic streptococci*

- Extension of a skin wound or ulcer
- Fungal infections
- Furuncles or carbuncles

ASSESSMENT FINDINGS

- Presence of one or more risk factors, including venous or lymphatic edema, diabetes mellitus, underlying skin lesion, or prior trauma
- Tenderness
- Pain at the site and, possibly, the surrounding area
- Erythema with indistinct margins
- Warmth
- Edema
- Possible fever, chills, and malaise
- Regional lymph node enlargement and tenderness
- Red streaking visible in skin proximal to area of cellulitis

TEST RESULTS

- White blood cell count shows mild leukocytosis.
- Erythrocyte sedimentation rate is elevated.
- Culture and Gram stain may show the causative organism.

TREATMENT

- Immobilization and elevation of the affected extremity
- Moist heat
- Well-balanced diet
- Bed rest possibly needed in severe infection
- Antibiotics
- Topical antifungals
- Analgesics
- Tracheostomy possibly needed for severe cellulitis of head and neck
- Possible abscess drainage
- Amputation (with gas-forming cellulitis [gangrene])

KEY PATIENT OUTCOMES

The patient will:
- avoid injury
- express feelings of increased comfort
- remain free from signs and symptoms of infection
- verbalize feelings and concerns.

NURSING INTERVENTIONS

- Administer prescribed drugs.
- Elevate the affected extremity.
- Apply moist heat as ordered.
- Encourage a well-balanced diet.
- Encourage adequate fluid intake.
- Encourage verbalization of feelings and concerns.
- Institute safety precautions.
- Monitor vital signs.
- Monitor for edema.
- Assist with pain control.
- Monitor laboratory results.
- Observe for signs and symptoms of infection.
- Assess for complications and cellulitis progression.
- Refer the patient for management of diabetes mellitus, if indicated.

PATIENT TEACHING

Be sure to cover:
- the disorder, diagnosis, and treatment
- medications and possible adverse reactions
- when to notify the physician
- use of warm compresses
- signs and symptoms of infection
- prevention of injury and trauma
- infection control procedures
- signs and symptoms of deep vein thrombosis.

Cholelithiasis, cholecystitis, and related disorders

DESCRIPTION

Cholelithiasis
- Leading biliary tract disease
- Formation of calculi (gallstones) in the gallbladder
- Prognosis usually good with treatment unless infection occurs

Cholecystitis
- Related disorder that arises from formation of gallstones
- Acute or chronic inflammation of gallbladder
- Usually caused by a gallstone lodged in the cystic duct
- Acute form most common during middle age

■ Chronic form most common among elderly persons
■ Prognosis good with treatment

Choledocholithiasis
■ Related disorder that arises from formation of gallstones
■ Partial or complete biliary obstruction due to gallstones lodged in the common bile duct
■ Prognosis good unless infection occurs

Cholangitis
■ Related disorder that arises from formation of gallstones
■ Infected bile duct
■ Commonly linked to choledocholithiasis
■ Rapid response of nonsuppurative type to antibiotic treatment
■ Poor prognosis of suppurative type unless surgery to correct obstruction and drain infected bile is performed promptly

Gallstone ileus
■ Related disorder that arises from formation of gallstones
■ Obstruction of the small bowel by a gallstone
■ Most common in elderly persons
■ Prognosis good with surgery

PATHOPHYSIOLOGY

■ Calculi formation in the biliary system causes obstruction.
■ Obstruction of hepatic duct leads to intrahepatic retention of bile; increased release of bilirubin into the bloodstream occurs.
■ Obstruction of cystic duct leads to inflammation of the gallbladder; increased gallbladder contraction and peristalsis occur.
■ Obstruction of bile causes impairment of digestion and absorption of lipids.

CAUSES

■ Acute cholecystitis also a result of conditions that alter gallbladder's ability to fill or empty (trauma, reduced blood supply to the gallbladder, prolonged immobility, chronic dieting, adhesions, prolonged anesthesia, opioid abuse)
■ Calculi formation (type of disorder that develops depends on where in the gallbladder or biliary tract the calculi collect)
■ Risk factors: diabetes mellitus, ileal disease, hemolytic disorders, hepatic disease (cirrhosis), and pancreatitis
■ Rapid weight loss

ASSESSMENT FINDINGS

- Possibly no symptoms (even when X-rays reveal gallstones)
- History of sudden onset of severe steady or aching pain in the mid-epigastric region or the right upper abdominal quadrant
- Pain radiating to the back, between the shoulder blades or over the right shoulder blade, or just to the shoulder area
- History of attacks occurring after fatty meals or, after fasting for an extended time, large meals
- History of attacks occurring in the middle of the night
- Nausea, vomiting, and chills
- History of milder GI symptoms that preceded the acute attack; indigestion, vague abdominal discomfort, belching, and flatulence after eating meals or snacks rich in fats
- Pallor
- Diaphoresis
- Low-grade fever (high in cholangitis)
- Exhaustion
- Jaundice (chronic disease)
- Dark-colored urine and clay-colored stools
- Tachycardia
- Tenderness over the gallbladder, which increases on inspiration (Murphy's sign)
- Palpable, painless, sausagelike mass (calculus-filled gallbladder without ductal obstruction)
- Hypoactive bowel sounds

TEST RESULTS

- Blood studies may reveal elevated levels of serum alkaline phosphatase, lactate dehydrogenase, aspartate aminotransferase, icteric index, and total bilirubin.
- White blood cell count is slightly elevated during cholecystitis attack.
- Abdominal X-rays show gallstones (if they contain enough calcium to be radiopaque), porcelain gallbladder, limy bile, and gallstone ileus.
- Ultrasonography of the gallbladder confirms cholelithiasis in most patients and distinguishes between obstructive and nonobstructive jaundice (calculi as small as 2 mm can be detected).
- Oral cholecystography confirms the presence of gallstones. (This test is gradually being replaced by ultrasonography.)
- Technetium-labeled iminodiacetic acid scan of the gallbladder reveals cys-

tic duct obstruction and acute or chronic cholecystitis if the gallbladder can't be seen.
- Percutaneous transhepatic cholangiography (imaging performed under fluoroscopic guidance) supports the diagnosis of obstructive jaundice and visualizing calculi in the ducts.

TREATMENT

- Endoscopic retrograde cholangiopancreatography (to visualize and re-move calculi)
- Lithotripsy
- Low-fat diet
- Nothing by mouth, if surgery required
- Activity as tolerated
- Gallstone dissolution therapy
- Bile salts
- Analgesics
- Antispasmodics
- Anticholinergics
- Antiemetics
- Antibiotics
- Cholecystectomy (laparoscopic or abdominal), cholecystectomy with op-erative cholangiography, choledochostomy, or exploration of the common bile duct

KEY PATIENT OUTCOMES

The patient will:
- express feelings of increased comfort
- show no signs of infection
- have laboratory values that return to within normal parameters
- avoid complications.

NURSING INTERVENTIONS

- Administer prescribed drugs.
- Check vital signs and intake and output.
- Ensure pain control.
- Monitor for postoperative signs and symptoms of bleeding, infection, or atelectasis.
- Inspect the wound site.
- Maintain T-tube patency and drainage.

PATIENT TEACHING

Be sure to cover:
- the disease, diagnosis, and treatment
- how to breathe deeply, cough, expectorate, and perform leg exercises that are necessary after surgery
- dietary modifications
- medication administration, dosage, and possible adverse effects
- wound care.

Cirrhosis

DESCRIPTION

- Chronic hepatic disease
- Several types

PATHOPHYSIOLOGY

- Diffuse destruction and fibrotic regeneration of hepatic cells occurs.
- Necrotic tissue yields to fibrosis.
- Liver structure and normal vasculature are altered.
- Blood and lymph flow is impaired.
- Hepatic insufficiency occurs. (See *Understanding cirrhosis.*)

CAUSES

Laënnec's or micronodular cirrhosis (alcoholic or portal cirrhosis)

- Chronic alcoholism
- Malnutrition

Postnecrotic or macronodular cirrhosis

- Complication of viral hepatitis
- Possible after exposure to such liver toxins as arsenic, carbon tetrachloride, and phosphorus

Biliary cirrhosis

- Prolonged biliary tract obstruction or inflammation

Idiopathic cirrhosis (cryptogenic)

- No known cause
- Chronic inflammatory bowel disease
- Sarcoidosis

FOCUS IN

UNDERSTANDING CIRRHOSIS

Cirrhosis is a chronic liver disease characterized by widespread destruction of hepatic cells. The destroyed cells are replaced by fibrotic cells in a process called *fibrotic regeneration*. As necrotic tissue yields to fibrosis, regenerative nodules form and the liver parenchyma undergo extensive and irreversible fibrotic changes. The disease alters normal liver structure and vasculature, impairs blood and lymphatic flow and, ultimately, causes hepatic insufficiency.

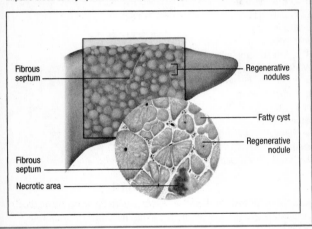

Fibrous septum — Regenerative nodules

— Fatty cyst

— Regenerative nodule

Fibrous septum —

Necrotic area —

ASSESSMENT FINDINGS

- History of chronic alcoholism, malnutrition, viral hepatitis, exposure to liver toxins (such as arsenic) and certain medications, or prolonged biliary tract obstruction or inflammation

Early stage
- Vague signs and symptoms
- Abdominal pain
- Diarrhea, constipation
- Fatigue
- Nausea, vomiting
- Muscle cramps
- Palpable, large, firm liver with a sharp edge

Later stage

- Chronic dyspepsia
- Constipation
- Pruritus
- Weight loss
- Bleeding tendency, such as frequent nosebleeds, easy bruising, and bleeding gums
- Telangiectasis on the cheeks and spider angiomas on the face, neck, arms, and trunk
- Gynecomastia
- Umbilical hernia
- Distended abdominal blood vessels
- Ascites and thigh and leg edema
- Testicular atrophy
- Menstrual irregularities
- Palmar erythema
- Clubbed fingers
- Anemia
- Jaundice
- Enlarged spleen
- Asterixis
- Slurred speech, paranoia, and hallucinations

TEST RESULTS

- Levels of liver enzymes, such as alanine aminotransferase, aspartate aminotransferase, total serum bilirubin, and indirect bilirubin are elevated.
- Total serum albumin and protein levels decrease.
- Prothrombin time is prolonged.
- Hematocrit and hemoglobin and serum electrolyte levels decrease.
- Levels of vitamins A, C, and K are deficient.
- Urine levels of bilirubin and urobilinogen increase; fecal urobilinogen level decreases.
- Abdominal X-rays show possible increase in liver and spleen size and cysts or gas in the biliary tract or liver; liver calcification; and massive ascites.
- Computed tomography and liver scans show possible increase in liver size, reveal liver masses, and visualize hepatic blood flow or obstruction.
- Radioisotope liver scans show possible increase in liver size and visualize blood flow or obstruction.

- Liver biopsy (definitive test for cirrhosis) reveals hepatic tissue destruction and fibrosis.
- Esophagogastroduodenoscopy reveals bleeding esophageal varices, stomach irritation or ulceration, and duodenal bleeding and irritation.

TREATMENT

- Removal or alleviation of underlying cause
- Paracentesis
- Esophageal balloon tamponade
- Sclerotherapy
- I.V. fluids
- Blood transfusion
- Restricted sodium consumption
- Restricted fluid intake
- No alcohol intake
- High-calorie diet
- Frequent rest periods as needed
- Vitamin and nutritional supplements
- Antacids
- Potassium-sparing diuretics
- Beta-adrenergic blockers and vasopressin (Pitressin)
- Ammonia detoxicant
- Antiemetics
- Peritoneovenous shunt, if ascites must be diverted into venous circulation
- Portal-systemic shunts

KEY PATIENT OUTCOMES

The patient will:
- maintain caloric intake as required
- maintain normal fluid volume
- incur no injuries
- exhibit no bleeding.

NURSING INTERVENTIONS

- Administer prescribed I.V. fluids and blood products.
- Administer prescribed drugs.
- Encourage verbalization and provide support.
- Provide appropriate skin care.
- Check vital signs, abdominal girth, and weight.

- Monitor laboratory values, ammonia level, and bleeding tendencies.
- Evaluate hydration and nutritional status.
- Help maintain skin integrity.
- Monitor for changes in mentation and behavior.
- Refer the patient for psychological counseling, if needed.

▶ **COLLABORATION** *Psychologic evaluation and interventions, along with dietary consultation, can enhance the patient's quality of life by focusing on behavior modifications.*

PATIENT TEACHING

Be sure to cover:
- the disorder, diagnosis, and treatment
- over-the-counter medications that may increase bleeding tendencies
- dietary modifications, including high-calorie diet and small, frequent meals
- need to avoid infections and abstain from alcohol
- need to avoid sedatives and acetaminophen (hepatotoxic)
- how to access Alcoholics Anonymous, if appropriate.

Colorectal cancer

DESCRIPTION

- Malignant tumors of colon or rectum almost always adenocarcinomas (About one-half are sessile lesions of rectosigmoid area; all others are polypoid lesions.)
- Slow progression
- Five-year survival rate of 50%; potentially curable in 75% of patients if early diagnosis allows resection before nodal involvement
- Second most common visceral neoplasm in United States and Europe

PATHOPHYSIOLOGY

- Most lesions of the large bowel are moderately differentiated adenocarcinomas.
- Tumors tend to grow slowly and remain asymptomatic for long periods.
- Tumors in the sigmoid and descending colon undergo circumferential growth and constrict the intestinal lumen.
- Tumors in the ascending colon are usually large at diagnosis and are palpable on physical examination.

CAUSES

- Unknown
- Risk factors: intake of excessive saturated animal fat, diseases of the digestive tract, age older than 40, history of ulcerative colitis, and familial polyposis

ASSESSMENT FINDINGS

- Right colon tumors: no signs and symptoms in early stages because stool is liquid in that part of colon
- History of black, tarry stools
- Abdominal aching, pressure, or dull cramps
- Weakness
- Diarrhea, anorexia, obstipation, weight loss, and vomiting
- Rectal bleeding
- Intermittent abdominal fullness
- Rectal pressure
- Urgent need to defecate on awakening
- Abdominal distention or visible masses
- Enlarged abdominal veins
- Enlarged inguinal and supraclavicular nodes
- Abnormal bowel sounds
- Abdominal masses (right-side tumors that usually feel bulky; tumors of transverse portion more easily detected)
- Generalized abdominal tenderness

TEST RESULTS

- Fecal occult blood test may show blood in stools, a warning sign of rectal cancer.
- Carcinoembryonic antigen measurement stages and monitors the treatment.
- Excretory urography verifies bilateral renal function and allows inspection for displacement of the kidneys, ureters, or bladder by a tumor pressing against these structures.
- Barium enema studies reveal location of lesions that aren't detectable manually or visually.

  ALERT *Barium examination shouldn't precede colonoscopy or excretory urography because barium sulfate interferes with these tests.*

- Computed tomography scan allows better visualization if a barium enema yields inconclusive results or if metastasis to the pelvic lymph nodes is suspected.

- Proctoscopy or sigmoidoscopy permits visualization of the lower GI tract (can detect up to 66% of colorectal cancers).
- Colonoscopy permits visual inspection and photography of the colon up to the ileocecal valve and provides access for polypectomies and biopsies of suspected lesions.
- Digital rectal examination detects colorectal cancers (specifically, rectal and perianal lesions).

TREATMENT

- Radiation preoperatively and postoperatively to induce tumor regression
- High-fiber diet
- After surgery, avoidance of heavy lifting and contact sports
- Chemotherapy for metastasis, residual disease, or recurrent inoperable tumor
- Analgesics
- Resection or right hemicolectomy for advanced disease (Surgery may include resection of the terminal segment of the ileum, cecum, ascending colon, and right half of the transverse colon with corresponding mesentery.)
- Right colectomy that includes the transverse colon and mesentery corresponding to midcolon vessels, or segmental resection of the transverse colon and associated midcolon vessels
- Resection surgery (usually limited to the sigmoid colon and mesentery)
- Anterior or low anterior resection (newer method, using a stapler; allows for much lower resections than previously possible)
- Abdominoperineal resection requiring permanent sigmoid colostomy

KEY PATIENT OUTCOMES

The patient will:
- maintain normal fluid volume
- maintain intact mucous membranes
- report feeling less pain
- express increased sense of well-being
- use support systems and employ coping strategies.

NURSING INTERVENTIONS

- Provide support and encourage verbalization.
- Administer prescribed drugs.
- Monitor hydration and nutritional status.
- Monitor vital signs, intake and output, and bowel function.
- Monitor electrolyte levels.

- Inspect wound site for infection and bleeding.

▶ **COLLABORATION** *Consult with enterostomal therapist, home care services for proper choice of ostomy products and ongoing patient teaching and follow-up.*

- Assess for postoperative complications.
- Assist with pain control.
- Monitor the patient's psychological status.
- Refer the patient to support services, such as the Colon Cancer Alliance or the American Cancer Society.

PATIENT TEACHING

Be sure to cover:
- the disease process, treatment, and postoperative course
- stoma care
- avoidance of heavy lifting
- need for keeping follow-up appointments
- risk factors and signs of recurrence.

Coronary artery disease

DESCRIPTION

- Heart disease that results from narrowing of coronary arteries over time as a result of atherosclerosis
- Primary effect: loss of oxygen and nutrients to myocardial tissue because of diminished coronary blood flow

PATHOPHYSIOLOGY

- Increased blood levels of low-density lipoprotein (LDL) irritate or damage the inner layer of coronary vessels.
- After damaging the protective barrier, LDL enters the vessel, accumulates, and forms a fatty streak.
- Smooth-muscle cells move to the inner layer to engulf the fatty substance, produce fibrous tissue, and stimulate calcium deposition.
- The cycle continues, resulting in transformation of the fatty streak into fibrous plaque; eventually, a coronary artery disease (CAD) lesion evolves.
- Oxygen deprivation forces the myocardium to shift from aerobic to anaerobic metabolism, leading to accumulation of lactic acid and reduction of cellular pH.
- The combination of hypoxia, reduced energy availability, and acidosis rapidly impairs left ventricular function.

- The strength of contractions in the affected myocardial region is reduced as the fibers shorten inadequately, resulting in less force and velocity.
- Wall motion is abnormal in the ischemic area, resulting in less blood being ejected from the heart with each contraction.

CAUSES

- Atherosclerosis
- Congenital defects
- Coronary artery spasm
- Dissecting aneurysm
- Infectious vasculitis
- Syphilis

ASSESSMENT FINDINGS

- Angina that may radiate to the left arm, neck, jaw, or shoulder blade
  - Commonly occurs after physical exertion but may also follow emotional excitement, exposure to cold, or a large meal
  - May develop during sleep, with symptoms awakening the patient
- Angina
  - *Stable* (predictable and relieved by rest or nitrates)
  - *Unstable* (increases in frequency and duration, is more easily induced, and generally indicates extensive or worsening disease; untreated, may progress to myocardial infarction)
  - *Prinzmetal's or variant* (severe non-effort-produced pain occurring at rest without provocation)
- Nausea and vomiting
- Fainting
- Sweating
- Cool extremities
- Xanthoma
- Arteriovenous nicking of the eye
- Obesity
- Hypertension
- Positive Levine sign (holding fist to chest)
- Decreased or absent peripheral pulses

TEST RESULTS

- Myocardial perfusion imaging with thallium 201 during treadmill exercise reveals ischemic areas of the myocardium, visualized as "cold spots."
- Pharmacologic myocardial perfusion imaging in arteries with stenosis reveals a decrease in blood flow proportional to the percentage of occlusion.

PREVENTING CORONARY ARTERY DISEASE

Because coronary artery disease is so widespread, prevention is important. Dietary restrictions aimed at reducing the intake of calories (in obesity) and of salt, fats, and cholesterol minimize the risk, especially when supplemented with regular exercise. Abstention from smoking and reduction of stress are also essential.

Other preventive actions include control of hypertension (with diuretics or sympathetic beta-adrenergic blockers), control of elevated serum cholesterol or triglyceride levels (with antilipemics such as HMG-CoA reductase inhibitors, including atorvastatin [Lipitor], pravastatin [Pravachol], or simvastatin [Zocor]), and measures to minimize platelet aggregation and the danger of blood clots (with aspirin, for example).

- Multiple-gated acquisition scanning reveals cardiac wall motion and reflects injury to cardiac tissue.
- Electrocardiography shows ischemic changes during angina (may be normal between anginal episodes).
- Exercise testing reveals ST-segment changes during exercise, indicating ischemia, and allows determination of a safe exercise prescription.
- Coronary angiography reveals the location and degree of coronary artery stenosis or obstruction, collateral circulation, and the condition of the artery beyond the narrowing.
- Stress echocardiography may reveal abnormal wall motion.

TREATMENT

- Stress-reduction techniques essential, especially if known stressors precipitate pain
- Lifestyle modifications, such as smoking cessation and maintaining ideal body weight (see *Preventing coronary artery disease*)
- Low-fat, low-sodium diet
- Activity restrictions possible
- Regular exercise
- Aspirin
- Nitrates
- Beta-adrenergic blockers
- Calcium channel blockers
- Antiplatelets
- Antilipemics
- Antihypertensives
- Coronary artery bypass graft

- "Keyhole" or minimally invasive surgery
- Angioplasty
- Endovascular stent placement
- Laser angioplasty
- Atherectomy

 ALERT *Advise patient that stopping nitrates abruptly causes coronary artery spasm.*

KEY PATIENT OUTCOMES

The patient will:
- maintain hemodynamic stability
- plan menus appropriate to prescribed diet
- demonstrate understanding of the disease process
- express concern about self-concept, self-esteem, and body image
- express feelings of increased comfort and decreased pain.

NURSING INTERVENTIONS

- Ask the patient to grade the severity of his pain on a scale of 1 to 10.
- Keep nitroglycerin available for immediate use. Instruct the patient to call immediately whenever he feels pain and before taking nitroglycerin.
- Observe for signs and symptoms that may signify worsening of condition.
- Guide the patient in pulmonary self-care.
- Check vital signs and intake and output.
- Determine effectiveness of pain medication during anginal episodes.
- Monitor for abnormal bleeding and distal pulses following intervention procedures.
- Assess breath sounds and cardiac rate and rhythm.
- Determine chest tube drainage after surgery.
- Refer the patient to a weight-loss program, if needed.
- Refer the patient to a smoking-cessation program, if needed.
- Refer the patient to a cardiac rehabilitation program, if indicated.

PATIENT TEACHING

Be sure to cover:
- risk factors for CAD
- avoidance of activities that precipitate episodes of pain
- effective coping mechanisms to deal with stress
- need to follow the prescribed drug regimen
- low-sodium and low-calorie diet
- importance of regular, moderate exercise.

Cushing's syndrome

DESCRIPTION

- Clinical manifestations of glucocorticoid excess, particularly cortisol
- May also reflect excess secretion of mineralocorticoids and androgens
- Classified as primary, secondary, or iatrogenic, depending on etiology
- Prognosis dependent on early diagnosis, identification of underlying cause, and effective treatment

PATHOPHYSIOLOGY

- Normal feedback inhibition by cortisol is lost.
- Elevated levels of cortisol don't suppress hypothalamic and anterior pituitary secretion of corticotropin-releasing hormone and adrenal corticotropic hormone (ACTH).
- The result is excessive levels of circulating cortisol.

CAUSES

- Chronic use of synthetic glucocorticoids or corticotropin
- Corticotropin-producing tumor in another organ
- Cortisol-secreting adrenal tumor
- Excess production of corticotropin
- Pituitary microadenoma

ASSESSMENT FINDINGS

- History revealing use of synthetic steroids
- Complaints of fatigue, muscle weakness, and sleep disturbances
- Polyuria, thirst, and other symptoms resembling those of hyperglycemia
- Frequent infections
- Water retention
- Amenorrhea
- Decreased libido and impotence
- Irritability and emotional instability
- Headache
- Alopecia of scalp hair in women and hirsutism of the face
- Moon-shaped face
- Buffalo-humplike back
- Central obesity
- Thin extremities and muscle wasting and weakness
- Petechiae, ecchymoses, and purplish striae
- Delayed wound healing

- Swollen ankles
- Hypertension
- Acne

TEST RESULTS

- Free cortisol level in the saliva and in urine is elevated.
- ACTH level decreases and excess pituitary or ectopic secretion of ACTH increases in adrenal disease.
- Blood chemistry may show hypernatremia, hypokalemia, hypocalcemia, and elevated blood glucose level.
- Serum cortisol is elevated in the morning.
- Glycosuria develops.
- Ultrasonography, computed tomography scan, and magnetic resonance imaging may show location of a pituitary or adrenal tumor.
- Low-dose dexamethasone suppression test shows failure of plasma cortisol levels to be suppressed.

TREATMENT

- Management to restore hormone balance and reverse Cushing's syndrome, including radiation, drug therapy, or surgery
- High-protein, high-potassium, low-calorie, low-sodium diet
- Activity as tolerated
- Aminoglutethimide
- Antifungal agents
- Antihypertensives
- Diuretics
- Glucocorticoids

ALERT *Glucocorticoid administration on the morning of surgery can help prevent acute adrenal insufficiency during surgery. Cortisol therapy is essential during and after surgery to help the patient tolerate the physiologic stress caused by removal of the pituitary or adrenal glands.*

- Potassium supplements
- Antineoplastic, antihormone agents
- Possible hypophysectomy or pituitary irradiation
- Bilateral adrenalectomy
- Excision of nonendocrine, corticotropin-producing tumor, followed by drug therapy

KEY PATIENT OUTCOMES

The patient will:
- maintain skin integrity
- remain free from infection
- perform activities of daily living within the confines of the disorder
- express positive feelings about self
- express understanding of disorder.

NURSING INTERVENTIONS

- Administer prescribed drugs.
- Consult a dietitian.
- Use protective measures to reduce the risk of infection.
- Use meticulous hand-washing technique.
- Schedule adequate rest periods.
- Institute safety precautions.
- Provide meticulous skin care.
- Encourage verbalization of feelings.
- Offer emotional support.
- Help to develop effective coping strategies.
- Refer the patient to a mental health professional for additional counseling, if necessary.

With transsphenoidal approach to hypophysectomy

- Keep the head of the bed elevated at least 30 degrees.
- Maintain nasal packing.
- Provide frequent mouth care.
- Avoid activities that increase intracranial pressure (ICP).
- Obtain vital signs, intake and output, and daily weight.
- Obtain serum electrolyte results.

After bilateral adrenalectomy and hypophysectomy

- Monitor neurologic and behavioral status.
- Watch for severe nausea, vomiting, and diarrhea.
- Assess bowel sounds.
- Monitor for adrenal hypofunction, hypopituitarism, transient diabetes insipidus, hemorrhage, and shock.
- Observe for increased ICP.

After transsphenoidal approach to hypophysectomy

- Monitor patient for cerebrospinal fluid leak.

PATIENT TEACHING

Be sure to cover:
- the disorder, diagnosis, and treatment
- medications and potential adverse effects
- when to notify the physician
- life-long steroid replacement
- signs and symptoms of adrenal crisis
- medical identification bracelet
- prevention of infection
- stress reduction strategies.

Diabetes insipidus

DESCRIPTION

- Disorder of water balance regulation characterized by excessive fluid intake and hypotonic polyuria
- Two types: primary and secondary
- May occur transiently during pregnancy, usually after the 5th or 6th month of gestation
- Impaired or absent thirst mechanism increases risk of complications
- If uncomplicated, prognosis good
- If complicated by underlying disorder, such as cancer, prognosis variable
- Also referred to as *DI*

PATHOPHYSIOLOGY

- Vasopressin (antidiuretic hormone) is synthesized in the hypothalamus and stored by the posterior pituitary gland.
- Following release into the general circulation, vasopressin acts on the distal and collecting tubules of the kidneys.
- Vasopressin increases the water permeability of the tubules and causes water reabsorption.
- The absence of vasopressin allows filtered water to be excreted in the urine instead of being reabsorbed.

CAUSES

- Certain medications such as lithium
- Congenital malformation of the central nervous system (CNS)
- Damage to hypothalamus or pituitary gland
- Failure of the kidneys to respond to vasopressin (called *nephrogenic DI*)
- Failure of vasopressin secretion in response to normal physiologic stimuli
- Familial

- Granulomatous disease
- Idiopathic
- Infection
- Neurosurgery, skull fracture, or head trauma
- Pregnancy (called *gestational DI*)
- Psychogenic
- Trauma
- Tumors
- Vascular lesions

ASSESSMENT FINDINGS

- Abrupt onset of extreme polyuria; nocturia
- Extreme thirst, extraordinarily large oral fluid intake
- Weight loss
- Dizziness, weakness, and fatigue
- Constipation
- Signs of dehydration, poor skin turgor
- Fever
- Dyspnea
- Pale, voluminous urine
- Tachycardia
- Decreased muscle strength
- Hypotension

TEST RESULTS

- Urinalysis shows colorless urine with low osmolality and specific gravity.
- Serum sodium is increased.
- Serum osmolality is increased.
- Serum vasopressin is decreased.
- 24-hour urine test shows decreased specific gravity and increased volume.
- Blood urea nitrogen (BUN) and creatinine levels increase.
- Dehydration test or water deprivation test shows an increase in urine osmolality after vasopressin administration exceeding 9%.

TREATMENT

- Identification and treatment of underlying cause
- Control of fluid balance
- Dehydration prevention
- Free access to oral fluids
- With nephrogenic DI, low-sodium diet

- Vasopressin; synthetic vasopressin analogue
- Vasopressin stimulant
- Thiazide diuretics in nephrogenic DI
- I.V. fluids:
    - If serum sodium greater than 150 mEq/L: 5% dextrose in water
    - If serum sodium less than 150 mEq/L: normal saline solution
- Surgery not indicated, unless required to treat underlying cause such as a tumor

KEY PATIENT OUTCOMES

The patient will:
- demonstrate balanced fluid volume
- display adaptive coping behaviors
- avoid complications
- demonstrate normal laboratory values.

NURSING INTERVENTIONS

- Administer medications as ordered.

   ALERT *Use caution when administering vasopressin to a patient with coronary artery disease because it can cause coronary artery constriction.*

- Provide meticulous skin and mouth care.
- Encourage verbalization of feelings.
- Offer encouragement while providing a realistic assessment of the situation.
- Help the patient develop effective coping strategies.
- Check vital signs, intake and output, and daily weight.
- Monitor urine specific gravity, serum electrolytes, and BUN.
- Watch for signs and symptoms of hypovolemic shock.
- Assess for changes in mental or neurologic status.
- Monitor the patient's cardiac rhythm.
- Refer the patient to a mental health professional for additional counseling, if indicated.

PATIENT TEACHING

Be sure to cover:
- the disorder, diagnosis, and treatment
- medication and potential adverse effects
- when to notify the physician
- signs and symptoms of dehydration
- importance of weighing himself daily

- intake and output
- use of a hydrometer to measure urine specific gravity
- need for medical identification jewelry
- need for ongoing medical care.

Diabetes mellitus

DESCRIPTION

- Chronic disease of absolute or relative insulin deficiency or resistance
- Characterized by disturbances in carbohydrate, protein, and fat metabolism
- Two primary forms:
  - Type 1, characterized by absolute insufficiency
  - Type 2, characterized by insulin resistance with varying degrees of insulin secretory defects

PATHOPHYSIOLOGY

- The effects of diabetes mellitus (DM) result from insulin deficiency or resistance to endogenous insulin. (See *Understanding diabetes mellitus*, page 96.)
- Insulin allows glucose transport into the cells for use as energy or storage as glycogen.
- Insulin also stimulates protein synthesis and free fatty acid storage in the adipose tissues.
- Insulin deficiency compromises the body tissues' access to essential nutrients for fuel and storage.

CAUSES

- Autoimmune disease (type 1)
- Genetic factors

ASSESSMENT FINDINGS

Type 1
- Rapidly developing symptoms
- Polyuria, nocturia
- Dehydration
- Polydipsia
- Dry mucous membranes, poor skin turgor
- Weight loss and hunger; muscle wasting and loss of subcutaneous fat
- Weakness, fatigue

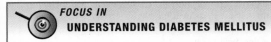

FOCUS IN
UNDERSTANDING DIABETES MELLITUS

Diabetes affects the way the body uses food to make the energy for life.

Type 1 diabetes
- The pancreas makes little or no insulin.
- In genetically susceptible patients, a triggering event (possibly a viral infection) causes production of autoantibodies against the beta cells of the pancreas.
- The resultant destruction of beta cells leads to a decline in and ultimate lack of insulin secretion.
- Insulin deficiency leads to hyperglycemia, enhanced lipolysis, and protein catabolism. These occur when more than 90% of the beta cells have been destroyed.

Type 2 diabetes
- Genetic factors are significant, and onset is accelerated by obesity and a sedentary lifestyle. The pancreas produces some insulin, but it's either too little or ineffective.
- Factors that contribute to type 2 diabetes development include:
    - impaired insulin secretion
    - inappropriate hepatic glucose production
    - peripheral insulin receptor insensitivity.

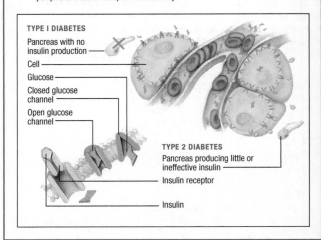

TYPE I DIABETES
Pancreas with no insulin production
Cell
Glucose
Closed glucose channel
Open glucose channel

TYPE 2 DIABETES
Pancreas producing little or ineffective insulin
Insulin receptor
Insulin

- Vision changes
- Frequent skin and urinary tract infections
- Dry, itchy skin
- Sexual problems
- Numbness or pain in the hands or feet
- Postprandial feeling of nausea or fullness
- Nocturnal diarrhea

Type 2
- Vague, long-standing symptoms that develop gradually
- Family history of DM
- Pregnancy
- Severe viral infection
- Other endocrine diseases
- Recent stress or trauma
- Use of drugs that increase blood glucose levels
- Obesity, particularly in the abdominal area

Both types
- Retinopathy or cataract formation
- Skin changes, especially on the legs and feet
- Dry mucous membranes
- Decreased peripheral pulses
- Cool skin temperature
- Diminished deep tendon reflexes
- Orthostatic hypotension
- Characteristic "fruity" breath odor in ketoacidosis
- Possible hypovolemia and shock in ketoacidosis and hyperosmolar hyperglycemic state

TEST RESULTS
- Fasting plasma glucose level is greater than or equal to 126 mg/dl on at least two occasions.
- Random blood glucose level is greater than or equal to 200 mg/dl.
- Two-hour postprandial blood glucose level is greater than or equal to 200 mg/dl.
- Glycosylated hemoglobin (Hb A_{1c}) level is increased.
- Urinalysis may show acetone or glucose.
- Ophthalmologic examination may show diabetic retinopathy.

TARGET NUMBERS FOR DIABETES MELLITUS

To help patients reduce their risk of complications from diabetes, the American Diabetes Association has recommended important target numbers. Teach your patient to monitor his target numbers for blood glucose, Hb A_{1c}, blood lipids, and blood pressure.

- Blood glucose: Some meters and test strips report blood glucose as plasma glucose values which are 10% to 15% higher than whole blood glucose values. Be sure to find out whether the meter and strips provide whole blood or plasma results.
  - The target glucose range for most people using whole blood is 80 to 120 mg/dl before meals and 100 to 140 mg/dl at bedtime.
  - The target glucose range for most people using plasma is 90 to 130 mg/dl before meals and 110 to 150 mg/dl at bedtime.
- Hb A_{1c}: measures how well blood glucose has been controlled over the previous 3 months; it should be performed twice per year.
  - The target: Hb A_{1c} for most people with diabetes is less than 7%.
- Blood lipids: low-density lipoprotein (LDL) is the cholesterol that causes the vessels to narrow and harden, which can lead to a heart attack.
  - The target LDL cholesterol for most people with diabetes is less than 100 mg/dl.
- Blood pressure: High blood pressure makes the heart work harder and can lead to strokes and kidney disease. Blood pressure should be checked at every physician visit.
  - The target blood pressure for most people with diabetes is less than 130/80 mm Hg.

From: National Institute of Health *www.ndep.nih.gov/diabetes/control/ principles/html.*

TREATMENT

COLLABORATION *Consult with a dietitian and a diabetes educator, who can assist in teaching the patient ways to gain dietary control.*

- Tight glycemic control for prevention of complications
- Modest caloric restriction for weight loss or maintenance
- American Diabetes Association recommendations for reaching target glucose, Hb A_{1c}, lipid, and blood pressure levels (see *Target numbers for diabetes mellitus*)
- Regular aerobic exercise
- Exogenous insulin (type 1 and possibly type 2)

- Oral antihyperglycemic drugs (type 2)
- Pancreas transplantation (rare)

KEY PATIENT OUTCOMES

The patient will:
- maintain optimal body weight
- remain free from infection
- avoid complications
- verbalize understanding of the disorder and treatment
- demonstrate adaptive coping behaviors.

NURSING INTERVENTIONS

- Administer prescribed drugs.
- Give rapidly absorbed carbohydrates for hypoglycemia or, if the patient is unconscious, glucagon or I.V. dextrose, as ordered.
- Administer I.V. fluids and insulin replacement for hyperglycemic crisis, as ordered.
- Provide meticulous skin care, especially to the feet and legs.
- Treat all injuries, cuts, and blisters immediately.
- Avoid constricting hose, slippers, or bed linens.
- Encourage adequate fluid intake.
- Encourage verbalization of feelings.
- Offer emotional support.
- Help to develop effective coping strategies.
- Check vital signs, intake and output, and daily weight.
- Monitor laboratory values, especially serum glucose and urine acetone.
- Assess renal and cardiovascular status, as needed.
- Watch for signs and symptoms of hypoglycemia, hyperglycemia, hyperosmolar coma, urinary tract and vaginal infections, and diabetic neuropathy.

ALERT *Watch for signs and symptoms of acute complications from diabetic therapy: altered thinking, dizziness, weakness, pallor, tachycardia, diaphoresis, seizures, and coma. If the patient is conscious, he must immediately receive carbohydrates in the form of fruit juice, hard candy, or honey. If he's unconscious, he must receive glucagon or dextrose I.V.*

- Refer the patient to a podiatrist, if indicated.
- Refer the patient to an ophthalmologist.
- Refer adult diabetic patients who are planning families for preconception counseling.

PATIENT TEACHING

Be sure to cover:
- the disorder, diagnosis, and treatment
- medication and potential adverse effects
- when to notify the physician
- prescribed meal plan
- prescribed exercise program
- signs and symptoms of infection, hypoglycemia, hyperglycemia, and diabetic neuropathy
- self-monitoring of blood glucose
- complications of hyperglycemia
- foot care
- annual ophthalmologic examinations
- safety precautions
- proper management of diabetes during illness
- how to access the Juvenile Diabetes Research Foundation, the American Association of Diabetes Educators, and the American Diabetes Association to obtain additional information.

Disseminated intravascular coagulation

DESCRIPTION

- Syndrome of activated coagulation characterized by bleeding or thrombosis
- Complicates diseases and conditions that accelerate clotting, causing occlusion of small blood vessels, organ necrosis, depletion of circulating clotting factors and platelets, and activation of the fibrinolytic system
- Also known as *DIC, consumption coagulopathy,* and *defibrination syndrome*

PATHOPHYSIOLOGY

- Typical accelerated clotting results in generalized activation of prothrombin and a consequent excess of thrombin.
- Excess thrombin converts fibrinogen to fibrin, producing fibrin clots in the microcirculation.
- This process consumes exorbitant amounts of coagulation factors (especially platelets, factor V, prothrombin, fibrinogen, and factor VIII), causing thrombocytopenia, deficiencies in factors V and VIII, hypoprothrombinemia, and hypofibrinogenemia.

- Circulating thrombin activates the fibrinolytic system, which lyses fibrin clots into fibrinogen degradation products (FDPs).
- The hemorrhage that occurs may be caused by the anticoagulant activity of FDPs and depletion of plasma coagulation factors.

CAUSES

- Acute respiratory distress syndrome
- Cardiac arrest
- Diabetic ketoacidosis
- Disorders that produce necrosis, such as extensive burns and trauma
- Drug reactions
- Heatstroke
- Incompatible blood transfusion
- Infection, sepsis
- Neoplastic disease
- Obstetric complications
- Pulmonary embolism
- Sickle cell anemia
- Shock
- Surgery necessitating cardiopulmonary bypass

ASSESSMENT FINDINGS

- Abnormal bleeding *without* a history of a serious hemorrhagic disorder, from any body orifice
- Signs of bleeding into the skin, such as cutaneous oozing, petechiae, ecchymoses, and hematomas
- Bleeding from surgical or invasive procedure sites, such as incisions or venipuncture sites
- Nausea and vomiting, epistaxis, or GI bleeding
- Severe muscle, back, chest, or abdominal pain
- Hematuria or oliguria
- Acrocyanosis
- Dyspnea, tachypnea, and possible hemoptysis
- Mental status changes, including confusion; seizures

TEST RESULTS

- Serum platelet count is less than $150,000/mm^3$.
- Serum fibrinogen level is less than 170 mg/dl.
- Prothrombin time is longer than 19 seconds.
- Partial thromboplastin time is longer than 40 seconds.

- FDPs are greater than 45 mcg/ml or positive at less than 1:100 dilution.
- Result of D-dimer test (specific fibrinogen test for DIC) is positive at less than 1:8 dilution.
- Thrombin time is prolonged.
- Blood clotting factors V and VIII are diminished.
- Complete blood count shows decreased hemoglobin levels (less than 10 g/dl).
- Blood urea nitrogen level is greater than 25 mg/dl, and serum creatinine level is greater than 1.3 mg/dl.

TREATMENT

 ALERT *Successful management of DIC necessitates prompt recognition and adequate treatment of the underlying disorder.*

- Possibly, supportive care alone if the patient isn't actively bleeding
- Activity as tolerated
  If the patient is actively bleeding:
- Administration of blood, fresh frozen plasma, platelets, or packed red blood cells
- Cryoprecipitate
- Antithrombin III and gabexate mesilate
- Fluid replacement

KEY PATIENT OUTCOMES

The patient will:
- maintain balanced intake and output
- maintain adequate ventilation
- express feelings of increased comfort and decreased pain
- have laboratory values return to normal
- use available support systems to assist in coping with fears.

NURSING INTERVENTIONS

- Provide emotional support.
- Provide adequate rest periods.
- Give prescribed analgesics as needed.
- Reposition the patient every 2 hours, and provide meticulous skin care.
- Give prescribed oxygen therapy.
- Protect the patient from injury.

 ALERT *To prevent clots from dislodging and causing fresh bleeding, don't vigorously rub the affected areas when bathing.*

- If bleeding occurs, use pressure and topical hemostatic agents to control bleeding.
- Limit venipunctures whenever possible.
- Watch for transfusion reactions and signs of fluid overload.
- Measure the amount of blood lost, weigh dressings and linen, and record drainage.
- Weigh the patient daily, particularly if there's renal involvement.
- Check vital signs and intake and output, especially when administering blood products.
- Evaluate results of serial blood studies.
- Watch for signs of shock.

PATIENT TEACHING

Be sure to cover (with the patient and his family):
- an explanation of the disorder
- the signs and symptoms of the problem, diagnostic procedures required, and treatment that the patient will receive.

Diverticular disease

DESCRIPTION

- Bulging pouches (diverticula) in GI wall pushing the mucosal lining through surrounding muscle
- Sigmoid colon most common site but may develop anywhere, from proximal end of the pharynx to the anus
- Other typical sites:
  - Duodenum, near the pancreatic border or the ampulla of Vater
  - Jejunum
- Diverticular disease of the ileum (Meckel's diverticulum) most common congenital anomaly of the GI tract
- Two clinical forms:
  - Diverticulosis: diverticula present but don't cause symptoms
  - Diverticulitis: diverticula becoming inflamed, possibly causing complications

PATHOPHYSIOLOGY

- Pressure in the intestinal lumen is exerted on weak areas, such as points where blood vessels enter the intestine, causing a break in the muscular continuity of the GI wall, creating a diverticulum. (See *How diverticular disease develops*, page 104.)

FOCUS IN
HOW DIVERTICULAR DISEASE DEVELOPS

Diverticula probably result from high intraluminal pressure on an area of weakness in the GI wall, where blood vessels enter.

In diverticulitis, retained undigested food and bacteria accumulate in the diverticular sac. This hard mass cuts off the blood supply to the thin walls of the sac, making them more susceptible to attack by colonic bacteria. Inflammation follows and may lead to perforation, abscess, peritonitis, obstruction, or hemorrhage.

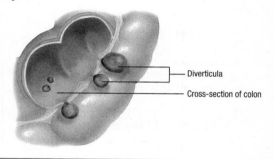

Diverticula

Cross-section of colon

- Inflammation follows bacterial infection, causing abdominal pain.
- Diverticulitis occurs when retained undigested food mixed with bacteria accumulates in the diverticulum, forming a hard mass (fecalith). This substance cuts off the blood supply to the diverticulum's thin walls, increasing its susceptibility to attack by colonic bacteria.

CAUSES

- Defects in colon wall strength
- Diminished colonic motility and increased intraluminal pressure

ASSESSMENT FINDINGS

Diverticulosis
- May be asymptomatic
- Occasional intermittent pain in the left lower abdominal quadrant, which may be relieved by defecation or the passage of flatus
- Alternating bouts of constipation and diarrhea

Diverticulitis
- History of diverticulosis
- Low fiber consumption
- Complaints of moderate dull or steady pain in the left lower abdominal quadrant, aggravated by straining, lifting, or coughing; tenderness in the area; palpable mass
- Mild nausea, gas, diarrhea, or intermittent bouts of constipation, sometimes accompanied by rectal bleeding
- Low-grade fever
- Guarding and rebound tenderness (signs of peritoneal irritation, if acute)

TEST RESULTS
- Complete blood count reveals leukocytosis.
- Erythrocyte sedimentation rate is elevated in diverticulitis.
- Stool test result is positive for occult blood in 25% of patients with diverticulitis.
- Barium studies reveal barium-filled diverticula or outlines (doesn't fill diverticula blocked by impacted stools).

> **ALERT** *Barium studies aren't performed for acute diverticulitis because of the risk of rupture.*

- Radiography may show colonic spasm, if irritable bowel syndrome accompanies diverticular disease.
- Abdominal X-rays rule out perforation.
- Colonoscopy or flexible sigmoidoscopy reveals diverticula or inflamed mucosa (not usually performed in the acute phase).
- Biopsy rules out cancer.
- Computed tomography scan of the abdomen checks for the presence of an abscess.

TREATMENT
- No treatment required for asymptomatic diverticulosis

If mild diverticulosis or diverticulitis (without fever, elevated white count, or signs of peritonitis or bleeding):
- Liquid diet for 2 days of bowel rest, followed by high-fiber diet (if patient experiencing pain)
- Stool softeners and fiber laxatives, if required
- Possible oral antibiotics

If severe diverticulitis:
- Nothing by mouth initially
- Nasogastric (NG) decompression
- Bed rest

- I.V. antibiotics
- Analgesics
- Antispasmodics
- I.V. therapy
- Colon resection for rupture or cases refractory to treatment
- Temporary colostomy possibly, to drain abscesses and rest the colon 6 to 8 weeks

KEY PATIENT OUTCOMES

The patient will:
- express feelings of increased comfort
- maintain normal fluid volume
- have bowel movements that return to normal
- verbalize understanding of the disease process and treatment regimen.

NURSING INTERVENTIONS

ALERT Remember that diverticulitis produces more serious signs and symptoms as well as complications, and requires more interventions than diverticulosis.
- Administer prescribed drugs.
- Maintain bed rest for acute diverticulitis.
- Maintain prescribed diet.
- Check vital signs and intake and output.
- If surgery is scheduled, provide routine preoperative care.
- Provide meticulous wound care.
- Encourage coughing and deep breathing.
- Provide colostomy care, if appropriate.
- Evaluate the effectiveness of pain control measures.
- Assess stools for color, consistency, and frequency.
- Set up NG drainage, if ordered.
- Monitor for signs and symptoms of infection, postoperative bleeding, and complications.
- Refer the patient to an enterostomal therapist if colostomy was required and to a dietitian if needed.

PATIENT TEACHING

Be sure to cover:
- the disorder, diagnosis, and treatment
- desired actions and possible adverse effects of prescribed medications
- bowel and dietary habits as well as characteristics of a high-fiber diet
- preoperative and postoperative teaching as appropriate.

Emphysema

DESCRIPTION

- Chronic lung disease characterized by permanent enlargement of air spaces distal to the terminal bronchioles and by exertional dyspnea
- One of several diseases usually labeled collectively as *chronic obstructive pulmonary disease* or *chronic obstructive lung disease*

PATHOPHYSIOLOGY

- Emphysema occurs when recurrent inflammation associated with the release of proteolytic enzymes from lung cells causes abnormal, irreversible enlargement of the air spaces distal to the terminal bronchioles.
- This enlargement leads to the destruction of alveolar walls, which results in a breakdown of elasticity.

CAUSES

- Cigarette smoking
- Genetic deficiency of alpha$_1$-antitrypsin

ASSESSMENT FINDINGS

- History of smoking
- Complaints of shortness of breath, chronic cough, and malaise
- Anorexia and weight loss
- Barrel chest
- Pursed-lip breathing, use of accessory muscles
- Cyanosis
- Clubbed fingers and toes
- Tachypnea; decreased tactile fremitus and chest expansion
- Hyperresonance
- Decreased breath sounds with crackles, inspiratory wheeze, and prolonged expiratory phase with grunting respirations
- Distant heart sounds

TEST RESULTS

- Arterial blood gas (ABG) analysis shows decreased partial pressure of oxygen; ABG analysis shows normal partial pressure of carbon dioxide until late in the disease, when it increases.
- Red blood cell count reveals an increased hemoglobin level late in the disease.

- Chest X-ray may show:
  - flattened diaphragm
  - reduced vascular markings at the lung periphery
  - overaeration of the lungs
  - vertical heart
  - enlarged anteroposterior chest diameter
  - large retrosternal air space.
- Pulmonary function tests reveal:
  - increased residual volume and total lung capacity
  - reduced diffusing capacity
  - increased inspiratory flow.
- Electrocardiography may show tall, symmetrical P waves in leads II, III, and aV$_F$; a vertical QRS axis; and signs of right ventricular hypertrophy late in the disease.

TREATMENT

COLLABORATION Many patients with emphysema receive outpatient treatment and need comprehensive instruction to help them comply with therapy.

- Chest physiotherapy
- Possible transtracheal catheterization and low-dose home oxygen therapy
- Adequate hydration
- High-protein, high-calorie diet
- Activity as tolerated
- Bronchodilators
- Anticholinergics
- Mucolytics
- Corticosteroids
- Antibiotics as needed
- Chest tube insertion for pneumothorax, if needed

KEY PATIENT OUTCOMES

The patient will:
- maintain a patent airway and adequate ventilation
- demonstrate energy conservation techniques
- express understanding of the illness
- demonstrate effective coping strategies.

NURSING INTERVENTIONS

- Administer prescribed medications.

- Provide supportive care.
- Help the patient adjust to lifestyle changes as needed.
- Encourage the patient to express his fears and concerns.
- Perform chest physiotherapy.
- Provide a high-calorie, protein-rich diet.
- Give small, frequent meals.
- Encourage daily activity and diversional activities.
- Provide frequent rest periods.
- Check vital signs, intake and output, and daily weight.
- Monitor for complications, respiratory status, and activity tolerance.
- Refer the family of patients with familial emphysema for alpha$_1$-antitrypsin deficiency screening, if interested.

PATIENT TEACHING

Be sure to cover:
- the disorder, diagnosis, and treatment
- medication and potential adverse effects
- when to notify the physician

> **ALERT** *Urge the patient to notify the physician if he experiences a sudden onset of worsening dyspnea or sharp pleuritic chest pain exacerbated by chest movement, breathing, or coughing.*

- avoidance of crowds and people with known infections
- avoidance of smoking and areas where smoking is permitted
- home oxygen therapy, if indicated
- transtracheal catheter care, if needed
- coughing and deep-breathing exercises
- proper use of handheld inhalers
- high-calorie, high-protein diet
- adequate oral fluid intake
- avoidance of respiratory irritants
- signs and symptoms of pneumothorax
- how to access a smoking-cessation program, if indicated
- need for influenza and pneumococcal pneumonia immunizations as needed.

Endocarditis

DESCRIPTION

- Infection of the endocardium, heart valves, or cardiac prosthesis

FOCUS IN

DEGENERATIVE CHANGES IN ENDOCARDITIS

This illustration shows typical vegetations on the endocardium produced by fibrin and platelet deposits on infection sites.

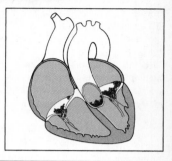

PATHOPHYSIOLOGY

- Fibrin and platelets cluster on valve tissue and engulf circulating bacteria or fungi. (See *Degenerative changes in endocarditis*.)
- This produces vegetation, which in turn may cover the valve surfaces, causing deformities and destruction of valvular tissue that may extend to the chordae tendineae, causing them to rupture, leading to valvular insufficiency.
- Vegetative growth on the heart valves, endocardial lining of a heart chamber, or endothelium of a blood vessel may embolize to the spleen, kidneys, central nervous system, and lungs.

CAUSES

- Asymmetrical septal hypertrophy
- Calcific aortic stenosis (in elderly patients)
- Cardiac valvular disease
- Congenital heart disease
- Degenerative heart disease
- I.V. drug use
- Long-term hemodialysis
- Marfan syndrome
- Mitral valve prolapse
- Prosthetic heart valves
- Rheumatic heart disease
- Syphilitic aortic valve

ASSESSMENT FINDINGS

- Nonspecific symptoms, such as weakness, fatigue, weight loss, anorexia, arthralgia, night sweats, and intermittent fever that may recur for weeks
- Petechiae on the skin (especially common on the upper anterior trunk) and on the buccal, pharyngeal, or conjunctival mucosa
- Splinter hemorrhages under the nails
- Clubbing of the fingers in patients with long-standing disease
- Heart murmur in all patients except those with early acute endocarditis and I.V. drug users with tricuspid valve infection
- Osler's nodes (painful red indurated areas in the pads of the fingers and toes)
- Roth's spots (small white spots surrounded by hemorrhage found in the eye)
- Janeway lesions (small hemorrhagic macular lesions on the palms and soles)
- Murmur that changes suddenly or a new murmur that develops in the presence of fever (classic physical sign)
- Splenomegaly in long-standing disease
- Dyspnea, tachycardia, and bibasilar crackles possible with left-sided heart failure
- Splenic infarction causing pain in the upper left quadrant, radiating to the left shoulder, and abdominal rigidity
- Renal infarction causing hematuria, pyuria, flank pain, and decreased urine output
- Cerebral infarction causing hemiparesis, aphasia, and other neurologic deficits
- Pulmonary infarction causing cough, pleuritic pain, pleural friction rub, dyspnea, and hemoptysis
- Peripheral vascular occlusion causing numbness and tingling in an arm, leg, finger, or toe or signs of impending peripheral gangrene

TEST RESULTS

- Three or more blood cultures during a 24- to 48-hour period identify the causative organism in up to 90% of patients.
- White blood cell count with differential is normal or elevated.
- Complete blood count and anemia panel show normocytic, normo-chromic anemia in subacute infective endocarditis.
- Erythrocyte sedimentation rate and serum creatinine level are elevated.
- Serum rheumatoid factor is positive in about one-half of all patients with endocarditis after the disease is present for 6 weeks.
- Urinalysis shows proteinuria and microscopic hematuria.

- Echocardiography may reveal valvular damage in up to 80% of patients with native valve disease.
- Electrocardiogram may show atrial fibrillation and other arrhythmias that accompany valvular disease.

TREATMENT

- Selection of anti-infective based on type of infecting organism and sensitivity studies start promptly and continue for 4 to 6 weeks
- If blood cultures negative (10% to 20% of subacute cases), possible I.V. antibiotic therapy (usually for 4 to 6 weeks) against probable infecting organism
- Adequate hydration
- Bed rest
- Aspirin
- With severe valvular damage, especially aortic insufficiency or infection of a cardiac prosthesis, possible corrective surgery if refractory heart failure develops or if an infected prosthetic valve must be replaced

KEY PATIENT OUTCOMES

The patient will:
- carry out activities of daily living without weakness or fatigue
- maintain hemodynamic stability with adequate cardiac output
- exhibit no arrhythmias
- maintain adequate ventilation
- express feelings about diminished capacity to perform usual roles.

NURSING INTERVENTIONS

- Stress the importance of bed rest.
- Provide a bedside commode.
- Allow the patient to express his concerns.
- Obtain a history of allergies.
- Administer antibiotics as ordered.
- Administer oxygen.

  ALERT *Watch for signs of embolization, a common occurrence during the first 3 months of treatment. Tell the patient to watch for and report these signs.*
- Monitor the patient's renal status.
- Perform cardiovascular status assessments every 1 to 2 hours, or more frequently as needed.
- Monitor arterial blood gas levels as ordered.

PATIENT TEACHING

Be sure to cover:
- the disorder, diagnosis, and treatment
- anti-infectives the patient needs to continue taking
- need to watch closely for fever, anorexia, and other signs of relapse about 2 weeks after treatment stops
- need for prophylactic antibiotics before dental work and some surgical procedures
- proper dental hygiene and avoiding flossing the teeth
- how to recognize symptoms of endocarditis and to notify the physician immediately if such symptoms occur
- need for follow-up care with a cardiologist.

Gastroesophageal reflux disease

DESCRIPTION

- Backflow of gastric or duodenal contents, or both, into the esophagus and past the lower esophageal sphincter (LES), without associated belching or vomiting
- Reflux of gastric acid, causing acute epigastric pain, usually after a meal
- Popularly called *heartburn*
- Also called *GERD*

PATHOPHYSIOLOGY

- Reflux occurs when LES pressure is deficient or when pressure in the stomach exceeds LES pressure. The LES relaxes, and gastric contents regurgitate into the esophagus.
- The degree of mucosal injury is based on the amount and concentration of refluxed gastric acid, proteolytic enzymes, and bile acids.

CAUSES

- Any condition or position that increases intra-abdominal pressure
- Hiatal hernia with incompetent sphincter
- Pyloric surgery (alteration or removal of the pylorus), which allows reflux of bile or pancreatic juice

ASSESSMENT FINDINGS

- Minimal or no symptoms in one-third of patients
- Heartburn that typically occurs 1 ½ to 2 hours after eating

- Heartburn that worsens with vigorous exercise, bending, lying down, wearing tight clothing, coughing, constipation, and obesity
- Reported relief by using antacids or sitting upright
- Regurgitation without associated nausea or belching
- Feeling of fluid accumulation in the throat without a sour or bitter taste
- Chronic pain radiating to the neck, jaws, and arms that may mimic angina pectoris
- Nocturnal hypersalivation and wheezing
- Odynophagia (sharp substernal pain on swallowing), possibly followed by a dull substernal ache
- Bright red or dark brown blood in vomitus
- Laryngitis and morning hoarseness
- Chronic cough

TEST RESULTS

- Barium swallow with fluoroscopy reveals evidence of recurrent reflux.
- Esophageal acidity test reveals degree of gastroesophageal reflux.
- Gastroesophageal scintillation test reveals reflux.
- Esophageal manometry reveals abnormal LES pressure and sphincter incompetence.
- Acid perfusion (Bernstein) test confirms esophagitis.
- Esophagoscopy and biopsy confirm pathologic changes in the mucosa.

TREATMENT

- Modification of lifestyle
- Positional therapy
- Removal of cause
- Weight reduction, if appropriate
- Avoidance of dietary causes
- Avoidance of eating 2 hours before sleep (see *Factors affecting LES pressure*)
- Parenteral nutrition or tube feeding
- Lifting restrictions for surgical treatment (no activity restrictions for medical treatment)
- Antacids
- Cholinergics
- Histamine-2 receptor antagonists
- Proton pump inhibitors
- Hiatal hernia repair
- Vagotomy or pyloroplasty
- Esophagectomy

FACTORS AFFECTING LES PRESSURE

Various dietary and lifestyle elements can increase or decrease lower esophageal sphincter (LES) pressure. Take these into account as you plan the patient's treatment program.

What increases LES pressure
- Carbohydrates
- Low-dose ethanol
- Nonfat milk
- Protein

What decreases LES pressure
- Antiflatulent (simethicone [Gas-X, Mylanta Gas, Phazyme])
- Chocolate
- Cigarette smoking
- Fat
- High-dose ethanol
- Lying on right or left side
- Orange juice
- Sitting
- Tomatoes

KEY PATIENT OUTCOMES

The patient will:
- state and demonstrate understanding of the disorder and its treatment
- express feelings of increased comfort
- show no signs of aspiration
- have minimal or no complications.

NURSING INTERVENTIONS

- Offer emotional and psychological support.
- Assist with diet modification.
- Use semi-Fowler's position for the patient with a nasogastric tube.
- Monitor respiratory status postoperatively.
- Ensure pain control.
- Check vital signs, intake and output, and bowel function.
- Measure chest tube drainage.

PATIENT TEACHING

Be sure to cover:
- the disorder, diagnosis, and treatment
- causes of gastroesophageal reflux
- prescribed antireflux regimen of medication, diet, and positional therapy
- how to develop a dietary plan
- need to identify situations or activities that increase intra-abdominal pressure
- need to refrain from using substances that reduce sphincter control
- signs and symptoms to watch for and report.

Glomerulonephritis

DESCRIPTION

- Bilateral inflammation of the glomeruli, typically following a streptococcal infection
- Also called *acute poststreptococcal glomerulonephritis*

PATHOPHYSIOLOGY

- Epithelial or podocyte layer of the glomerular membrane is disturbed, resulting in a loss of negative charge.
- Acute poststreptococcal glomerulonephritis results from the entrapment and collection of antigen-antibody complexes in the glomerular capillary membranes, after infection with group A beta-hemolytic streptococcus.
- Antigens stimulate the formation of antibodies.
- Circulating antigen-antibody complexes become lodged in the glomerular capillaries.
- Complexes initiate complement activation and the release of immunologic substances that lyse cells and increase membrane permeability.
- Antibody damage to basement membranes causes crescent formation.
- Antibody or antigen-antibody complexes in the glomerular capillary wall activate biochemical mediators of inflammation — complement, leukocytes, and fibrin.
- Activated complement attracts neutrophils and monocytes, which release lysosomal enzymes that damage the glomerular cell walls and cause a proliferation of the extracellular matrix, affecting glomerular blood flow.
- Membrane permeability increases, causing a loss of negative charge across the glomerular membrane as well as enhanced protein filtration.
- Membrane damage leads to platelet aggregation, and platelet degranulation releases substances that increase glomerular permeability.

CAUSES

- Immunoglobulin A nephropathy (Berger's disease)
- Impetigo
- Lipoid nephrosis
- Streptococcal infection of the respiratory tract

Chronic glomerulonephritis

- Focal glomerulosclerosis
- Goodpasture's syndrome
- Hemolytic uremic syndrome
- Membranoproliferative glomerulonephritis
- Membranous glomerulopathy
- Poststreptococcal glomerulonephritis
- Rapidly progressive glomerulonephritis
- Systemic lupus erythematosus

ALERT *The presenting features of glomerulonephritis in children may be encephalopathy with seizures and local neurologic deficits. An elderly patient with glomerulonephritis may report vague, nonspecific symptoms, such as nausea, malaise, and arthralgia.*

ASSESSMENT FINDINGS

- Complaints of decreased urination
- History of recent streptococcal infection of the respiratory tract
- Smoky or coffee-colored urine
- Dyspnea
- Periorbital edema
- Increased blood pressure

TEST RESULTS

- Throat culture reveals group A beta-hemolytic streptococcus.
- Electrolyte, blood urea nitrogen, and creatinine levels are elevated.
- Serum protein level decreases.
- Hemoglobin level decreases in chronic glomerulonephritis.
- Antistreptolysin-O titer is elevated.
- Streptozyme and anti-DNase B levels are elevated.
- Serum complement level is low.
- Urine testing reveals red blood cells, white blood cells, mixed cell casts, protein, fibrin-degradation products, and C3 protein.
- Kidney-ureter-bladder X-ray reveals bilateral kidney enlargement (acute glomerulonephritis).

- X-ray reveals symmetric contraction with normal pelves and calyces (chronic glomerulonephritis).
- Renal biopsy confirms diagnosis.

TREATMENT

- Treatment of the primary disease
- Bed rest
- Fluid restriction
- Sodium-restricted diet
- Correction of electrolyte imbalance
- Dialysis
- Plasmapheresis
- Antibiotics
- Anticoagulants
- Diuretics
- Vasodilators
- Corticosteroids
- Kidney transplant

KEY PATIENT OUTCOMES

The patient will:
- maintain adequate fluid balance
- identify risk factors that exacerbate the condition, and modify lifestyle accordingly
- maintain hemodynamic stability
- have laboratory values return to normal.

NURSING INTERVENTIONS

- Provide appropriate skin care and oral hygiene.
- Encourage the patient to express his feelings about the disorder.
- Administer prescribed drugs.
- Monitor vital signs, intake and output, and daily weight.
- Monitor laboratory studies.
- Watch for signs of renal failure.

PATIENT TEACHING

Be sure to cover:
- taking prescribed drugs
- how to assess ankle edema
- reporting signs of infection
- recording daily weight.

Heart failure

DESCRIPTION

- Fluid buildup in the heart and body from myocardium that can't provide sufficient cardiac output
- Usually occurs in a damaged left ventricle, but it may happen in right ventricle primarily, or secondary to left-sided heart failure

PATHOPHYSIOLOGY

Left-sided heart failure

- The pumping ability of the left ventricle fails and cardiac output falls.
- Blood backs up into the left atrium and lungs, causing pulmonary congestion.

Right-sided heart failure

- Ineffective contractile function of the right ventricle leads to blood backing up into the right atrium and the peripheral circulation, which results in peripheral edema and engorgement of the kidneys and other organs.

CAUSES

- Anemia
- Arrhythmias
- Cardiomyopathy
- Constrictive pericarditis
- Coronary artery disease
- Emotional stress
- Hypertension
- Increased salt or water intake
- Infections
- Mitral or aortic insufficiency
- Mitral stenosis secondary to rheumatic heart disease, constrictive pericarditis, or atrial fibrillation
- Myocardial infarction (MI)
- Myocarditis
- Pregnancy
- Pulmonary embolism
- Thyrotoxicosis
- Ventricular and atrial septal defects

ASSESSMENT FINDINGS

- Symptoms of any underlying disorder as precipitant
- Dyspnea or paroxysmal nocturnal dyspnea
- Peripheral edema
- Fatigue
- Weakness
- Insomnia
- Anorexia
- Nausea
- Sense of abdominal fullness (particularly in right-sided heart failure)
- Reduced cardiac output
- Cough that produces pink, frothy sputum
- Cyanosis of the lips and nail beds
- Pale, cool, clammy skin
- Diaphoresis
- Jugular vein distention
- Ascites
- Tachycardia
- Pulsus alternans
- Hepatomegaly and, possibly, splenomegaly
- Decreased pulse pressure
- S_3 and S_4 heart sounds
- Moist, bibasilar crackles, rhonchi, and expiratory wheezing
- Decreased pulse oximetry
- Decreased urinary output
- Anxiety
- Orthopnea
- Substance abuse (alcohol, drugs, tobacco)

TEST RESULTS

- B-type natriuretic peptide immunoassay is elevated.
- Blood urea nitrogen and creatinine levels are elevated.
- Chest X-rays show increased pulmonary vascular markings, interstitial edema, or pleural effusion and cardiomegaly.
- Electrocardiography reveals atrial enlargement, tachycardia, extrasystole, atrial fibrillation, prior MI, or left ventricular hypertrophy.
- Pulmonary artery pressure monitoring typically shows elevated pulmonary artery and pulmonary artery wedge pressures, left ventricular end-diastolic pressure in left-sided heart failure, and elevated right atrial or central venous pressure in right-sided heart failure.

- Echocardiography reveals wall motion abnormalities, decreased left ventricular function, valvular disease, cardiac tamponade, and constriction.

TREATMENT

- Antiembolism stockings
- Elevation of lower extremities
- Low-sodium, low-fat diet
- Fluid restriction
- Calorie restriction, if indicated
- Walking program, if indicated
- Activity, as tolerated
- Diuretics
- Oxygen
- Inotropic drugs
- Vasodilators
- Angiotensin-converting enzyme inhibitors
- Angiotensin receptor blockers
- Cardiac glycosides
- Nesiritide (Natrecor)
- Potassium supplements
- Beta-adrenergic blockers
- Anticoagulants
- Morphine sulfate (MSIR)
- For valvular dysfunction with recurrent acute heart failure, surgical replacement
- Heart transplantation
- Ventricular assist device
- Stent placement

KEY PATIENT OUTCOMES

The patient will:
- maintain hemodynamic stability
- maintain adequate cardiac output
- carry out activities of daily living without excess fatigue or decreased energy
- maintain adequate ventilation
- maintain adequate fluid balance.

NURSING INTERVENTIONS

- Place the patient in Fowler's position, and give supplemental oxygen.

- Provide continuous cardiac monitoring during acute and advanced episodes.
- Assist the patient with range-of-motion exercises.
- Apply antiembolism stockings; check for calf pain and tenderness.
- Obtain daily weight.
- Monitor the patient's cardiac rhythm.
- Monitor intake and output.
- Monitor the patient's response to treatment.
- Monitor vital signs.
- Monitor the patient's mental status.
- Assess for peripheral edema.
- Monitor the patient's blood urea nitrogen and serum creatinine, potassium, sodium, chloride, and magnesium levels.

 ALERT *Auscultate for abnormal heart and breath sounds, and report changes immediately.*

PATIENT TEACHING

Be sure to cover:
- the disorder, diagnosis, and treatment
- signs and symptoms of worsening heart failure
- when to notify the physician
- importance of follow-up care
- need to avoid high-sodium foods
- need to avoid fatigue
- instructions about fluid restrictions
- need to weigh himself every morning, at the same time, before eating and after urinating; keeping a record of his weight, and reporting a weight gain of 3 to 5 lb (1.5 to 2.5 kg) in 1 week
- importance of smoking cessation, if appropriate
- weight reduction, as needed
- medication dosage, administration, potential adverse effects, and monitoring needs.

Hepatitis, viral

DESCRIPTION

- Infection and inflammation of the liver caused by a virus
- Six types recognized (A, B, C, D, E, and G), and a seventh suspected
- Marked by hepatic cell destruction, necrosis, and autolysis, leading to anorexia, jaundice, and hepatomegaly

- In most patients, eventual regeneration of hepatic cells with little or no residual damage, allowing recovery
- Complications more likely with old age and serious underlying disorders
- Prognosis poor if edema and hepatic encephalopathy develop

PATHOPHYSIOLOGY

- Hepatic inflammation caused by a virus leads to diffuse injury and necrosis of hepatocytes.
- Hypertrophy and hyperplasia of Kupffer cells and sinusoidal lining cells occur.
- Bile obstruction may occur.

CAUSES

- Infection with the causative viruses for each of six major forms of viral hepatitis

Type A
- Ingestion of contaminated food, milk, or water
- Transmittal by the fecal-oral or parenteral route

Type B
- Transmittal by contact with contaminated human blood, secretions (such as saliva, tears, semen, or vaginal mucus), and stool

Type C
- Transmittal primarily by sharing of needles by I.V. drug users or through blood transfusions or tattoo needles

Type D
- Found only in patients with an acute or a chronic episode of hepatitis B

Type E
- Transmittal by parenteral route and commonly water-borne

Type G
- Thought to be blood-borne, with transmission similar to that of hepatitis B and C

ASSESSMENT FINDINGS

Prodromal stage
- Patient easily fatigued, with generalized malaise
- Anorexia, mild weight loss
- Depression

- Headache, photophobia
- Weakness
- Arthralgia, myalgia (hepatitis B)
- Nausea or vomiting
- Changes in the senses of taste and smell
- Fever (100° to 102° F [37.8° to 38.9° C])
- Dark-colored urine
- Clay-colored stools
- Irritability

Clinical jaundice stage

- Pruritus
- Abdominal pain or tenderness in right upper quadrant
- Indigestion
- Anorexia
- Possible jaundice of sclerae, mucous membranes, and skin
- Rashes, erythematous patches, or hives
- Enlarged and tender liver (see *Effect of viral hepatitis on the liver*)
- Splenomegaly
- Cervical adenopathy

Posticteric stage

- Most symptoms decreasing or subsided
- Decrease in liver enlargement

TEST RESULTS

- Routine hepatitis profile identifies antibodies specific to the causative virus and establishes the type of hepatitis:
  - Type A: detection of presence of an antibody to hepatitis A
  - Type B: detection of presence of hepatitis B surface antigens and hepatitis B antibodies confirming the diagnosis
  - Type C: diagnosis dependent upon serologic testing for the specific antibody one or more months after the onset of acute illness; until then, diagnosis principally established by obtaining negative test results for hepatitis A, B, and D
  - Type D: detection of intrahepatic delta antigens or immunoglobulin (Ig) M antidelta antigens in acute disease (or IgM and IgG in chronic disease)
  - Type E: detection of hepatitis E antigens supporting the diagnosis; however, diagnosis possibly also ruling out hepatitis C
  - Type G: detection of hepatitis G ribonucleic acid supporting the diagnosis (Serologic assays are being developed.)

FOCUS IN
EFFECT OF VIRAL HEPATITIS ON THE LIVER

On entering the body, the virus either kills hepatocytes directly or activates inflammatory and immune reactions that injure or destroy the hepatocytes by lysing the infected or neighboring cells. Later, direct antibody attack against the viral antigens causes further destruction of the infected cells. Edema and swelling of the interstitium lead to collapse of capillaries and decreased blood flow, tissue hypoxia, and scarring and fibrosis.

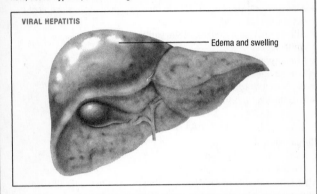

VIRAL HEPATITIS

Edema and swelling

- Additional findings from liver function studies support the diagnosis:
  - Serum aspartate aminotransferase and serum alanine aminotransferase levels are increased in the prodromal stage of acute viral hepatitis.
  - Serum alkaline phosphatase level is slightly increased.
  - Serum bilirubin level is elevated; level may stay elevated late in the disease, especially with severe disease.
  - Prothrombin time (PT) is prolonged (PT more than 3 seconds longer than normal indicates severe liver damage).
  - White blood cell count commonly reveals transient neutropenia and lymphopenia, followed by lymphocytosis.
- Liver biopsy shows chronic hepatitis.

TREATMENT

- No specific drug therapy exists for hepatitis, except for hepatitis C.

- Small, high-calorie, high-protein meals (reduced protein intake if signs of precoma — lethargy, confusion, mental changes — develop)
- Parenteral feeding, if appropriate
- Abstinence from alcohol use
- Frequent rest periods, as needed
- Avoidance of contact sports and strenuous activity
- Standard immunoglobulin
- Vaccine

For hepatitis C
- Aimed at clearing hepatitis C from the body, stopping or slowing of hepatic damage, and symptom relief
- Alfa-2b interferon (Roferon-A) (hepatitis B and C)
- Antiemetics
- Cholestyramine (Locholest)
- Lamivudine (Combivir) (hepatitis B)
- Ribavirin (Virazole) (hepatitis C)
- Possible liver transplant (hepatitis C)

KEY PATIENT OUTCOMES

The patient will:
- develop no complications
- maintain stable vital signs
- perform activities of daily living within the confines of the disease process
- express understanding of the disorder and treatment regimen.

NURSING INTERVENTIONS

- Observe standard precautions to prevent transmission of the disease.
- Provide rest periods throughout the day.
- Give prescribed medications.
- Encourage oral fluid intake.
- Monitor the patient's weight daily.
- Monitor intake and output.
- Assess stool for color, consistency, amount, and frequency.
- Observe for signs of complications.

PATIENT TEACHING

Be sure to cover:
- the disorder, diagnosis, and treatment
- measures to prevent the spread of disease

- importance of rest and a proper diet
- need to abstain from alcohol use and hepatotoxins such as acetaminophen
- medication administration, dosage, and possible adverse effects
- need to avoid over-the-counter medications unless approved by the physician
- need for follow-up care.

Hernia, inguinal

DESCRIPTION

- Part of an internal organ that protrudes through an abnormal opening in the wall of the cavity that surrounds it (see *Common sites of hernia*, pages 128 and 129)
- The most common type of hernia
- Two types: direct and indirect
  - Direct: occurs more commonly in middle-age and elderly people
  - Indirect: more common, may develop at any age, three times more common in males, and especially prevalent in infants
- Also called *ruptures*

PATHOPHYSIOLOGY

- In an inguinal hernia, the large or small intestine, omentum, or bladder protrudes into the inguinal canal.
- In a direct inguinal hernia, instead of entering the canal through the internal ring, the hernia passes through the posterior inguinal wall, protrudes directly through the transverse fascia of the canal (in an area known as *Hesselbach's triangle*), and comes out at the external ring.
- In an indirect hernia, abdominal viscera leave the abdomen through the inguinal ring and follow the spermatic cord (in males) or round ligament (in females); they emerge at the external ring and extend down into the inguinal canal, often into the scrotum or labia.
- In strangulated hernia, part of the herniated intestine becomes twisted or edematous, interfering with normal blood flow and peristalsis, and possibly leading to obstruction and necrosis.

CAUSES

- Direct — weakness in fascial floor of inguinal canal
- Indirect — weakness in fascial margin of internal inguinal ring
- Either — weak abdominal muscles (caused by congenital malformation,

COMMON SITES OF HERNIA

There are four common sites of hernia: umbilical, incisional, inguinal, and femoral. Here are descriptions of each type with an illustration demonstrating where each type is located.

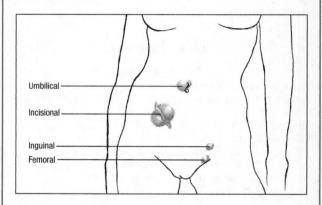

Umbilical
Umbilical hernia results from abnormal muscular structures around the umbilical cord. This hernia is quite common in neonates but also occurs in women who are obese or who have had several pregnancies. Because most umbilical hernias in infants close spontaneously, surgery is warranted only if the hernia persists for more than 4 or 5 years. Taping or binding the affected area or supporting it with a truss may relieve symptoms until the hernia closes. A severe congenital umbilical hernia, which allows the abdominal viscera to protrude outside the body, must be repaired immediately.

Incisional
Incisional (ventral) hernia develops at the site of previous surgery, usually along vertical incisions. This hernia may result from a weakness in the abdominal wall, caused by an infection, impaired wound healing, inadequate nutrition, extreme abdominal distention, or obesity. Palpation of an incisional hernia may reveal several defects in the surgical scar. Effective repair requires pulling the layers of the abdominal wall together without creating tension or, if this isn't possible, the use of Teflon, Marlex mesh, or tantalum mesh to close the opening.

COMMON SITES OF HERNIA *(continued)*

Inguinal

Inguinal hernia can be direct or indirect. An indirect inguinal hernia causes the abdominal viscera to protrude through the inguinal ring and follow the spermatic cord (in males) or round ligament (in females). A direct inguinal hernia results from a weakness in the fascial floor of the inguinal canal.

Femoral

Femoral hernia occurs where the femoral artery passes into the femoral canal. Typically, a fatty deposit within the femoral canal enlarges and eventually creates a hole big enough to accommodate part of the peritoneum and bladder. A femoral hernia appears as a swelling or bulge at the pulse point of the large femoral artery. It's usually a soft, pliable, reducible, nontender mass but commonly becomes incarcerated or strangulated.

---

trauma, or aging) or increased intra-abdominal pressure (caused by heavy lifting, pregnancy, ascites, obesity, or straining)

ASSESSMENT FINDINGS

- Sharp or "catching" pain when lifting or straining (see *Identifying a hernia*, page 130)
- Obvious swelling or lump in the inguinal area (large hernia)

TEST RESULTS

- White blood cell count is elevated with intestinal obstruction.

TREATMENT

- Manual reduction
- Truss
- Activity, as tolerated, avoiding lifting and straining
- Nothing by mouth if surgery is necessary
- Analgesics
- Antibiotics
- Electrolyte replacement
- Herniorrhaphy
- Hernioplasty
- Bowel resection (with strangulation or necrosis)

IDENTIFYING A HERNIA

Palpation of the inguinal area while the patient is performing Valsalva's maneuver confirms the diagnosis of inguinal hernia. To detect a hernia in a male patient, ask the patient to stand with his ipsilateral leg slightly flexed and his weight resting on the other leg. Insert an index finger into the lower part of the scrotum and invaginate the scrotal skin so the finger advances through the external inguinal ring to the internal ring (about ½" to 2" [1 to 5 cm] through the inguinal canal). Tell the patient to cough. If pressure is felt against the fingertip, an indirect hernia exists; if pressure is felt against the side of the finger, a direct hernia exists.

KEY PATIENT OUTCOMES

The patient will:
- express feelings of increased comfort
- have normal bowel function
- avoid complications.

NURSING INTERVENTIONS

- Apply a truss after a hernia has been reduced.
- Give all prescribed medications for pain.
- Encourage coughing and deep breathing, while you splint the incision with a pillow.
- Monitor vital signs.
- Assess pain control.
- Observe for signs of strangulation or incarceration.

PATIENT TEACHING

Be sure to cover:
- avoiding lifting heavy objects or straining during bowel movements
- signs and symptoms of infection (oozing, tenderness, warmth, and redness) at the incision site
- wound care
- after surgery, not resuming normal activity or returning to work without the surgeon's permission.

Herniated intervertebral disk

DESCRIPTION

- Rupture of fibrocartilaginous material that surrounds the intervertebral disk, allowing protrusion of the nucleus pulposus
- Results in pressure on spinal nerve roots or spinal cord that causes back pain and other symptoms of nerve root irritation
- Most common site for herniation: L4-L5 disk space; other sites include L5-S1, L2-L3, L3-L4, C6-C7, and C5-C6
- Clinical manifestations determined by:
  - location and size of the herniation into the spinal canal
  - amount of space that exists inside the spinal canal
- About 90% affecting lumbar (L) and lumbosacral spine; 8% cervical (C) spine; 1% to 2% thoracic (T) spine
- Lumbar herniation more common in people ages 20 to 45
- Cervical herniation more common in people ages 45 and older
- Herniated disks more common in men than in women
- Also known as *herniated nucleus pulposus, slipped disk,* or *ruptured disk*

PATHOPHYSIOLOGY

- The ligament and posterior capsule of the disk are usually torn, allowing the nucleus pulposus to extrude, compressing the nerve root.
- Occasionally, the injury tears the entire disk loose, causing protrusion onto the nerve root or compression of the spinal cord.
- Large amounts of extruded nucleus pulposus or complete disk herniation of the capsule and nucleus pulposus may compress the spinal cord. (See *How a herniated disk develops,* page 132.)

CAUSES

- Degenerative disk disease
- Direct injury
- Improper lifting or twisting

ASSESSMENT FINDINGS

- Previous traumatic injury or back strain
- Unilateral, lower back pain
- Pain that may radiate to the buttocks, legs, and feet
- Pain that may begin suddenly, subside in a few days, and then recur at shorter intervals with progressive intensity

FOCUS IN

HOW A HERNIATED DISK DEVELOPS

Physical stress (from severe trauma or strain) or joint degeneration may cause herniation of an intervertebral disk, as shown below.

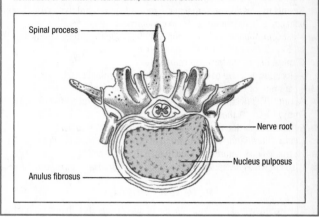

Spinal process

Nerve root

Nucleus pulposus

Anulus fibrosus

- Sciatic pain beginning as a dull ache in the buttocks, worsening with Valsalva's maneuver, coughing, sneezing, or bending
- Pain that may subside with rest
- Muscle spasms
- Chronic repetitive injury
- Limited ability to bend forward
- Posture favoring the affected side
- Muscle atrophy, in later stages
- Tenderness over the affected region
- Radicular pain with straight leg raising in lumbar herniation
- Increased pain with neck movement in cervical herniation
- Referred upper trunk pain with cervical neck compression

TEST RESULTS

- X-rays of the spine show degenerative changes.
- Myelography shows the level of the herniation.
- Computed tomography scan shows bone and soft-tissue abnormalities; it may also show spinal canal compression.

- Magnetic resonance imaging shows soft-tissue abnormalities.
- Electromyography measures muscle response to nerve stimulation.
- Nerve conduction studies show sensory and motor loss.

TREATMENT

- Initial treatment conservative and symptomatic, unless neurologic impairment progresses rapidly
- Possible traction
- Supportive devices such as a brace
- Heat or cold applications
- Transcutaneous electrical nerve stimulation
- Chemonucleolysis
- Avoidance of repetitive activity
- Diet, as tolerated
- Bed rest, initially
- Prescribed exercise program
- Physical therapy
- Nonsteroidal anti-inflammatory drugs
- Steroids
- Muscle relaxants
- Analgesics
- Laminectomy
- Spinal fusion
- Microdiskectomy

KEY PATIENT OUTCOMES

The patient will:
- express feelings of increased comfort
- demonstrate adequate joint mobility and range of motion
- perform activities of daily living within the confines of the disorder
- achieve the highest level of mobility possible
- demonstrate strategies to prevent self-injury.

NURSING INTERVENTIONS

- Give prescribed medications.
- Plan a pain control regimen.
- Offer the patient supportive care.
- Provide encouragement.
- Help the patient cope with chronic pain and impaired mobility.
- Include the patient and his family in all phases of his care.
- Encourage the patient to express his concerns.

- Encourage performance of self-care.
- Help the patient to identify activities that promote rest and relaxation.
- Prepare the patient for myelography, if indicated.
- Periodically remove traction to inspect the skin.
- Prevent deep vein thrombosis.
- Prevent footdrop.
- Ensure a consistent regimen of leg and back-strengthening exercises.
- Encourage adequate oral fluid intake.
- Encourage coughing and deep-breathing exercises.
- Provide meticulous skin care.
- Provide a fracture bedpan for the patient on complete bed rest.

ALERT *During conservative treatment, watch for a deterioration in neurologic status, especially during the first 24 hours after admission, which may indicate an urgent need for surgery.*

After surgery

COLLABORATION *Physical therapy may reduce pain and relax muscle spasms. Physical therapy may also be needed to strengthen muscles.*

- Enforce bed rest, as ordered.
- Use the logrolling technique to turn the patient.
- Assist the patient during his first attempt to walk.
- Provide a straightbacked chair for the patient to sit in briefly.
- Monitor vital signs.
- Measure and evaluate intake and output.
- Assess pain control.
- Assess mobility status and ability.
- Assess motor strength.
- Observe for deep vein thrombosis.
- Assess bowel and bladder function.
- Assess blood drainage system.
- Monitor drainage, incisions, and dressings.
- Assess neurovascular status.

PATIENT TEACHING

Be sure to cover:
- the disorder, diagnosis, and treatment
- prescribed medications and potential adverse effects
- when to notify the physician
- bed rest

- traction
- heat or cold application
- exercise program
- myelography, if indicated
- preoperative and postoperative care, if indicated
- relaxation techniques
- proper body mechanics
- skin care.

Hip fracture

DESCRIPTION

- Break in the head or neck of the femur (usually the head)
- Most common fall-related injury resulting in hospitalization
- Leading cause of disability among older adults
- May permanently change level of functioning and independence
- Almost 25% of patients die within 1 year following hip fracture
- Affects more than 200,000 people each year
- Occurs in one of five women by age 80, and is more common in females than in males

PATHOPHYSIOLOGY

- With bone fracture, the periosteum and blood vessels in the marrow, cortex, and surrounding soft tissues are disrupted.
- Disruption of the periosteum and blood vessels results in bleeding from the damaged ends of the bone and from the neighboring soft tissue.
- Clot formation occurs within the medullary canal, between the fractured bone ends, and beneath the periosteum.
- Bone tissue immediately adjacent to the fracture dies, and the necrotic tissue causes an intense inflammatory response.
- Vascular tissue invades the fracture area from surrounding soft tissue and marrow cavity within 48 hours, increasing blood flow to the entire bone.
- Bone-forming cells in the periosteum, endosteum, and marrow are activated to produce subperiosteal procallus along the outer surface of the shaft and over the broken ends of the bone.
- Collagen and matrix, which become mineralized to form callus, are synthesized by osteoblasts within the procallus.
- During the repair process, remodeling occurs; unnecessary callus is resorbed, and trabeculae are formed along stress lines.
- New bone, not scar tissue, is formed over the healed fracture.

CAUSES

- Cancer metastasis
- Falls
- Osteoporosis
- Skeletal disease
- Trauma

ASSESSMENT FINDINGS

- Falls or trauma to the bones
- Pain in the affected hip and leg
- Pain exacerbated by movement
- Outward rotation of affected extremity
- Affected extremity possibly appearing shorter
- Limited or abnormal range of motion (ROM)
- Edema and discoloration of the surrounding tissue
- In an open fracture, bone protruding through the skin

TEST RESULTS

- X-rays show the location of the fracture.
- Computed tomography scan shows abnormalities in complicated fractures.

TREATMENT

- Depends on age, comorbidities, cognitive functioning, support systems, and functional ability
- Possible skin traction
- Physical therapy
- Non–weight-bearing transfers
- Well-balanced diet
- Foods rich in vitamin C and A, calcium, and protein
- Adequate vitamin D
- Bed rest, initially
- Ambulation as soon as possible after surgery
- Analgesics
- Total hip arthroplasty
- Hemiarthroplasty
- Percutaneous pinning
- Internal fixation using a compression screw and plate

KEY PATIENT OUTCOMES

The patient will:
- identify factors that increase the potential for injury
- maintain muscle strength and tone and joint ROM
- verbalize feelings of increased comfort
- attain the highest degree of mobility possible within the confines of the injury
- maintain skin integrity.

NURSING INTERVENTIONS

- Give prescribed medications.
- Give prescribed prophylactic anticoagulation medications after surgery.
- Maintain traction.
- Maintain proper body alignment.
- Use logrolling techniques to turn the patient in bed.
- Maintain non–weight-bearing status.
- Increase the patient's activity level, as prescribed.

▶ **COLLABORATION** *To help the patient attain mobility and decrease complications, consult a physical therapist early in the patient's rehabilitation. Follow-up with home physical therapy referral to determine home safety. Teach the patient the home exercise program.*

- Assist with active ROM exercises to unaffected limbs, and monitor mobility and ROM.
- Encourage coughing and deep-breathing exercises.
- Keep the patient's skin clean and dry; prevent skin breakdown.
- Encourage good nutrition; offer high-protein, high-calorie snacks.
- Perform daily wound care.

✔ **ALERT** *Don't massage the patient's legs and feet to promote circulation because this could increase the risk of thromboembolism.*

- Monitor vital signs.
- Measure and evaluate intake and output.
- Assess level of pain.
- Assess incision and dressings and perform wound care.
- Observe for complications.
- Monitor coagulation study results.
- Observe for signs of bleeding.
- Assess neurovascular status.
- Assess skin integrity.
- Observe for signs and symptoms of infection.

ALERT *After surgery, assess the patient for complications, such as deep vein thrombosis, pulmonary embolus, and hip dislocation.*

PATIENT TEACHING

Be sure to cover:
- the disorder, diagnosis, and treatment
- prescribed medications and potential adverse effects
- ROM exercises
- meticulous skin care
- proper body alignment
- wound care
- signs of infection
- coughing and deep-breathing exercises and incentive spirometry
- assistive devices
- activity restrictions and lifestyle changes
- safe ambulation practices
- nutritious diet and adequate fluid intake.

Human immunodeficiency virus infection

DESCRIPTION

- Human immunodeficiency virus (HIV) type 1; retrovirus causing acquired immunodeficiency syndrome (AIDS)
- Causes patients to become susceptible to opportunistic infections, unusual cancers, and other abnormalities
- Marked by progressive failure of the immune system
- Transmitted by contact with infected blood or body fluids and associated with identifiable high-risk behaviors

PATHOPHYSIOLOGY

- HIV strikes helper T cells bearing the CD4 antigen.
- The antigen serves as a receptor for the retrovirus and lets it enter the cell.
- After invading a cell, HIV replicates, leading to cell death, or becomes latent.
- HIV infection leads to profound pathology, either directly, through destruction of CD4+ cells, other immune cells, and neuroglial cells, or indirectly, through the secondary effects of CD4+ T-cell dysfunction and resultant immunosuppression.

CAUSES

- Infection with HIV, a retrovirus

ASSESSMENT FINDINGS

- A high-risk exposure and inoculation, followed by a mononucleosis-like syndrome (patient then possibly asymptomatic for years)
- In the latent stage, laboratory evidence of seroconversion the only sign of HIV infection
- Persistent generalized adenopathy
- Nonspecific symptoms (weight loss, fatigue, night sweats, fevers)
- Neurologic symptoms resulting from HIV encephalopathy
- Opportunistic infection or cancer (Kaposi's sarcoma)

TEST RESULTS

- CD4$^+$ T-cell count is at least 200 cells/ml.
- Screening test enzyme-linked immunosorbent assay and confirmatory test (Western blot) detect the presence of HIV antibodies.
- Direct testing detects HIV itself; these tests include antigen testing, HIV cultures, nucleic acid probes of peripheral blood lymphocytes, and polymerase chain reaction tests.

TREATMENT

- Variety of therapeutic options for opportunistic infections (the leading cause of morbidity and mortality in patients infected with HIV)
- Disease-specific therapy for a variety of neoplastic and premalignant diseases and organ-specific syndromes
- Symptom management (fatigue and anemia)
- Well-balanced diet
- Regular exercise, as tolerated, with adequate rest periods
- Immunomodulatory agents
- Anti-infective agents
- Antineoplastic agents
- Highly active antiretroviral therapy
- Protease inhibitors
- Nucleoside reverse transcriptase inhibitors
- Nonnucleoside reverse transcriptase inhibitors

KEY PATIENT OUTCOMES

The patient will:
- achieve management of symptoms of illness

- demonstrate use of protective measures, including conservation of energy, maintenance of well-balanced diet, and getting adequate rest
- follow safer sex practices
- utilize available support systems to assist with coping
- voice feelings about changes in sexual identity and social response to disease
- develop no complications of illness
- comply with the treatment regimen.

NURSING INTERVENTIONS

- Help the patient to cope with an altered body image, the emotional burden of serious illness, and the threat of death.
- Avoid glycerin swabs for mucous membranes. Use normal saline or bicarbonate mouthwash for daily oral rinsing.
- Ensure adequate fluid intake during episodes of diarrhea.
- Provide meticulous skin care, especially in the debilitated patient.
- Encourage the patient to maintain as much physical activity as he can tolerate. Make sure his schedule includes time for exercise and rest.
- Monitor vital signs, especially temperature, noting any pattern.
- Observe the patient for signs of illness, such as cough, sore throat, or diarrhea.
- Assess for swollen, tender lymph nodes.
- Monitor laboratory values, including complete blood count; electrolyte, blood urea nitrogen, and creatinine levels; and chest X-rays.
- Record calorie intake.
- Monitor progression of lesions in Kaposi's sarcoma.
- Observe for opportunistic infections or signs of disease progression.
- Discuss and monitor compliance with medication regimen.
- Refer the patient to a local support group.
- Refer the patient to hospice care, as indicated.
- Provide information on community support services, resources, mental health counseling, or social service assistance.

PATIENT TEACHING

Be sure to cover:
- medication regimens
- importance of informing potential sexual partners, caregivers, and health care workers of HIV infection
- signs of impending infection and the importance of seeking immediate medical attention
- symptoms of AIDS dementia and its stages and progression.

CLINICAL EFFECTS OF HYPERCALCEMIA

Listed below are the effects of hypercalcemia on various body systems.

Body system	Effects
Cardiovascular	■ Signs of heart block, cardiac arrest, hypertension
Gastrointestinal	■ Anorexia, nausea, vomiting, constipation, dehydration, polydipsia
Musculoskeletal	■ Weakness, muscle flaccidity, bone pain, pathologic fractures
Neurologic	■ Drowsiness, lethargy, headaches, depression or apathy, irritability, confusion
Other	■ Renal polyuria, flank pain and, eventually, azotemia

Hypercalcemia

DESCRIPTION

■ Excessive serum levels of calcium

PATHOPHYSIOLOGY

■ Together with phosphorus, calcium is responsible for the formation and structure of bones and teeth.
■ Calcium helps to maintain cell structure and function by playing a role in cell membrane permeability and impulse transmission.
■ It affects the contraction of cardiac muscle, smooth muscle, and skeletal muscle and participates in the blood-clotting process.
■ Increased resorption of calcium from bone leads to increased rate of calcium entry into extracellular fluid.
■ Calcium in extracellular fluid becomes greater than calcium excretion by the kidneys. (See *Clinical effects of hypercalcemia.*)

CAUSES

■ Certain cancers, such as kidney, lung, ovarian, and parathyroid
■ Certain medications, such as calcium-containing antacids, lithium, and thiazide diuretics
■ Hyperparathyroidism
■ Hypervitaminosis D
■ Multiple fractures and prolonged immobilization

- Paget's disease
- Vitamin A and D supplementation

ASSESSMENT FINDINGS

- Underlying cause
- Lethargy
- Weakness
- Anorexia
- Constipation
- Nausea, vomiting
- Polyuria
- Confusion
- Muscle weakness
- Hyporeflexia
- Decreased muscle tone

TEST RESULTS

- Serum calcium level is greater than 10.5 mg/dl.
- Ionized calcium level is less than 5.3 mg/dl.
- Electrocardiogram shows shortened QT interval and ventricular arrhythmias.

TREATMENT

- Treatment of the underlying cause
- Activity, as tolerated
- Normal saline solution
- Loop diuretics

KEY PATIENT OUTCOMES

The patient will:
- maintain stable vital signs
- maintain adequate cardiac output
- express an understanding of the disorder and treatment regimen.

NURSING INTERVENTIONS

- Provide safety measures and institute seizure precautions, if appropriate.
- Give prescribed I.V. solutions.
- Observe patient for signs of heart failure.
- Monitor the patient's cardiac rhythm.
- Observe the patient for seizures.
- Monitor calcium levels.

PATIENT TEACHING

Be sure to cover:
- avoiding nonprescription medications that are high in calcium
- increasing fluid intake
- following a low-calcium diet.

Hyperkalemia

DESCRIPTION

- Excessive serum levels of the potassium anion
- Commonly induced by other treatments such as drugs

PATHOPHYSIOLOGY

- Potassium facilitates contraction of both skeletal and smooth muscles, including myocardial contraction. It also figures prominently in nerve impulse conduction, acid-base balance, enzyme action, and cell membrane function.
- Slight deviation in serum potassium levels can produce profound clinical consequences, such as muscle weakness and flaccid paralysis, because of an ionic imbalance in neuromuscular tissue excitability. (See *Clinical effects of hyperkalemia.*)

CLINICAL EFFECTS OF HYPERKALEMIA

Listed below are the effects of hyperkalemia on various body systems.

Body system	Effects
Cardiovascular	■ Tachycardia and later bradycardia, electrocardiogram changes (tented and elevated T waves, widened QRS complex, prolonged PR interval, flattened or absent P waves, depressed ST segment), cardiac arrest (with levels > 7 mEq/L)
Gastrointestinal	■ Nausea, diarrhea, abdominal cramps
Genitourinary	■ Oliguria, anuria
Musculoskeletal	■ Muscle weakness, flaccid paralysis
Neurologic	■ Hyperreflexia progressing to weakness, numbness, tingling, flaccid paralysis
Other	■ Metabolic acidosis

CAUSES

- Adrenal gland insufficiency
- Burns
- Certain medications, such as angiotensin-converting enzyme inhibitors, antibiotics, beta-adrenergic blockers, chemotherapeutic medications, nonsteroidal anti-inflammatory drugs, potassium supplements, and spironolactone
- Crushing injuries
- Decreased urinary excretion of potassium
- Dehydration
- Diabetic acidosis
- Digoxin toxicity
- Increased intake of potassium
- Large quantities of blood transfusions
- Renal dysfunction or failure
- Rhabdomyolysis
- Severe infection
- Use of potassium-sparing diuretics, such as triamterene (Dyrenium), by patients with renal disease

ASSESSMENT FINDINGS

- Irritability
- Paresthesia
- Muscle weakness
- Nausea
- Abdominal cramps
- Diarrhea
- Hypotension
- Irregular heart rate
- Cardiac arrhythmia (possible)
- Decreased deep tendon reflexes

TEST RESULTS

- Serum potassium level is greater than 5 mEq/L.
- Arterial pH is decreased.
- Electrocardiogram shows a tall, tented T wave.

TREATMENT

- Treatment of the underlying cause
- Hemodialysis or peritoneal dialysis

- Activity, as tolerated
- Rapid infusion of 10% calcium gluconate (decreases myocardial irritability)
- Insulin and 10% to 50% glucose I.V.
- Sodium polystyrene sulfonate (Kayexalate) with 70% sorbitol
- Diuretics

KEY PATIENT OUTCOMES

The patient will:
- maintain hemodynamic stability
- maintain a normal potassium level
- understand potential adverse effects of prescribed medications.

NURSING INTERVENTIONS

- Give prescribed medications.
- Insert an indwelling urinary catheter.
- Implement appropriate safety measures.
- Be alert for signs of hypokalemia after treatment.
- Monitor the patient's serum potassium levels.

   ALERT If your patient's laboratory test result indicates a high potassium level, but the result doesn't make sense, make sure it's a true result. If the sample was drawn using poor technique, the results may be falsely high. To avoid falsely high results consider the following causes:
   - *drawing the sample above an I.V. infusion containing potassium*
   - *using a recently exercised arm or leg for the venipuncture site*
   - *causing hemolysis (cell damage) as the specimen is obtained*
   - *delays in the processing of the blood leading to blood clotting in the collection tube and ultimately, hemolysis of the cells.*

- Monitor the patient's cardiac rhythm.
- Record and evaluate intake and output.

PATIENT TEACHING

Be sure to cover:
- prescribed medications and potential adverse effects
- monitoring intake and output
- preventing future episodes of hyperkalemia
- need for potassium-restricted diet.

Hyperlipidemia

DESCRIPTION

- Increased plasma concentrations of one or more lipoproteins
- Primary form includes at least five distinct and inherited metabolic disorders
- May occur secondary to other conditions such as diabetes mellitus
- Clinical changes ranging from relatively mild symptoms, managed by diet, to potentially fatal pancreatitis
- Also known as *hyperlipoproteinemia* and *hyperlipemia*

PATHOPHYSIOLOGY

- Increased low-density lipoprotein (LDL) and decreased high-density lipoprotein (HDL) levels
- Accelerated development of atherosclerosis

Type I
- Relatively rare and present at birth

Type II
- Onset between ages 10 and 30

Type III
- Uncommon; usually occurring after age 20

Type IV
- Relatively common, especially in middle-age men

Type V
- Uncommon; usually occurring in late adolescence or early adulthood

CAUSES

Primary hyperlipoproteinemia
- Types I and III transmitted as autosomal recessive traits
- Types II, IV, and V transmitted as autosomal dominant traits

Secondary hyperlipoproteinemia
- Diabetes mellitus
- Hypothyroidism
- Pancreatitis
- Renal disease

ASSESSMENT FINDINGS

Type I

- Papular or eruptive xanthomas over pressure points and extensor surfaces
- Ophthalmoscopic examination: lipemia retinalis (reddish white retinal vessels)
- Abdominal spasm, rigidity, or rebound tenderness
- Hepatosplenomegaly, with liver or spleen tenderness
- Fever possibly present

Type II

- Tendinous xanthomas on the Achilles tendons and tendons of the hands and feet
- Tuberous xanthomas, xanthelasma
- Juvenile corneal arcus

Type III

- Tuberoeruptive xanthomas over elbows and knees
- Palmar xanthomas on the hands, particularly the fingertips

Type IV

- Obesity
- Xanthomas possibly noted during exacerbations

Type V

- Eruptive xanthomas on extensor surface of arms and legs
- Ophthalmoscopic examination: lipemia retinalis
- Hepatosplenomegaly

TEST RESULTS

- Serum lipid profiles show elevated levels of total cholesterol, triglycerides, very-low-density lipoproteins, LDLs, or decreased levels of HDL.

TREATMENT

- Weight reduction
- Elimination or treatment of aggravating factors, such as diabetes mellitus, alcoholism, and hypothyroidism
- Reduction of risk factors for atherosclerosis
- Smoking cessation
- Treatment of hypertension

- Avoidance of hormonal and estrogen-containing contraceptive medications
- Restriction of cholesterol and saturated animal fat intake
- Avoidance of alcoholic beverages to decrease plasma triglyceride levels
- Inclusion of polyunsaturated vegetable oils (reduces plasma LDLs) and omega-3 oils
- Maintenance of exercise and physical fitness program
- Nicotinic acid (Nicobid)
- Clofibrate (Atromid-S)
- Gemfibrozil (Lopid)
- If unable to tolerate drug therapy, surgical creation of an ileal bypass
- For severely affected homozygote children, portacaval shunt as a last resort to reduce plasma cholesterol levels

Type I
- Restricted fat intake (less than 20 g/day); 20- to 40-g/day, medium-chain triglyceride diet to supplement calorie intake

Type II
- Restriction of cholesterol intake to less than 300 mg/day for adults and less than 150 mg/day for children; restricted triglyceride intake (to less than 100 mg/day for children and adults); and diet high in polyunsaturated fats

Type III
- Restricted cholesterol intake (to less than 300 mg/day) and carbohydrates; increased polyunsaturated fats

Type IV
- Restricted cholesterol intake; increased polyunsaturated fats

Type V
- Long-term maintenance of a low-fat diet; 20- to 40-g/day medium-chain triglyceride diet

KEY PATIENT OUTCOMES

The patient will:
- develop no complications
- maintain lipid levels within acceptable range
- verbalize understanding of the disorder and treatment regimen.

NURSING INTERVENTIONS

- Give prescribed antilipemics.
- Prevent or minimize adverse reactions.
- Urge the patient to adhere to the prescribed diet.
- Assist the patient with additional lifestyle changes.
- Encourage verbalization of fears related to premature coronary artery disease (CAD).
- Monitor vital signs.
- Assess for adverse reactions.
- Monitor serum lipoproteins.
- Evaluate the response to treatment.
- Assess for signs and symptoms related to CAD or its sequelae.
- Refer the patient for a medically supervised exercise program, a smoking-cessation program, if indicated, and a dietitian, if necessary.

PATIENT TEACHING

Be sure to cover:
- the disorder, diagnosis, and treatment
- need to maintain a steady weight and strictly adhere to the prescribed diet (for the 2 weeks preceding serum cholesterol and serum triglyceride tests), and to fast for 12 hours before the test
- need to avoid excessive sugar intake and alcoholic beverages
- need to minimize intake of saturated fats (higher in meats and coconut oil)
- increased intake of polyunsaturated fats (vegetable oils)
- avoiding hormonal contraceptives or medications that contain estrogen
- avoiding foods high in cholesterol and saturated fats
- prescribed drug regimen and potential adverse effects
- signs and symptoms requiring medical evaluation.

Hypertension

DESCRIPTION

- Intermittent or sustained elevation of diastolic or systolic blood pressure
- Usually begins as benign disease, slowly progressing to accelerated or malignant state
- Two major types: essential (also called *primary* or *idiopathic*) hypertension and secondary hypertension, which results from renal disease or another identifiable cause

FOCUS IN
UNDERSTANDING HYPERTENSION

Arterial blood pressure is a product of total peripheral resistance (TPR) and cardiac output (CO). CO is increased by conditions that increase heart rate, stroke volume, or both. TPR is increased by factors that increase blood viscosity or reduce the lumen size of vessels, especially the arterioles.

Several theories help explain how hypertension develops, including:

■ changes in the arteriolar bed, causing increased TPR

■ abnormally increased tone in the sympathetic nervous system, causing increased TPR

■ increased blood volume resulting from renal or hormonal dysfunction

■ increased arteriolar thickening caused by genetic factors, leading to increased TPR

■ abnormal renin release, resulting in formation of angiotensin II, which constricts the arteriole and increases blood volume.

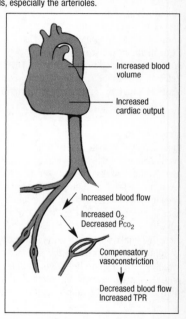

Increased blood volume

Increased cardiac output

Increased blood flow

Increased O_2
Decreased P_{CO_2}

Compensatory vasoconstriction

Decreased blood flow
Increased TPR

■ Malignant hypertension: a severe, fulminant form and a medical emergency; commonly arises from both types

PATHOPHYSIOLOGY

■ There are several theories on how hypertension develops. (See *Understanding hypertension*.)

CAUSES

- Unknown
- Risk factors: family history; African-American heritage; stress; obesity; high-sodium, high–saturated fat diet; sedentary lifestyle; aging; tobacco use; excessive alcohol intake

ASSESSMENT FINDINGS

- In many cases, no symptoms, and disorder revealed incidentally during evaluation for another disorder or during a routine blood pressure screening program
- Symptoms that reflect the effect of hypertension on the organ systems
- Awakening with a headache in the occipital region, which subsides spontaneously after a few hours
- Dizziness, fatigue, and confusion
- Palpitations, chest pain, dyspnea
- Epistaxis
- Hematuria
- Blurred vision
- Bounding pulse
- S_4
- Peripheral edema in late stages
- Hemorrhages, exudates, and papilledema of the eye in late stages
- Pulsating abdominal mass, suggesting an abdominal aneurysm
- Elevated blood pressure on at least two consecutive occasions after initial screenings
- Serial blood pressure measurements:
  - prehypertension: systolic blood pressure (SBP) 120 to 139 mm Hg or diastolic blood pressure (DBP) 80 to 89 mm Hg
  - stage 1: SBP 140 to 159 mm Hg or DBP 90 to 99 mm Hg
  - stage 2: SBP greater than 160 mm Hg or DBP greater than 100 mm Hg
- Bruits over the abdominal aorta and femoral arteries or the carotids

TEST RESULTS

- Urinalysis may show protein, red blood cells, or white blood cells, suggesting renal disease, or glucose, suggesting diabetes mellitus.
- Serum potassium levels less than 3.5 mEq/L may indicate adrenal dysfunction (primary hyperaldosteronism).
- Blood urea nitrogen levels are normal or elevated to more than 20 mg/dl and serum creatinine levels are normal or elevated to more than 1.5 mg/dl, suggesting renal disease.

- Excretory urography reveals renal atrophy and indicate chronic renal disease; one kidney more than 5⁄8″ (1.6 cm) shorter than the other suggests unilateral renal disease.
- Chest X-rays demonstrate cardiomegaly.
- Renal arteriography shows renal artery stenosis.
- Electrocardiography may show left ventricular hypertrophy or ischemia.
- Oral captopril (Capoten) challenge testing for renovascular hypertension may indicate renal disease.
- Ophthalmoscopy reveals arteriovenous nicking and, in hypertensive encephalopathy, edema.

TREATMENT

- Lifestyle modification, such as weight control, limiting alcohol, regular exercise, and smoking cessation
- For a patient with secondary hypertension, correction of the underlying cause and control of hypertensive effects
- Low-saturated fat and low-sodium diet
- Adequate calcium, magnesium, and potassium in diet
- Regular exercise program
- Diuretics
- Beta-adrenergic blockers
- Calcium channel blockers
- Angiotensin-converting enzyme inhibitors
- Alpha-receptor antagonists
- Vasodilators
- Angiotensin-receptor blockers
- Aldosterone antagonist

KEY PATIENT OUTCOMES

The patient will:
- maintain adequate cardiac output
- maintain hemodynamic stability
- develop no arrhythmias
- express feelings of increased energy
- comply with the therapy regimen.

NURSING INTERVENTIONS

- Give prescribed medications.
- Encourage dietary changes, as appropriate.
- Help the patient identify risk factors and modify his lifestyle, as appropriate.

- Monitor vital signs, especially blood pressure.
- Observe for signs and symptoms of target end-organ damage.
- Assess for complications.
- Monitor and evaluate response to treatment.
- Discuss risk factor modification.
- Discuss and monitor adverse effects of antihypertensive agents.

PATIENT TEACHING

Be sure to cover:
- the disorder, diagnosis, and treatment
- how to use a self-monitoring blood pressure cuff and to record the reading in a journal for review by the physician
- importance of compliance with antihypertensive therapy and establishing a daily routine for taking prescribed medications
- need to report adverse effects of medications
- need to avoid high-sodium antacids and over-the-counter cold and sinus medications containing harmful vasoconstrictors
- examining and modifying lifestyle, including diet
- need for a routine exercise program, particularly aerobic walking
- dietary restrictions
- importance of follow-up care.

Hypokalemia

DESCRIPTION

- Deficient serum levels of the potassium anion
- Normal range for a serum potassium level narrow (3.5 to 5 mEq/L); slight decrease can have a profound consequence

PATHOPHYSIOLOGY

- Potassium facilitates contraction of both skeletal and smooth muscles, including myocardial contraction.
- Potassium figures prominently in nerve impulse conduction, acid-base balance, enzyme action, and cell membrane function.
- Inadequate potassium intake or excessive loss of potassium (from prolonged suctioning, vomiting, gastric lavage, osmotic diuresis, or high level of magnesium)
- Leads to shifting of potassium from extracellular to intracellular space
- Movement of potassium ions into cell as hydrogen ions move out possibly causing alkalosis. (See *Clinical effects of hypokalemia*, page 154.)

CLINICAL EFFECTS OF HYPOKALEMIA

Listed below are the effects of hypokalemia on various body systems.

Body system	Effects
Cardiovascular	■ Dizziness, hypotension, arrhythmias, electrocardiogram changes (flattened T waves, elevated U waves, decreased ST segments), cardiac arrest (with levels < 2.5 mEq/L)
Gastrointestinal	■ Nausea, vomiting, anorexia, diarrhea, abdominal distention, paralytic ileus, decreased peristalsis
Genitourinary	■ Polyuria
Musculoskeletal	■ Muscle weakness and fatigue, leg cramps
Neurologic	■ Malaise, irritability, confusion, mental depression, speech changes, decreased reflexes, respiratory paralysis
Other	■ Metabolic alkalosis

CAUSES

- Acid-base imbalances
- Certain medications, especially potassium-wasting diuretics, steroids, and certain sodium-containing antibiotics (carbenicillin)
- Chronic renal disease, with tubular potassium wasting
- Cushing's syndrome
- Excessive GI or urinary losses, such as through vomiting, gastric suction, diarrhea, dehydration, anorexia, or chronic laxative abuse
- Excessive ingestion of licorice
- Hyperglycemia
- Low-potassium diet
- Primary hyperaldosteronism
- Prolonged potassium-free I.V. therapy
- Severe serum magnesium deficiency
- Trauma (injury, burns, or surgery)

ASSESSMENT FINDINGS

- Muscle weakness
- Paresthesia
- Abdominal cramps
- Anorexia

- Nausea, vomiting
- Constipation
- Polyuria
- Hyporeflexia
- Weak, irregular pulse
- Orthostatic hypotension
- Decreased bowel sounds
- Arrhythmias

TEST RESULTS

- Serum potassium level is less than 3.5 mEq/L.
- pH and bicarbonate levels are elevated.
- Serum glucose level is slightly elevated.
- Characteristic ECG changes include flattened T wave and depressed ST segment and U wave.

TREATMENT

- Treatment of the underlying cause
- High-potassium diet
- Activity, as tolerated
- Potassium chloride (I.V. or orally)

ALERT *A patient taking a diuretic may be switched to a potassium-sparing diuretic to prevent excessive urinary loss of potassium.*

KEY PATIENT OUTCOMES

The patient will:
- maintain hemodynamic stability
- maintain a normal potassium level
- understand potential adverse effects of medications
- express understanding of high-potassium foods.

NURSING INTERVENTIONS

- Administer prescribed medications.

ALERT *A patient taking a cardiac glycoside, especially if he's also taking a diuretic, should be monitored closely for hypokalemia, which can potentiate the action of the cardiac glycoside and cause toxicity.*

- Insert an indwelling urinary catheter.
- Implement appropriate safety measures.

- Be alert for signs of hyperkalemia after treatment.
- Administer I.V. fluids.
- Monitor the patient's serum potassium levels.
- Monitor the patient's cardiac rhythm.
- Measure and evaluate the patient's intake and output.
- Monitor all vital signs.
- Assess the patient's respiratory status.

PATIENT TEACHING

Be sure to cover:
- the disorder and treatment
- prescribed medications and potential adverse effects
- monitoring intake and output
- preventing future episodes of hypokalemia
- need for a high-potassium diet
- warning signs and symptoms to report to the physician.

Hypopituitarism

DESCRIPTION

- Partial or complete failure of the anterior pituitary gland to produce its vital hormones: corticotropin, thyroid-stimulating hormone (TSH), luteinizing hormone (LH), follicle-stimulating hormone (FSH), growth hormone (GH), and prolactin
- May be primary or secondary, resulting from dysfunction of the hypothalamus
- Development of clinical features typically slow and not apparent until 75% of the pituitary gland is destroyed
- Total loss of all hormones fatal without treatment
- Prognosis good with adequate replacement therapy and correction of the underlying causes
- Panhypopituitarism: absence of all hormones

PATHOPHYSIOLOGY

- The pituitary gland is extremely vulnerable to ischemia and infarction because it's highly vascular.
- Any event that leads to circulatory collapse and compensatory vasospasm may result in gland ischemia, tissue necrosis, or edema.
- Expansion of the pituitary within the fixed compartment of the sella turcica further impedes blood supply to the pituitary.

CAUSES

- Congenital defects
- Deficiency of hypothalamus-releasing hormones
- Granulomatous disease
- Idiopathic
- Infection
- Partial or total hypophysectomy by surgery, irradiation, or chemical agents
- Pituitary gland hypoplasia or aplasia
- Pituitary infarction
- Trauma
- Tumor

ASSESSMENT FINDINGS

Signs and symptoms depend on which pituitary hormones are deficient, patient's age, and severity of disorder.

GH deficiency
- Physical signs possibly not apparent in neonate
- Growth retardation usually apparent at age 6 months

In children
- Chubbiness from fat deposits in the lower trunk
- Short stature
- Delayed secondary tooth eruption
- Delayed puberty
- Average height of 4′ (1.2 m), with normal proportions
- More subtle signs in adults (fine wrinkles near the mouth and eyes)

Gonadotropin (FSH and LH) deficiency
In women
- Amenorrhea
- Dyspareunia
- Infertility
- Reduced libido
- Breast atrophy
- Sparse or absent axillary and pubic hair
- Dry skin
- Osteoporosis

In men
- Impotence
- Reduced libido
- Decreased muscle strength
- Testicular softening and shrinkage
- Retarded secondary sexual hair growth

TSH deficiency
- Cold intolerance
- Constipation
- Menstrual irregularity
- Lethargy
- Severe growth retardation in children despite treatment
- Dry, pale, puffy skin
- Slow thought processes
- Bradycardia

Corticotropin deficiency
- Fatigue
- Nausea, vomiting, anorexia
- Weight loss
- Depigmentation of skin and nipples
- Hypothermia and hypotension during periods of stress

Prolactin deficiency
- Absent postpartum lactation
- Amenorrhea
- Sparse or absent growth of pubic and axillary hair

Panhypopituitarism
- Mental abnormalities, including lethargy and psychosis
- Physical abnormalities, including orthostatic hypotension and brady-cardia

TEST RESULTS
- Serum thyroxine levels are decreased in diminished thyroid gland function due to lack of TSH.
- Radioimmunoassay shows decreased plasma levels of some or all of the pituitary hormones.
- Increased prolactin levels may indicate a lesion in the hypothalamus or pituitary stalk.
- Computed tomography scans, magnetic resonance imaging, or cerebral angiography may show the presence of intrasellar or extrasellar tumors.

- Oral administration of metyrapone may show the source of low hydroxy-corticosteroid levels.
- Insulin administration revealing low levels of corticotropin, indicating pituitary or hypothalamic failure.
- Dopamine antagonist administration for evaluating prolactin secretory reserve may reveal elevated prolactin from decreased pituitary function.
- I.V. administration of gonadotropin-releasing hormone may distinguish pituitary and hypothalamic causes of gonadotropin deficiency.
- Provocative testing shows persistently low GH and insulin-like growth factor-1 levels, confirming GH deficiency.

TREATMENT

- If caused by a lesion or tumor, removal, radiation, or both, followed by possible lifelong hormone replacement therapy
- Endocrine substitution therapy for affected organs
- High-calorie, high-protein diet
- Regular exercise program
- Rest periods for fatigue
- Hormone replacement
- Surgery for pituitary tumor

KEY PATIENT OUTCOMES

The patient will:
- maintain body weight
- maintain normal body temperature
- demonstrate age-appropriate skills and behavior to the extent possible
- verbalize feelings of positive self-esteem.

NURSING INTERVENTIONS

- Administer prescribed medications.
- Encourage maintenance of adequate calorie intake.
- Offer the patient small, frequent meals.
- Keep the patient warm.
- Institute safety precautions.
- Provide emotional support.
- Encourage the patient to express his feelings.
- Evaluate laboratory tests for hormonal deficiencies.
- Record calorie intake.
- Check and evaluate daily weight.
- Monitor vital signs.
- Assess neurologic status.

- Assess for signs and symptoms of pituitary apoplexy, a medical emergency (sudden, severe headache, vomiting, and visual changes)
- Assess for signs and symptoms of hypoglycemia.

PATIENT TEACHING

Be sure to cover:
- the disorder, diagnosis, and treatment
- long-term hormonal replacement therapy and adverse reactions
- when to notify the physician
- regular follow-up appointments
- energy-conservation techniques
- need for adequate rest
- need for a balanced diet.

Hypothyroidism

DESCRIPTION

- Clinical condition characterized by either decreased circulating levels of or resistance to free thyroid hormone (TH)
- Classified as primary or secondary
- Severe hypothyroidism known as *myxedema*

PATHOPHYSIOLOGY

- In primary hypothyroidism, a decrease in TH production is a result of the loss of thyroid tissue.
- Loss of thyroid tissue results in an increased secretion of thyroid-stimulating hormone (TSH) that leads to a goiter.
- In secondary hypothyroidism, the pituitary typically fails to synthesize or secrete adequate amounts of TSH, or target tissues fail to respond to normal blood levels of TH.
- Either type may progress to myxedema, which is clinically more severe and considered a medical emergency.

CAUSES

- Amyloidosis
- Antithyroid medications
- Autoimmune thyroiditis (Hashimoto's) (most common cause)
- Congenital defects
- Endemic iodine deficiency
- External radiation to the neck

- Hypothalamic failure to produce thyrotropin-releasing hormone
- Idiopathic
- Inflammatory conditions
- Medications, such as iodides and lithium
- Pituitary failure to produce TSH
- Pituitary tumor
- Postpartum pituitary necrosis
- Radioactive iodine therapy
- Sarcoidosis
- Thyroid gland surgery

ASSESSMENT FINDINGS

- Vague and varied symptoms that developed slowly over time
- Energy loss, fatigue
- Forgetfulness
- Sensitivity to cold
- Unexplained weight gain
- Constipation
- Anorexia
- Decreased libido
- Menorrhagia
- Paresthesia
- Joint stiffness
- Muscle cramping
- Slight mental slowing to severe obtundation
- Thick, dry tongue
- Hoarseness; slow, slurred speech
- Dry, flaky, inelastic skin
- Puffy face, hands, and feet
- Periorbital edema; drooping upper eyelids
- Dry, sparse hair with patchy hair loss
- Loss of outer third of eyebrow
- Thick, brittle nails with transverse and longitudinal grooves
- Ataxia, intention tremor, nystagmus
- Doughy skin that feels cool
- Weak pulse and bradycardia
- Muscle weakness
- Sacral or peripheral edema
- Delayed reflex relaxation time
- Possible goiter
- Absent or decreased bowel sounds

- Hypotension
- A gallop or distant heart sounds
- Adventitious breath sounds
- Abdominal distention or ascites

TEST RESULTS

- Radioimmunoassay shows decreased serum levels of T_3 and T_4.
- Serum TSH level is increased with thyroid insufficiency and decreased with hypothalamic or pituitary insufficiency.
- Serum cholesterol, alkaline phosphatase, and triglycerides levels are elevated.
- Serum electrolytes show low serum sodium levels in myxedema coma.
- Arterial blood gases show decreased pH and increased partial pressure of carbon dioxide in myxedema coma.
- Skull X-rays, computed tomography scan, and magnetic resonance imaging may show pituitary or hypothalamic lesions.

TREATMENT

- Long-term thyroid replacement
- Low-fat, low-cholesterol, high-fiber, low-sodium diet
- Possibly fluid restriction
- Activity, as tolerated
- Synthetic hormone levothyroxine (Levothroid)
- Synthetic liothyronine (Cytomel)
- Surgery for underlying cause such as pituitary tumor

KEY PATIENT OUTCOMES

The patient will:
- maintain adequate cardiac output
- maintain stable vital signs
- demonstrate normal laboratory values
- maintain balanced fluid volume status
- consume adequate daily calorie requirements
- express positive feelings about self.

NURSING INTERVENTIONS

- Administer prescribed medications.
- Provide adequate rest periods.
- Apply antiembolism stockings.
- Encourage coughing and deep-breathing exercises.

■ Maintain fluid restrictions and a low-sodium diet.
■ Provide a high-bulk, low-calorie diet.
■ Reorient the patient, as needed.
■ Offer support and encouragement.
■ Provide meticulous skin care.
■ Keep the patient warm, as needed.
■ Encourage the patient to express his feelings.
■ Help the patient develop effective coping strategies.
■ Monitor vital signs.
■ Record and evaluate intake and output.
■ Check daily weight.
■ Assess the patient's cardiovascular status.
■ Assess the patient's pulmonary status.
■ Assess for the presence of edema.
■ Monitor the patient's bowel sounds, abdominal distention, and frequency of bowel movements.
■ Monitor the patient's mental and neurologic status.
■ Observe for signs and symptoms of hyperthyroidism.

PATIENT TEACHING

Be sure to cover:
■ the disorder, diagnosis, and treatment
■ prescribed medications and possible adverse effects
■ when to notify the physician
■ physical and mental changes
■ signs and symptoms of myxedema
■ need for life-long hormone replacement therapy
■ need to wear a medical identification bracelet
■ importance of keeping accurate records of daily weight
■ need to adhere to a well-balanced, high-fiber, low-sodium diet
■ energy-conservation techniques.

Intestinal obstruction

DESCRIPTION

■ Partial or complete blockage of the lumen of the small or large bowel
■ Commonly a medical emergency
■ Most likely after abdominal surgery or with congenital bowel deformities
■ Without treatment, may cause death within hours from shock and vascular collapse

PATHOPHYSIOLOGY

- Mechanical or nonmechanical (neurogenic) blockage of the lumen occurs.
- Fluid, air, or gas collects near the site.
- Peristalsis increases temporarily in an attempt to break through the blockage.
- Intestinal mucosa is injured, and distention at and above the site of obstruction occurs.
- Venous blood flow is impaired, and normal absorptive processes cease.
- Water, sodium, and potassium are secreted by the bowel into the fluid pooled in the lumen.

CAUSES

Mechanical obstruction
- Adhesions
- Carcinomas
- Compression of the bowel wall from stenosis, intussusception, volvulus of the sigmoid or cecum, tumors, and atresia
- Foreign bodies
- Strangulated hernias

Nonmechanical obstruction
- Electrolyte imbalances
- Neurogenic abnormalities
- Paralytic ileus
- Thrombosis or embolism of mesenteric vessels
- Toxicity, such as that associated with uremia or generalized infection

ASSESSMENT FINDINGS

- Recent change in bowel habits
- Hiccups

Mechanical obstruction
- Colicky pain
- Nausea, vomiting
- Constipation
- Distended abdomen
- Borborygmi and rushes (occasionally loud enough to be heard without a stethoscope)
- Abdominal tenderness
- Rebound tenderness

Title: Medical-Surgical Nursing
            (Lippincott Manual of Nursing
            Practice Pocket Guides)
Cond: Good
Date: 2024-06-26 21:48:28 (UTC)
mSKU: ZWM.YFG
vSKU: ZWV.1582558973.G
unit_id: 16534450
Source: CATALINA

ZWV.1582558973.G

delist unit# 16534450

XXXXX

Nonmechanical obstruction
■ Diffuse abdominal discomfort
■ Frequent vomiting
■ Severe abdominal pain (if obstruction results from vascular insufficiency or infarction)
■ Abdominal distention
■ Decreased bowel sounds (early), then absent bowel sounds

TEST RESULTS
■ Serum sodium, chloride, and potassium levels are decreased.
■ White blood cell count is elevated.
■ Serum amylase level is increased if pancreas is irritated by a bowel loop.
■ Blood urea nitrogen is increased with dehydration.
■ Abdominal X-rays reveal the presence and location of intestinal gas or fluid. (In small-bowel obstruction, a typical "stepladder" pattern emerges, with alternating fluid and gas levels apparent in 3 to 4 hours.)
■ Barium enema reveals a distended, air-filled colon or a closed loop of sigmoid with extreme distention (in sigmoid volvulus).

TREATMENT
■ Correction of fluid and electrolyte imbalances
■ Decompression of the bowel to relieve vomiting and distention
■ Treatment of shock and peritonitis
■ Nothing by mouth if surgery scheduled
■ Parenteral nutrition until bowel is functioning
■ High-fiber diet when obstruction is relieved and peristalsis returns
■ Bed rest during acute phase
■ Postoperatively, avoidance of lifting and contact sports
■ Broad-spectrum antibiotics
■ Analgesics
■ Blood replacement
■ Surgery is usually the treatment of choice (exception is paralytic ileus in which nonoperative therapy usually attempted first)
■ Type of surgery dependent on cause of blockage

KEY PATIENT OUTCOMES
The patient will:
■ express feelings of increased comfort
■ maintain normal fluid volume

- return to normal bowel function
- maintain caloric requirement
- maintain stable vital signs.

NURSING INTERVENTIONS

- Insert a nasogastric (NG) tube and attach to low-pressure, intermittent suction.
- Maintain the patient in semi-Fowler's position.
- Provide mouth and nose care.
- Begin and maintain I.V. therapy, as ordered.
- Administer prescribed medications.
- Monitor vital signs.
- Assess for signs and symptoms of shock.
- Assess bowel sounds and signs of returning peristalsis.
- Monitor NG tube function and drainage.
- Assess pain control and provide comfort measures.
- Measure the abdominal girth to detect progressive distention.
- Assess hydration and nutritional status.
- Monitor electrolytes and signs and symptoms of metabolic derangements.
- Assess the wound site (postoperatively) and provide wound care.
- Refer the patient to an enterostomal therapist, if indicated, and home health care services.

PATIENT TEACHING

Be sure to cover:
- the disorder (focusing on the patient's type of intestinal obstruction), diagnosis, and treatment
- techniques for coughing and deep breathing and incentive spirometry
- colostomy or ileostomy care, if appropriate
- incision care
- postoperative activity limitations and why these are necessary
- proper use of prescribed medications, focusing on their correct administration, desired effects, and possible adverse reactions
- importance of following a structured bowel regimen, particularly if the patient had a mechanical obstruction from fecal impaction.

Latex allergy

DESCRIPTION

- An immunoglobulin (Ig) E–mediated immediate hypersensitivity reaction to products that contain natural latex
- Can range from local dermatitis to life-threatening anaphylactic reaction
- Present in 1% to 5% of population of the United States
- Affects 10% to 30% of health care workers
- Most prevalent (20% to 68%) in patients with spina bifida and urogenital abnormalities
- Affects males and females equally

PATHOPHYSIOLOGY

- Mast cells release histamine and other secretory products.
- Vascular permeability increases and vasodilation and bronchoconstriction occur.
- Chemical sensitivity dermatitis is a type IV delayed hypersensitivity reaction to the chemicals used in processing rather than the latex itself.
- In a cell-mediated allergic reaction, sensitized T lymphocytes are triggered, stimulating the proliferation of other lymphocytes and mononuclear cells, resulting in tissue inflammation and contact dermatitis.

CAUSES

- Frequent contact with latex-containing products

ASSESSMENT FINDINGS

- Exposure to latex
- Signs of anaphylaxis
- Rash
- Angioedema and urticaria
- Conjunctivitis
- Wheezing, stridor

TEST RESULTS

- Radioallergosorbent test shows specific IgE antibodies to latex (safest for use in patients with history of type I hypersensitivity).
- Patch test results in hives with itching or redness as a positive response.

TREATMENT

- Prevention of exposure, including use of latex-free products to decrease possible exacerbation of hypersensitivity
- Maintenance of patent airway
- Corticosteroids
- Antihistamines
- Histamine-2 receptor blockers
- Epinephrine 1:1,000
- Oxygen therapy
- Volume expanders
- I.V. vasopressors
- Aminophylline and albuterol (Proventil)

KEY PATIENT OUTCOMES

The patient will:
- maintain a patent airway
- remain hemodynamically stable
- identify latex products in order to avoid exposure.

NURSING INTERVENTIONS

- Maintain airway, breathing, and circulation.
- Administer prescribed medications.

   ALERT *When adding medication to an I.V. bag, inject the drug through the spike port, not the rubber latex port.*
- Monitor vital signs.
- Assess and continue to monitor respiratory status.
- Keep the patient's environment latex free.

PATIENT TEACHING

Be sure to cover:
- the disorder, diagnosis, and treatment
- potential for life-threatening reaction
- wearing medical identification jewelry that identifies allergy
- how to use an epinephrine autoinjector.

Leukemia, acute

DESCRIPTION

- Malignant proliferation of white blood cell (WBC) precursors, or blasts, in bone marrow or lymph tissue; blasts accumulate in peripheral blood, bone marrow, and body tissues
- Most common form of cancer among children
- Common forms:
  - Acute lymphoblastic (lymphocytic) leukemia (ALL), characterized by abnormal growth of lymphocyte precursors (lymphoblasts)
  - Acute myeloblastic (myelogenous) leukemia (AML); causes rapid accumulation of myeloid precursors (myeloblasts)
  - Acute monoblastic (monocytic) leukemia, or *Schilling's type*, results in marked increase in monocyte precursors (monoblasts)

PATHOPHYSIOLOGY

- Immature, nonfunctioning WBCs appear to accumulate first in the tissue where they originate, such as lymphocytes in lymph tissue and granulocytes in bone marrow.
- The immature, nonfunctioning WBCs spill into the bloodstream and overwhelm red blood cells (RBCs) and platelets; from there, they infiltrate other tissues. (See *Understanding leukemia*, page 170.)

CAUSES

- Unknown
- Risk factors: radiation exposure, drugs, genetic abnormalities, toxins, and viruses

ASSESSMENT FINDINGS

- Sudden onset of high fever
- Abnormal bleeding or bruising
- Fatigue and night sweats
- Weakness, lassitude, recurrent infections, and chills
- Abdominal or bone pain in patients with ALL, AML, or acute monoblastic leukemia
- Tachycardia, palpitations, and a systolic ejection murmur
- Decreased ventilation
- Pallor
- Lymph node enlargement
- Liver or spleen enlargement

FOCUS IN
UNDERSTANDING LEUKEMIA

Leukemias cause an abnormal proliferation of white blood cells (WBC) and suppression of other blood components. A rapidly progressing disease, acute
leukemia is characterized by the malignant proliferation of WBC precursors
(blasts) in bone marrow or lymph tissue and by their accumulation in peripheral
blood, bone marrow, and body tissues. In chronic forms of leukemia, disease
onset occurs more insidiously, commonly with no symptoms.

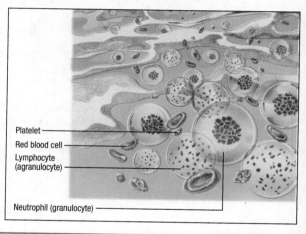

Platelet
Red blood cell
Lymphocyte
(agranulocyte)

Neutrophil (granulocyte)

TEST RESULTS

- Blood counts show thrombocytopenia and neutropenia, and a WBC differential shows the cell type.
- Computed tomography scan shows the affected organs, and cerebrospinal
  fluid analysis shows abnormal WBC invasion of the central nervous system.
- Bone marrow aspiration shows a proliferation of immature WBCs (confirming acute leukemia).

  ALERT *If aspirate is dry or free from leukemic cells but the
  patient has other typical signs of leukemia, a bone marrow
  biopsy, usually of the posterior superior iliac spine, must be performed.*

- Lumbar puncture detects meningeal involvement.

TREATMENT

- Transfusions of platelets to prevent bleeding
- Transfusions of RBCs to prevent anemia
- Bone marrow transplantation in some patients
- Radiation therapy in case of brain or testicular infiltration
- Chemotherapeutic and radiation treatment, depending on diagnosis
- Well-balanced diet
- Frequent rest periods
- Consultation with a mental health professional or spiritual counseling should be considered.

▶ **COLLABORATION** *The care of the patient will involve a multi-disciplinary team including an oncologist, oncology and staff nurses, pharmacists, phlebotomists, dietitians, and social workers.*

For meningeal infiltration

- Intrathecal instillation of methotrexate (Rheumatrex) or cytarabine (Tarabine PFS) with cranial radiation

For ALL

- Vincristine (Oncovin), prednisone (Orasone), high-dose cytarabine, and daunorubicin
- Intrathecal methotrexate or cytarabine because ALL carries 40% risk of meningeal infiltration
- Induces remission in 90% of children (with best survival rate among children ages 2 to 8) and in 65% of adults

For AML

- A combination of I.V. daunorubicin and cytarabine
- If combination of I.V. daunorubicin and cytarabine fails to induce remission, some or all of the following medications: a combination of cyclophosphamide, vincristine, prednisone, or methotrexate; high-dose cytarabine alone or with other drugs; amsacrine; etoposide; and 5-azacytidine and mitoxantrone
- Average survival time 1 year after diagnosis, even with aggressive treatment (remissions lasting 2 to 10 months in 50% of children)

For acute monoblastic leukemia

- Cytarabine and thioguanine with daunorubicin or doxorubicin
- Anti-infective agents, such as antibiotics, antifungals, and antiviral drugs and granulocyte injections

KEY PATIENT OUTCOMES

The patient will:

- have no further weight loss
- exhibit intact mucous membranes
- experience no chills, fever, or other signs and symptoms of illness
- express feelings of increased comfort
- utilize available support systems.

NURSING INTERVENTIONS

- Encourage verbalization and provide comfort.
- Provide adequate hydration.
- After bone marrow transplantation, keep the patient in a sterile room, administer antibiotics, and transfuse packed RBCs as necessary.
- Administer prescribed medications.
- Control mouth ulceration by checking often for obvious ulcers and gum swelling and by providing frequent mouth care and saline rinses.
- Observe for complications from treatment.
- Assess the patient's hydration and nutritional status.
- Test urine pH (should be above 7.5).
- Monitor vital signs.
- Observe for signs and symptoms of bleeding.
- The patient and family should be referred to community support groups and services.

PATIENT TEACHING

Be sure to cover:

- the disorder, diagnosis, and treatment
- medication administration, dosage, and possible adverse effects
- use of a soft toothbrush and avoidance of hot, spicy foods and commercial mouthwashes
- signs and symptoms of infection
- signs and symptoms of abnormal bleeding
- planned rest periods during the day.

Leukemia, chronic lymphocytic

DESCRIPTION

- Most benign and slowly progressive form of leukemia
- Prognosis poor if anemia, thrombocytopenia, neutropenia, bulky lymphadenopathy, and severe lymphocytosis develop

- Most common in elderly people; nearly all afflicted are men older than age 50
- Accounts for almost one-third of new leukemia cases annually
- Higher incidence recorded within families
- Typically, can be an incidental finding of other miscellaneous blood tests

PATHOPHYSIOLOGY

- Chronic lymphocytic leukemia is a generalized, progressive disease marked by an uncontrollable spread of abnormal, small lymphocytes in lymphoid tissue, blood, and bone marrow.
- Once these cells infiltrate bone marrow, lymphoid tissue, and organ systems, clinical signs begin to appear.
- Gross bone marrow replacement by abnormal lymphocytes is the most common cause of death, usually within 4 to 5 years of diagnosis.

CAUSES

- Exact cause unknown

ASSESSMENT FINDINGS

- Fatigue, malaise, fever, weight loss, and frequent infections
- Weakness, palpitations
- Macular or nodular eruptions and evidence of skin infiltration
- Enlarged lymph nodes, liver, and spleen
- Bone tenderness and edema from lymph node obstruction
- Pallor, dyspnea, tachycardia, bleeding, and infection from bone marrow involvement
- Signs of opportunistic fungal, viral, or bacterial infections

TEST RESULTS

- A complete blood count reveals numerous abnormal lymphocytes.
  - In the early stages, white blood cell (WBC) count is mildly but persistently elevated; granulocytopenia is the rule, although WBC count climbs as disease progresses.
  - Hemoglobin level is under 11g/dl.
  - WBC differential shows neutropenia (less than 1,500/μl) or lymphocytosis (more than 10,000/μl).
  - Platelet count shows thrombocytopenia (less than 150,000/μl).
  - Serum protein electrophoresis shows hypogammaglobulinemia.
- Computed tomography scan shows affected organs.
- Bone marrow aspiration and biopsy show lymphocytic invasion.

TREATMENT

- Radiation therapy to relieve symptoms (generally for patient with enlarged lymph nodes, painful bony lesions, or massive splenomegaly)
- High-calorie, high-protein diet
- Avoidance of hot and spicy foods for patient with impaired oral membranes
- Frequent rest periods
- Systemic chemotherapy
- Prednisone

KEY PATIENT OUTCOMES

The patient will:
- have no further weight loss
- have intact mucous membranes
- experience no chills, fever, or other signs and symptoms of illness
- express feelings of increased comfort and energy
- utilize available support systems.

NURSING INTERVENTIONS

- Help establish an appropriate rehabilitation program during remission.
- Place the patient in reverse isolation, if necessary.
- Administer prescribed medications.
- Encourage verbalization and provide support.
- Administer blood component therapy, as necessary.
- Observe for signs and symptoms of bleeding and thrombocytopenia.
- Monitor for adverse effects of treatment.
- Assess pain control and provide comfort measures.
- Monitor vital signs.

PATIENT TEACHING

Be sure to cover:
- the disorder, diagnosis, and treatment
- use of a soft toothbrush and avoidance of commercial mouthwashes to prevent irritating the mouth ulcers that result from chemotherapy
- medication administration, dosage, and possible adverse effects
- signs and symptoms of infection, bleeding, and recurrence
- staying away from anyone with an infection
- importance of follow-up care.

Liver cancer

DESCRIPTION

- Malignant cells growing in the tissues of the liver
- Rapidly fatal, usually within 6 months
- After cirrhosis, the leading cause of fatal hepatic disease
- Liver metastasis: Solitary or multiple discrete lesions occurring secondary to cancer in another organ

PATHOPHYSIOLOGY

- Most (90%) primary liver tumors originate in the parenchymal cells and are hepatomas. Others originate in the intrahepatic bile ducts (cholangiomas).
- Approximately 30% to 70% of patients with hepatomas also have cirrhosis.
- Rare tumors include a mixed-cell type, Kupffer cell sarcoma, and hepatoblastoma.
- The liver is one of the most common sites of metastasis from other primary cancers. Cells metastasize to gallbladder, mesentery, peritoneum, and diaphragm by direct extension.

CAUSES

- Immediate cause unknown
- Environmental exposure to carcinogens
- Hepatitis B virus
- Hepatitis C virus
- Hepatitis D virus
- Possibly androgens and oral estrogens

ASSESSMENT FINDINGS

- Weight loss
- Weakness, fatigue, and fever
- Initially, dull aching abdominal pain
- Severe pain in the epigastrium or right upper quadrant
- Jaundice
- Dependent edema
- Abdominal bruit, hum, or rubbing sound
- Tender, nodular, enlarged liver
- Ascites
- Palpable mass in the right upper quadrant

TEST RESULTS

- Serum glutamic-oxaloacetic transaminase, serum glutamic-pyruvic transaminase, alkaline phosphatase, lactic dehydrogenase, and bilirubin reveal abnormal liver function.
- Alpha-fetoprotein levels are greater than 500 mcg/ml.
- Electrolyte results indicate retention of sodium, causing functional renal failure.
- Liver scan may show filling defects and lesions in the liver.
- Arteriography may define large tumors.
- Ultrasound and computed tomography scans may reveal lesions in the liver.
- Liver biopsy by needle or open biopsy reveals cancerous cells.

TREATMENT

- Radiation therapy (alone or with chemotherapy)
- High-calorie, low-protein diet
- Frequent rest periods
- Postoperative avoidance of heavy lifting and contact sports
- Chemotherapeutic drugs
- Liver transplantation
- Resection (lobectomy or partial hepatectomy)

KEY PATIENT OUTCOMES

The patient will:
- maintain hemodynamic stability
- maintain adequate cardiac output
- exhibit adequate coping behaviors
- maintain normal fluid volume
- express feelings of increased comfort.

NURSING INTERVENTIONS

- Administer prescribed medications.
- Provide meticulous skin care.
- Encourage verbalization and provide support.
- Monitor vital signs.
- Assess the patient's hydration and nutritional status.
- Obtain daily weight.
- Assess pain control and provide comfort measures.
- Assess the patient's neurologic status.
- Monitor complete blood count and liver function tests.
- Observe for postoperative complications.

- Assess the wound site and provide wound care.
- Refer the patient to community resource and support services and hospice care, if indicated.

PATIENT TEACHING

Be sure to cover:
- the disorder, diagnosis, and treatment
- dietary restrictions
- relaxation techniques
- medication administration, dosage, and possible adverse effects
- end-of-life issues.

Lung cancer

DESCRIPTION

- Malignant tumors arising from the respiratory epithelium
- Most common types: epidermoid (squamous cell), adenocarcinoma, small-cell (oat cell), and large-cell (anaplastic)
- Most common site: wall or epithelium of bronchial tree
- For most patients, poor prognosis, depending on extent of cancer when diagnosed and cells' growth rate (13% of patients survive 5 years after diagnosis)

PATHOPHYSIOLOGY

- Individuals with lung cancer demonstrate bronchial epithelial changes progressing from squamous cell alteration or metaplasia to carcinoma in situ.
- Tumors originating in the bronchi are thought to be more mucus producing.
- Partial or complete obstruction of the airway occurs with tumor growth, resulting in lobar collapse distal to the tumor.
- Early metastasis occurs to other thoracic structures, such as hilar lymph nodes or the mediastinum.
- Distant metastasis occurs to the brain, liver, bone, and adrenal glands. (See *How lung cancer develops,* page 178.)

CAUSES

- Exact cause unknown
- Risk factors: tobacco smoking, exposure to carcinogens, genetic predisposition

FOCUS IN
HOW LUNG CANCER DEVELOPS

Lung cancer usually begins with the transformation of one epithelial cell within the patient's airway. Although the exact cause of such change remains unclear, some lung cancers originating in the bronchi may be more vulnerable to injuries from carcinogens.

As the tumor grows, it can partially or completely obstruct the airway, resulting in lobar collapse distal to the tumor. Early metastasis may occur to other thoracic structures as well.

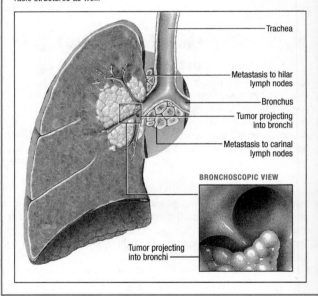

Trachea

Metastasis to hilar lymph nodes

Bronchus

Tumor projecting into bronchi

Metastasis to carinal lymph nodes

BRONCHOSCOPIC VIEW

Tumor projecting into bronchi

ASSESSMENT FINDINGS

- Possibly no symptoms
- Exposure to carcinogens
- Coughing
- Hemoptysis
- Hoarseness

- Fatigue
- Dyspnea on exertion
- Finger clubbing
- Edema of the face, neck, and upper torso
- Dilated chest and abdominal veins (superior vena cava syndrome)
- Weight loss
- Enlarged lymph nodes
- Enlarged liver
- Decreased breath sounds
- Wheezing
- Pleural friction rub
- Recurrent bronchitis or pneumonia

TEST RESULTS

- Cytologic sputum analysis shows diagnostic evidence of pulmonary malignancy.
- Liver function test results are abnormal, especially with metastasis.
- Chest X-rays may show size and location of advanced lesions (possibly as old as 2 years).
- Contrast studies of the bronchial tree (chest tomography, bronchography) demonstrate size, location, and spread of lesion.
- Bone scan detects metastasis.
- Computed tomography (CT) of the chest detects malignant pleural effusion.
- CT of the brain detects metastasis.
- Positron emission tomography aids in the diagnosis of primary and metastatic sites.
- Bronchoscopy identifies tumor site (bronchoscopic washings provide material for cytologic and histologic study).
- Needle biopsy of the lungs (relies on biplanar fluoroscopic visual control to locate peripheral tumors before withdrawing a tissue specimen for analysis) allows firm diagnosis in 80% of patients.
- Tissue biopsy of metastatic sites, including supraclavicular and mediastinal nodes and pleura, is used to assess disease extent (based on histologic findings; staging describes disease's extent and prognosis and is used to direct treatment).
- Thoracentesis allows chemical and cytologic examination of pleural fluid.
- Gallium scans of the liver and spleen detect metastasis.
- Exploratory thoracotomy is used to obtain a biopsy specimen.

TREATMENT

- Various combinations of surgery, radiation therapy, and chemotherapy to improve prognosis
- Palliative (most treatments)
- Preoperative and postoperative radiation therapy
- Laser therapy (experimental)
- Well-balanced diet
- Activity, as tolerated per breathing capacity
- Chemotherapy drug combinations
- Immunotherapy (investigational)
- Partial removal of lung (wedge resection, segmental resection, lobectomy, radical lobectomy)
- Total removal of lung (pneumonectomy, radical pneumonectomy)

▶ **COLLABORATION** *Optimal management of the lung cancer patient will include consultation with a radiation oncologist, social worker, dietitian, and physical therapist.*

KEY PATIENT OUTCOMES

The patient will:
- maintain normal fluid volume
- maintain adequate ventilation
- maintain a patent airway
- express feelings of increased comfort and decreased pain.

NURSING INTERVENTIONS

- Provide supportive care.
- Encourage verbalization.
- Administer prescribed medications.
- Assess chest tube function and drainage.
- Observe for postoperative complications.
- Assess wound site and provide wound care.
- Monitor vital signs.
- Assess sputum production.
- Monitor and record hydration and nutrition.
- Monitor oxygenation.
- Assess pain control and provide comfort measures.
- Refer smokers to local branches of the American Cancer Society or Smokenders.
- Provide information about group therapy, individual counseling, and hypnosis to end smoking.

PATIENT TEACHING

Be sure to cover:
- the disorder, diagnosis, and treatment
- postoperative procedures and equipment
- chest physiotherapy
- exercises to prevent shoulder stiffness
- medication administration, dosage, and possible adverse effects
- risk factors for recurrent cancer.

Lyme disease

DESCRIPTION

- A multisystem disorder caused by a spirochete

PATHOPHYSIOLOGY

- A tick injects spirochete laden saliva into the bloodstream or deposits fecal matter on the skin.
- After incubating for 3 to 32 days, the spirochetes migrate outward on the skin, causing a rash, and disseminate to other skin sites or organs through the bloodstream or lymph system.
- Spirochetes may survive for years in the joints or die after triggering an inflammatory response in the host.

CAUSES

- The spirochete *Borrelia burgdorferi*, carried by the minute tick *Ixodes dammini* (also called *I. scapularis*) or another tick in the Ixodidae family

ASSESSMENT FINDINGS

- Recent exposure to ticks
- Onset of symptoms in warmer months
- Severe headache and stiff neck with rash eruption
- Fever (up to 104° F [40° C]) and chills
- Regional lymphadenopathy
- Tenderness in the skin lesion site or the posterior cervical area
- Tachycardia or irregular heartbeat
- Mild dyspnea
- Erythema migrans
- Headache
- Myalgia

DIFFERENTIATING LYME DISEASE

Lyme disease, or *chronic neuroborreliosis,* needs to be differentiated from chronic fatigue syndrome or fibromyalgia, which is difficult late in the disease because of chronic pain and fatigue. The other diseases produce more generalized and disabling symptoms; also, patients lack evidence of joint inflammation, have normal neurologic tests, and have a greater degree of anxiety and depression than patients with Lyme disease.

- Arthralgia
- Neurologic signs and symptoms, such as memory impairment and myelitis
- Bell's palsy
- Intermittent arthritis (see *Differentiating Lyme disease*)
- Cardiac symptoms, such as heart failure, pericarditis, and dyspnea
- Fibromyalgia
- Ocular signs such as conjunctivitis

TEST RESULTS

- Assays for anti–*B. burgdorferi* (anti-B) show evidence of previous or current infection.
- Enzyme-linked immunosorbent technology or indirect immunofluorescence microscopy shows immunoglobulin (Ig) M levels that peak 3 to 6 weeks after infection; IgG antibodies detected several weeks after infection may continue to develop for several months and generally persist for years.
- Positive Western blot assay shows serologic evidence of past or current infection with *B. burgdorferi.*

  ALERT Serologic testing isn't useful early in the course of Lyme disease because of its low sensitivity. However, it may be more useful in later disease stages, when sensitivity and specificity of the test are improved.
- Lumbar puncture with analysis of cerebrospinal fluid may show antibodies to *B. burgdorferi.*
- Skin biopsy may detect *B. burgdorferi.*

TREATMENT

- Prompt tick removal using proper technique
- Rest periods when needed
- I.V. or oral antibiotics (initiated as soon as possible after infection)

▶ **COLLABORATION** *Consult with a dermatologist, neurologist, cardiologist, and infectious disease specialist to obtain the best functional outcome for the patient.*

KEY PATIENT OUTCOMES

The patient will:
- maintain hemodynamic stability
- maintain adequate cardiac output
- express relief from pain
- attain the highest degree of mobility possible.

NURSING INTERVENTIONS

- Plan care to provide adequate rest.
- Administer prescribed medications.
- Assist with range-of-motion and strengthening exercises (with arthritis).
- Encourage verbalization and provide support.
- Assess for skin lesions and healing of the lesions.
- Observe response to treatment.
- Monitor for adverse drug reactions.
- Observe for complications.

PATIENT TEACHING

Be sure to cover:
- the disorder, diagnosis, and treatment
- medication administration, dosage, and possible adverse effects
- importance of follow-up care and reporting recurrent or new symptoms to the physician
- prevention of Lyme disease, such as avoiding tick-infested areas, covering the skin with clothing, using insect repellents, inspecting exposed skin for attached ticks at least every 4 hours, and removing ticks
- information about the vaccine for persons at risk for contracting Lyme disease.

Lymphoma, non-Hodgkin's

DESCRIPTION

- Heterogeneous group of malignant diseases that originate in lymph glands and other lymphoid tissue
- Usually classified according to histologic, anatomic, and immunomorphic

characteristics developed by the National Cancer Institute (Rappaport histologic and Lukes and Collins classifications also used in some facilities)

- New categories of non-Hodgkin's lymphoma, called *mantle zone lymphoma* and *marginal zone lymphoma*, identified recently
- Also called *malignant lymphoma* and *lymphosarcoma*
- Three times more common than Hodgkin's disease
- Incidence increasing, especially in patients with autoimmune disorders and those receiving immunosuppressant treatment or those with acquired immunodeficiency syndrome
- Uses same staging system as Hodgkin's disease

PATHOPHYSIOLOGY

- Non-Hodgkin's lymphoma seems to be similar to Hodgkin's disease, but Reed-Sternberg cells aren't present, and the lymph node destruction is different.
- Lymphoid tissue is defined by the pattern of infiltration as diffuse or nodular. Nodular lymphomas yield a better prognosis than the diffuse form, but in both the prognosis is less hopeful than in Hodgkin's disease.

CAUSES

- Exact cause unknown

ASSESSMENT FINDINGS

- Symptoms mimic those of Hodgkin's disease
- Painless, swollen lymph glands (swelling may have appeared and disappeared over several months)
- Complaints of fatigue, malaise, weight loss, fever, and night sweats
- Difficulty breathing, cough (usually children)
- Enlarged tonsils and adenoids
- Rubbery nodes in the cervical and supraclavicular areas

TEST RESULTS

- Complete blood count shows anemia.
- Uric acid level is normal or elevated.
- Calcium level is elevated because of bone lesions.
- Miscellaneous scans (chest X-rays; lymphangiography; liver, bone, and spleen scans; a computed tomography scan of the abdomen; and excretory urography) show disease progression.
- Biopsies of lymph nodes; of tonsils, bone marrow, liver, bowel, or skin; or, as needed, of tissue removed during exploratory laparotomy help differentiate non-Hodgkin's lymphoma from Hodgkin's disease.

TREATMENT

■ Radiation therapy mainly during the localized stage of the disease
■ Total nodal irradiation usually effective in nodular and diffuse lymphomas
■ Well-balanced, high-calorie, high-protein diet
■ Increased fluid intake
■ Small, frequent meals
■ Limited activity
■ Frequent rest periods
■ Chemotherapy in combinations
■ Perforation (common in patients with gastric lymphomas) usually necessitates debulking procedure (such as subtotal or, in some cases, total gastrectomy) before chemotherapy

KEY PATIENT OUTCOMES

The patient will:
■ have no further weight loss
■ demonstrate effective coping mechanisms
■ express feelings of increased comfort and decreased pain.

NURSING INTERVENTIONS

■ Administer prescribed medications.
■ Provide time for rest periods.
■ Encourage verbalization and provide support.
■ Observe for adverse effects of treatment.
■ Monitor vital signs.
■ Assess pain control and provide comfort measures.
■ Assess hydration and nutritional status.

PATIENT TEACHING

Be sure to cover:
■ the disorder, diagnosis, and treatment
■ preoperative and postoperative procedures
■ dietary plan
■ mouth care using a soft-bristled toothbrush and avoidance of commercial mouthwashes
■ relaxation and comfort measures
■ medication administration, dosage, and possible adverse effects
■ symptoms that require immediate attention.

Melanoma, malignant

DESCRIPTION

- Neoplasm that arises from melanocytes
- Potentially the most lethal of the skin cancers
- Common sites: head and neck in men, legs in women, and back in people exposed to excessive sunlight
- Four types:
  - Superficial spreading melanoma — most common type; usually develops between ages 40 and 50
  - Nodular melanoma — grows vertically, invades the dermis, and metastasizes early; usually develops between ages 40 and 50
  - Acral-lentiginous melanoma — occurs on the palms and soles and under the tongue; most common among Hispanics, Asians, and Blacks
  - Lentigo maligna melanoma — relatively rare; most benign, slowest growing, and least aggressive of the four types; most commonly occurs in areas heavily exposed to the sun; arises from a lentigo maligna on an exposed skin surface; usually occurs between ages 60 and 70

PATHOPHYSIOLOGY

- Melanomas arise as a result of malignant degeneration of melanocytes located either along the basal layer of the epidermis or in a benign melanocytic nevus.
- Up to 70% of malignant melanomas arise from a preexisting nevus.
- Malignant melanoma spreads through the lymphatic and vascular systems and metastasizes to the regional lymph nodes, skin, liver, lungs, and central nervous system.
- Malignant melanoma follows an unpredictable course; recurrence and metastasis may not appear for more than 5 years after resection of the primary lesion.

CAUSES

- Ultraviolet rays from the sun (damage the skin)

ASSESSMENT FINDINGS

- A sore that doesn't heal, a persistent lump or swelling, and changes in preexisting skin markings, such as moles, birthmarks, scars, freckles, or warts

- Preexisting skin lesion or nevus that enlarges, changes color, becomes inflamed or sore, itches, ulcerates, bleeds, changes texture, or shows signs of surrounding pigment regression
- Lesions on the ankles or the inside surfaces of the knees
- Uniformly discolored nodule on knee or ankle
- Small, elevated tumor nodules that may ulcerate and bleed
- Palpable polypoid nodules that resemble the surface of a blackberry
- Pigmented lesions on the palms and soles or under the nails
- Long-standing lesion that has ulcerated
- Flat nodule with smaller nodules scattered over the surface

TEST RESULTS

- Complete blood count with differential shows anemia.
- Erythrocyte sedimentation rate is elevated.
- Platelet count is abnormal if metastasis is present.
- Liver function studies are abnormal if metastasis is present.
- Chest X-ray assists in staging.
- Excisional biopsy and full-depth punch biopsy with histologic examination show tumor thickness and disease stage.

TREATMENT

- Close, long-term follow-up care to detect metastasis and recurrences
- Radiation therapy (usually for metastatic disease)
- Well-balanced diet
- Avoidance of sun exposure
- Chemotherapy
- Biotherapy
- Immunotherapy
- Immunostimulants
- Surgical resection to remove tumor and 3- to 5-cm margin
- Regional lymphadenectomy

KEY PATIENT OUTCOMES

The patient will:
- have no further weight loss
- express positive feelings about self
- demonstrate effective coping mechanisms
- experience healing of wound without signs of infection
- express feelings of increased comfort.

NURSING INTERVENTIONS

- Encourage verbalization and provide support.
- Provide appropriate wound care.
- Give prescribed medications.
- Provide a high-protein, high-calorie diet.
- Monitor complications of treatment.
- Assist with pain control.
- Inspect the wound site.
- Monitor patient for postoperative complications.

PATIENT TEACHING

Be sure to cover:
- the disorder, diagnosis, and treatment
- preoperative and postoperative care
- need for close follow-up care to detect recurrences early
- signs and symptoms of recurrence, including asymmetry, border irregularities, color variation, and diameter larger than 5 mm (ABCD rule)
- detrimental effects of overexposure to solar radiation and benefits of regular use of a sunblock or a sunscreen and protective clothing
- how to access the American Cancer Society.

Methicillin-resistant *Staphylococcus aureus*

DESCRIPTION

- A mutation of a common bacterium easily spread by direct person-to-person contact
- Also known as *MRSA*

PATHOPHYSIOLOGY

- When natural defense systems break down (after invasive procedures, trauma, or chemotherapy), the usually benign bacteria can invade tissue, proliferate, and cause infection.
- 90% of *Staphylococcus aureus* isolates or strains are penicillin-resistant, and about 27% of all *S. aureus* isolates are resistant to methicillin, a penicillin derivative. These strains may also resist cephalosporins, aminoglycosides, erythromycin, tetracycline, and clindamycin.
- The most frequent colonization site is the anterior nares (40% of adults and most children become transient nasal carriers). The groin, armpits, and intestines are less common colonization sites.

CAUSES

- Methicillin-resistant *S. aureus* that enters a health care facility through an infected or colonized patient (symptom-free carrier of the bacteria) or colonized health care worker
- Transmitted mainly by health care workers' hands

ASSESSMENT FINDINGS

- Possible risk factors for methicillin-resistant *S. aureus*, including immunosuppression, prolonged stays in health care facility, extended antibiotic therapy, and proximity to others who are colonized or infected with MRSA
- Carrier patient commonly asymptomatic
- In symptomatic patients, signs and symptoms related to the primary diagnosis (respiratory, cardiac, or other major system symptoms)

TEST RESULTS

- Cultures from suspicious wounds, skin, urine, or blood show methicillin-resistant *S. aureus*.

TREATMENT

- Transmission precautions: contact isolation for wound, skin, and urine infection; respiratory isolation for sputum infection
- No treatment needed for patient with colonization only
- High-protein diet
- Rest periods, as needed
- Vancomycin (Vancocin), imipenem-cilastatin (Primaxin), or tigecycline (Tygacil) for documented infections

KEY PATIENT OUTCOMES

The patient will:
- maintain collateral circulation
- attain hemodynamic stability
- maintain adequate cardiac output
- remain afebrile
- have an adequate fluid volume.

NURSING INTERVENTIONS

- Provide emotional support to the patient and his family.
- Consider grouping infected patients together and having the same nursing staff care for them.

- Use proper hand-washing technique.
- Use contact precautions and standard precautions.
- Monitor vital signs.
- Monitor culture results.
- Observe the patient for response to treatment.
- Observe the patient for adverse drug reactions.
- Monitor patient for complications.
- Refer the patient to an infectious disease specialist, if indicated.

PATIENT TEACHING

Be sure to cover:
- the disorder, diagnosis, and treatment
- difference between methicillin-resistant *S. aureus* infection and colonization
- prevention of methicillin-resistant *S. aureus* spread
- proper hand-washing technique
- need for family and friends to wear protective garb (and to dispose of it properly) when they visit the patient
- medication administration, dosage, and possible adverse effects
- need to take antibiotics for the full prescription period, even if the patient begins to feel better.

Mitral stenosis

DESCRIPTION

- Narrowing of the mitral valve orifice, which is normally 3 to 6 cm
- Mild mitral stenosis: valve orifice of 2 cm
- Severe mitral stenosis: valve orifice of 1 cm

PATHOPHYSIOLOGY

- Valve leaflets become diffusely thickened by fibrosis and calcification. (See *Understanding mitral stenosis*.)
- The mitral commissures and the chordae tendineae fuse and shorten, the valvular cusps become rigid, and the valve's apex becomes narrowed.
- The narrowing of the apex obstructs blood flow from the left atrium to the left ventricle, resulting in incomplete emptying.
- Left atrial volume and pressure increase, and the atrial chamber dilates.
- Increased resistance to blood flow causes pulmonary hypertension, right ventricular hypertrophy and, eventually, right-sided heart failure and reduced cardiac output.

FOCUS IN
UNDERSTANDING MITRAL STENOSIS

Narrowing of the valve by valvular abnormalities, fibrosis, or calcification obstructs blood flow from the left atrium to the left ventricle. Left atrial volume and pressure rise and the chamber dilates. Greater resistance to blood flow causes pulmonary hypertension, right ventricular hypertrophy, and right-sided heart failure. Inadequate filling of the left ventricle results in low cardiac output.

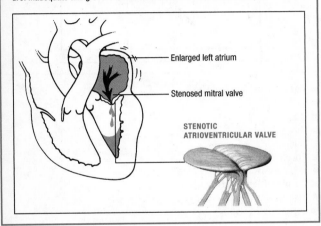

Enlarged left atrium

Stenosed mitral valve

STENOTIC ATRIOVENTRICULAR VALVE

CAUSES

- Atrial myxoma
- Congenital anomalies
- Endocarditis
- Rheumatic fever
- Adverse effect of fenfluramine and phentermine (Fen-phen) diet-drug combination (Fen-phen was removed from the market in 1997.)

ASSESSMENT FINDINGS

Mild mitral stenosis
- Asymptomatic

Moderate to severe mitral stenosis
- Gradual decline in exercise tolerance
- Dyspnea on exertion; shortness of breath

IDENTIFYING THE MURMUR OF MITRAL STENOSIS

A low, rumbling crescendo-decrescendo murmur in the mitral valve area characterizes mitral stenosis.

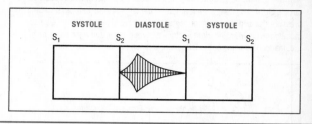

- Paroxysmal nocturnal dyspnea
- Orthopnea
- Weakness
- Fatigue
- Palpitations
- Cough
- Hemoptysis
- Peripheral and facial cyanosis
- Malar rash
- Jugular vein distention
- Ascites
- Peripheral edema
- Hepatomegaly
- Loud S_1 or opening snap
- Diastolic murmur at the apex (see *Identifying the murmur of mitral stenosis*)
- Crackles over lung fields
- Right ventricular lift
- Resting tachycardia; irregularly irregular heart rhythm

TEST RESULTS

- Chest X-rays show left atrial and ventricular enlargement (in severe mitral stenosis), straightening of the left border of the cardiac silhouette, enlarged pulmonary arteries, dilation of the upper lobe pulmonary veins, and mitral valve calcification.
- Echocardiography discloses thickened mitral valve leaflets and left atrial enlargement.

- Cardiac catheterization shows a diastolic pressure gradient across the valve, elevated pulmonary artery wedge pressure (greater than 15 mm Hg), and pulmonary artery pressure in the left atrium with severe pulmonary hypertension.
- Electrocardiography reveals left atrial enlargement, right ventricular hypertrophy, right-axis deviation, and (in 40% to 50% of cases) atrial fibrillation.

TREATMENT

- Synchronized electrical cardioversion to correct atrial fibrillation
- Sodium-restricted diet
- Activity, as tolerated
- Digoxin
- Diuretics
- Oxygen
- Beta-adrenergic blockers
- Calcium channel blockers
- Anticoagulants
- Infective endocarditis antibiotic prophylaxis
- Nitrates
- Commissurotomy or valve replacement
- Percutaneous balloon valvuloplasty

KEY PATIENT OUTCOMES

The patient will:
- carry out activities of daily living without weakness or fatigue
- maintain hemodynamic stability and adequate cardiac output
- have no complications from fluid excess
- exhibit adequate coping mechanisms.

NURSING INTERVENTIONS

- Check for hypersensitivity reaction to antibiotics.
- If the patient needs bed rest, stress its importance.
- Provide a bedside commode.
- Allow the patient to express concerns over his inability to meet responsibilities because of activity restrictions.
- Place the patient in an upright position to relieve dyspnea, if needed.
- Provide a low-sodium diet.
- Check vital signs, hemodynamics, and intake and output.
- Monitor the patient for signs and symptoms of heart failure, pulmonary edema, and thromboembolism.

- Observe for adverse drug reactions.
- Monitor the patient for cardiac arrhythmias.
- Assess postoperatively for hypotension, arrhythmias, and thrombus formation.

PATIENT TEACHING

Be sure to cover:
- the disorder, diagnosis, and treatment
- need to plan for periodic rest in daily routine
- how to check the pulse
- dietary restrictions
- prescribed medications and potential adverse effects
- signs and symptoms to report
- importance of consistent follow-up care
- when to notify the physician
- use of prophylactic antibiotics for procedures.

Mitral valve prolapse

DESCRIPTION

- Prolapse of a portion of the mitral valve into the left atrium during ventricular contraction (systole)

PATHOPHYSIOLOGY

- Myxomatous degeneration of mitral valve leaflets with redundant tissue leads to prolapse of the mitral valve into the left atrium during systole.
- In some patients, this results in leakage of blood into the left atrium from the left ventricle.

CAUSES

- Acquired heart disease, such as coronary artery disease and rheumatic heart disease
- Congenital heart disease
- Connective tissue disorders, such as systemic lupus erythematosus and Marfan syndrome

ASSESSMENT FINDINGS

- Usually asymptomatic
- Possible fatigue, syncope, palpitations, chest pain, or dyspnea on exertion

- Orthostatic hypotension
- Mid-to-late systolic click and late systolic murmur

TEST RESULTS

- Echocardiography may reveal mitral valve prolapse (MVP) with or without mitral insufficiency.
- Electrocardiography (ECG) is usually normal but may reveal atrial or ventricular arrhythmia.
- Signal-averaged ECG may show ventricular and supraventricular arrhythmias.
- Holter monitor worn for 24 hours may show an arrhythmia.

TREATMENT

- Usually requires no treatment; only regular monitoring
- Decreased caffeine intake
- Fluid intake to maintain hydration
- Antibiotic prophylaxis
- Beta-adrenergic blockers
- Anticoagulants
- Antiarrhythmics

KEY PATIENT OUTCOMES

The patient will:
- carry out activities of daily living without fatigue or decreased energy
- maintain adequate cardiac output, without arrhythmias
- exhibit adequate coping mechanisms.

NURSING INTERVENTIONS

- Provide reassurance and comfort if the patient experiences anxiety.
- If fatigue is a concern, plan rest periods.
- Discuss the patient's drug therapy including dosage, adverse reactions, and when to notify the physician if a problem arises.
- Discuss the importance of adequate hydration.
- Check vital signs including blood pressure while lying, sitting, and standing and heart sounds.
- Monitor patient for signs and symptoms of mitral insufficiency.
- Obtain serial echocardiograms.
- Monitor ECG for arrhythmias.

PATIENT TEACHING

Be sure to cover:
- the disorder, diagnosis, and treatment
- need to perform the most important activities of the day when energy levels are highest
- need for antibiotic prophylaxis therapy before dental or surgical procedures as indicated (not all patients with MVP require antibiotic prophylaxis)
- need to avoid foods and beverages high in caffeine
- importance of documenting activities throughout the monitoring process if patient is being discharged with a Holter monitor
- how to access an MVP support group.

Multiple sclerosis

DESCRIPTION

- Progressive demyelination of white matter of brain and spinal cord
- Characterized by exacerbations and remissions
- Years of testing and observation possibly required for diagnosis
- Prognosis varied (70% of patients with multiple sclerosis lead active lives with prolonged remissions), but may progress rapidly, causing death within months
- Also known as *MS*

PATHOPHYSIOLOGY

- Sporadic patches of demyelination occur in the central nervous system, resulting in widespread and varied neurologic dysfunction. (See *How myelin breaks down.*)

CAUSES

- Exact cause unknown
- Allergic response
- Autoimmune response of the nervous system
- Events preceding onset:
  - Acute respiratory tract infections
  - Emotional stress
  - Fatigue
  - Overwork
  - Pregnancy
- Genetic factors possibly involved
- Slow-acting viral infection

FOCUS IN
HOW MYELIN BREAKS DOWN

Myelin speeds electrical impulses to the brain for interpretation. This lipoprotein complex (formed of glial cells or oligodendrocytes) protects the neuron's axon much like the insulation on an electrical wire. Its high electrical resistance and low capacitance allow the myelin to conduct nerve impulses from one node of Ranvier to the next.

Myelin is susceptible to injury (for example, by hypoxemia, toxic chemicals, vascular insufficiencies, or autoimmune responses). The sheath becomes inflamed, and the membrane layers break down into smaller components that become well-circumscribed plaques (filled with microglial elements, macroglia, and lymphocytes). This process is called *demyelination*.

The damaged myelin sheath can't conduct normally. The partial loss or dispersion of the action potential causes neurologic dysfunction.

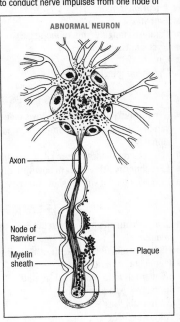

ABNORMAL NEURON

Axon

Node of
Ranvier

Plaque

Myelin
sheath

ASSESSMENT FINDINGS

■ Symptoms related to extent and site of myelin destruction, extent of remyelination, and adequacy of subsequent restored synaptic transmission
■ Symptoms possibly transient or last for hours or weeks
■ Symptoms unpredictable and difficult to describe
■ Visual problems and sensory impairment (the first signs)
■ Blurred vision or diplopia
■ Urinary problems

- Emotional lability
- Dysphagia
- Bowel disturbances (involuntary evacuation or constipation)
- Fatigue (typically the most disabling symptom)
- Poor articulation
- Muscle weakness of the involved area
- Spasticity; hyperreflexia
- Intention tremor
- Gait ataxia
- Paralysis, ranging from monoplegia to quadriplegia
- Nystagmus; scotoma
- Optic neuritis
- Ophthalmoplegia

TEST RESULTS

- Cerebrospinal fluid analysis shows mononuclear cell pleocytosis, an elevation in the level of total immunoglobulin (Ig) G, and presence of oligoclonal Ig.
- Magnetic resonance imaging detects multiple sclerosis focal lesions.
- EEG abnormalities occur in one-third of patients with MS.
- Evoked potential studies show slowed conduction of nerve impulses.

TREATMENT

- Symptomatic treatment for acute exacerbations and related signs and symptoms
- High fluid and fiber intake in case of constipation
- Frequent rest periods
- I.V. steroids followed by oral steroids
- Immunosuppressants
- Antimetabolites
- Alkylating drugs
- Biological response modifiers

▶ **COLLABORATION** *A physical therapy program that includes active resistive and stretching exercises helps maintain muscle tone and joint mobility, decrease spasticity, and improve coordination.*

KEY PATIENT OUTCOMES

The patient will:
- perform activities of daily living
- remain free from infection

- maintain joint mobility and range of motion
- express feelings of increased energy and decreased fatigue
- develop regular bowel and bladder habits
- use available support systems and coping mechanisms.

NURSING INTERVENTIONS

- Provide emotional and psychological support.
- Assist with physical therapy program.
- Provide adequate rest periods.
- Promote emotional stability.
- Keep the bedpan or urinal readily available because the need to void is immediate.
- Provide bowel and bladder training, if indicated.
- Administer prescribed medications.
- Monitor the patient for response to medications and adverse drug reactions.
- Assess the patient for sensory impairment, muscle dysfunction, and energy level.
- Observe for signs and symptoms of infection.
- Monitor the patient for speech and vision changes.
- Record elimination patterns.
- Monitor appropriate laboratory values.

PATIENT TEACHING

Be sure to cover:
- the disease process
- medication and adverse effects
- avoidance of stress, infections, and fatigue
- maintaining independence
- avoiding exposure to bacterial and viral infections
- nutritional management
- adequate fluid intake and regular urination
- how to access the National Multiple Sclerosis Society.

 Life-threatening disorder

Myocardial infarction

DESCRIPTION

- Reduced blood flow through one or more coronary arteries causing myocardial ischemia and necrosis

- Infarction site dependent on the vessels involved
- Also called *MI* and *heart attack*

PATHOPHYSIOLOGY

- One or more coronary arteries become occluded.
- If coronary occlusion causes ischemia lasting longer than 30 to 45 minutes, irreversible myocardial cell damage and muscle death occur.
- Every MI has a central area of necrosis surrounded by an area of hypoxic injury. This injured tissue is potentially viable and may be salvaged if circulation is restored, or it may progress to necrosis.

CAUSES

- Atherosclerosis
- Coronary artery stenosis or spasm
- Platelet aggregation
- Thrombosis

ASSESSMENT FINDINGS

- Possible coronary artery disease with increasing anginal frequency, severity, or duration
- Cardinal symptom of MI: persistent, crushing substernal pain or pressure possibly radiating to the left arm, jaw, neck, and shoulder blades, and possibly persisting for 12 or more hours
- In elderly patient or patient with diabetes, pain possibly absent; in others, pain possibly mild and confused with indigestion
- A feeling of impending doom
- Sudden death (may be the first and only indication of MI)
- Extreme anxiety and restlessness
- Dyspnea
- Diaphoresis
- Tachycardia
- Hypertension
- Bradycardia and hypotension, in inferior MI
- An S_4, an S_3, and paradoxical splitting of S_2 with ventricular dysfunction
- Systolic murmur of mitral insufficiency
- Pericardial friction rub with transmural MI or pericarditis
- Low-grade fever during the next few days
- Fatigue
- Shortness of breath
- Nausea and vomiting

TEST RESULTS

- Serum creatine kinase (CK) level, especially the CK-MB isoenzyme, the cardiac muscle fraction of CK, is elevated.
- Serum lactate dehydrogenase (LD) level is elevated; LD_1 isoenzyme (found in cardiac tissue) is higher than LD_2 isoenzyme (found in serum).
- White blood cell count is elevated usually starting on the second day and lasting 1 week.
- Myoglobin, the hemoprotein in cardiac and skeletal muscle that's released with muscle damage, is detected as soon as 2 hours after MI.
- Troponin I, a structural protein found in cardiac muscle, is elevated with only cardiac muscle damage; more specific than the CK-MB level. (Troponin levels increase within 4 to 6 hours of myocardial injury and may remain elevated for 5 to 11 days.)
- Nuclear medicine scans, using I.V. technetium 99m pertechnetate, identify acutely damaged muscle by picking up accumulations of radioactive nucleotide, which appear as a "hot spot" on the film.
- Myocardial perfusion imaging with thallium 201 reveals a "cold spot" in most patients during first few hours after a transmural MI.
- Echocardiography shows ventricular wall dyskinesia with a transmural MI and helps to evaluate the ejection fraction.
- Serial 12-lead electrocardiography (ECG) readings are normal or inconclusive during the first few hours after an MI.
- Characteristic 12-lead ECG abnormalities include serial ST-segment depression in subendocardial MI and ST-segment elevation and Q waves, representing scarring and necrosis, in transmural MI.
- Pulmonary artery catheterization may be performed to detect left- or right-sided heart failure and to monitor response to treatment.

TREATMENT

- For arrhythmias, a pacemaker or electrical cardioversion
- Intraaortic balloon pump for cardiogenic shock
- Low-fat, low-cholesterol diet
- Calorie restriction, if indicated
- Bed rest with bedside commode
- Gradual increase in activity, as tolerated
- I.V. thrombolytic therapy started within 3 hours of the onset of symptoms
- Aspirin
- Antiarrhythmics, antianginals
- Calcium channel blockers
- Heparin I.V.

- Morphine I.V.
- Inotropic drugs
- Beta-adrenergic blockers
- Angiotensin-converting inhibitors
- Stool softeners
- Oxygen
- Surgical revascularization
- Percutaneous revascularization

KEY PATIENT OUTCOMES

The patient will:
- maintain adequate cardiac output
- maintain hemodynamic stability
- develop no arrhythmias
- develop no complications of fluid volume excess
- express feelings of increased comfort and decreased pain
- exhibit adequate coping skills.

NURSING INTERVENTIONS

- Assess pain and give prescribed analgesics. Record the severity, location, type, and duration of pain. Avoid I.M. injections.
- Check the patient's blood pressure before and after giving nitroglycerin.
- During episodes of chest pain, obtain ECG.
- Organize patient care and activities.
- Provide a low-cholesterol, low-sodium diet with caffeine-free beverages.
- Allow the patient to use a bedside commode.
- Assist with range-of-motion exercises.
- Provide emotional support, and help to reduce stress and anxiety.
- If the patient has undergone percutaneous transluminal coronary angioplasty, sheath care is necessary. Watch for bleeding. Keep the leg with the sheath insertion site immobile. Maintain strict bed rest. Check peripheral pulses in the affected leg frequently.
- Obtain serial ECGs and cardiac enzyme results.
- Monitor the appropriate coagulation studies.
- Monitor vital signs and heart and breath sounds.

  ALERT *Watch for crackles, cough, tachypnea, and edema, which may indicate impending left-sided heart failure.*
- Monitor daily weight and intake and output.
- Monitor cardiac rhythm for reperfusion arrhythmias (treat according to facility protocol).

- Refer the patient to a cardiac rehabilitation program.
- Refer the patient to a smoking-cessation program, if needed.
- Refer the patient to a weight-reduction program, if needed.

PATIENT TEACHING

Be sure to cover:
- procedures (answering questions for the patient and family members)
- medication dosages, adverse reactions, and signs of toxicity to watch for and report
- dietary restrictions
- progressive resumption of sexual activity
- appropriate responses to new or recurrent symptoms
- typical or atypical chest pain to report.

Obesity

DESCRIPTION

- An excess of body fat, generally 20% above ideal body weight
- Body mass index (BMI) of 30 or greater (see *BMI measurements*)
- Second-leading cause of preventable deaths
- Affects over one-third of U.S. residents
- Affects one in five children

PATHOPHYSIOLOGY

- Fat cells increase in size in response to dietary intake.
- When the cells can no longer expand, they increase in number.

BMI MEASUREMENTS

Use these steps to calculate body mass index (BMI):
- Multiply weight in pounds by 705.
- Divide this number by height in inches.
- Then divide this by height in inches again.
- Compare results to these standards:
  - 18.5 to 24.9: normal
  - 25.0 to 29.9: overweight
  - 30 to 39.9: obese
  - 40 or greater: morbidly obese.

- With weight loss, the size of the fat cells decreases, but the number of cells doesn't.

CAUSES

- Excessive caloric intake combined with inadequate energy expenditure
- Theories include:
  - abnormal absorption of nutrients
  - environmental factors
  - genetic predisposition
  - hypothalamic dysfunction of hunger and satiety centers
  - impaired action of GI and growth hormones and of hormonal regulators such as insulin
  - psychological factors
  - socioeconomic status

ASSESSMENT FINDINGS

- Increasing weight
- Complications of obesity, including type 2 diabetes, hypertension, osteoarthritis, sleep apnea, gallbladder disease, and liver disease
- BMI of 30 or greater

TEST RESULTS

- Waist measurement is over 35″ in women or 40″ in men.
- Anthropometric arm measurement over the 95th percentile may indicate overweight or obesity (see *Taking anthropometric arm measurements*)
- Elevated blood glucose and glycosylated hemoglobin.

TREATMENT

- Hypnosis and behavior modification techniques
- Psychological counseling
- Reduction in daily caloric intake
- Increase in daily activity level
- Vertical banded gastroplasty
- Gastric bypass

▶ **COLLABORATION** *Promote weight loss by coordinating care with a weight-reduction program that includes dietary counseling and psychological counseling or support. A physical trainer may also be consulted, if not contraindicated by comorbid conditions.*

TAKING ANTHROPOMETRIC ARM MEASUREMENTS

Follow these steps to determine triceps skin-fold thickness, midarm circumference, and midarm muscle circumference.

Triceps skin-fold thickness

- Find the midpoint circumference of the arm by placing the tape measure halfway between the axilla and the elbow. Grasp the patient's skin with your thumb and forefinger, about 3/8" (1 cm) above the midpoint, as shown below.
- Place calipers at the midpoint, and squeeze for 3 seconds.
- Record the measurement to the nearest millimeter.
- Take two more readings, and use the average.

Midarm circumference and midarm muscle circumference

- At the midpoint, measure the midarm circumference, as shown below. Record the measurement in centimeters.
- Calculate the midarm muscle circumference by multiplying the triceps skin-fold thickness — measured in millimeters — by 3.14.
- Subtract this number from the midarm circumference.

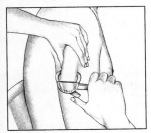

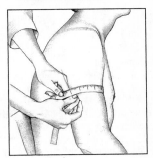

Recording the measurements

Record all three measurements as a percentage of the standard measurements (see table below), using this formula: $\dfrac{\text{Actual measurement}}{\text{Standard measurement}} \times 100\%$

Remember, a measurement less than 90% of the standard indicates caloric deprivation. A measurement over 90% indicates adequate or more-than-adequate energy reserves.

Measurement	Standard	90%
Triceps skin-fold thickness	Men: 12.5 mm Women: 16.5 mm	Men: 11.3 mm Women: 14.9 mm
Midarm circumference	Men: 29.3 cm Women: 28.5 cm	Men: 26.4 cm Women: 25.7 cm
Midarm muscle circumference	Men: 25.3 cm Women: 23.3 cm	Men: 22.8 cm Women: 20.9 cm

KEY PATIENT OUTCOMES

The patient will:
- reduce BMI to normal level
- safely reduce weight
- demonstrate effective coping mechanisms to deal with long-term compliance.

NURSING INTERVENTIONS

- Obtain an accurate diet history to identify the patient's eating habits and the importance of food to his lifestyle.
- Promote increased physical activity as appropriate.
- Monitor dietary intake and compliance with dietary restrictions.
- Record and evaluate intake and output.
- Monitor vital signs.
- Obtain height, weight and BMI.

PATIENT TEACHING

Be sure to cover:
- need for long-term maintenance after desired weight is achieved
- dietary guidelines
- safe weight loss practices.

Ovarian cancer

DESCRIPTION

- Malignancy arising from the ovary; a rapidly progressing cancer that's difficult to diagnose
- Prognosis varying with histologic type and stage
- 90% primary epithelial tumors
- Stromal and germ cell tumors also important tumor types
- More common after age 50 and in women living in industrialized nations

PATHOPHYSIOLOGY

- Ovarian cancer spreads rapidly intraperitoneally by local extension or surface seeding and, occasionally, through the lymphatics and the bloodstream.
- Metastasis to the ovary can occur from breast, colon, gastric, and pancreatic cancers.

CAUSES

- Exact cause unknown

ASSESSMENT FINDINGS

- Lack of obvious signs, or signs and symptoms that vary with tumor size and extent of metastasis (disease usually metastasized before diagnosis is made)
- In later stages, urinary frequency, constipation, pelvic discomfort, distention, weight loss, abdominal pain
- Gaunt appearance
- Grossly distended abdomen accompanied by ascites
- Palpable abdominal mass with rocky hardness or rubbery or cystlike quality

TEST RESULTS

- Laboratory tumor marker studies (such as ovarian carcinoma antigen, carcinoembryonic antigen, and human chorionic gonadotropin) show abnormalities that may indicate complications.
- Abdominal ultrasonography, computed tomography scan, or X-rays delineate tumor size.
- Aspiration of ascitic fluid reveals atypical cells.
- Exploratory laparotomy, including lymph node evaluation and tumor resection, provides accurate diagnosis and staging.

TREATMENT

- Radiation therapy (not commonly used because it causes myelosuppression, which limits effectiveness of chemotherapy)
- Radioisotopes as adjuvant therapy
- High-protein diet
- Small, frequent meals
- Chemotherapy after surgery
- Immunotherapy (investigational)
- Hormone replacement therapy in prepubertal girls who had bilateral salpingo-oophorectomy
- Total abdominal hysterectomy and bilateral salpingo-oophorectomy with tumor resection
- Omentectomy, appendectomy, lymph node palpation with probable lymphadenectomy, tissue biopsies, and peritoneal washings
- Resection of involved ovary

- Biopsies of omentum and uninvolved ovary
- Peritoneal washings for cytologic examination of pelvic fluid

KEY PATIENT OUTCOMES

The patient will:
- show no further evidence of weight loss
- express feelings about the potential loss of childbearing ability
- express feelings of increased comfort and decreased pain
- establish effective coping mechanisms.

NURSING INTERVENTIONS

- Encourage verbalization and provide support.
- Give prescribed medications.
- Provide abdominal support, and be alert for abdominal distention.
- Encourage coughing and deep breathing.
- Monitor vital signs.
- Record and evaluate intake and output.
- Assess the wound site and provide wound care.
- Monitor pain control and provide comfort measures.
- Monitor the effects of medications.
- Assess the hydration and nutrition status.

PATIENT TEACHING

Be sure to cover:
- the disorder, diagnosis, and treatment
- dietary needs
- relaxation techniques
- importance of preventing infection, emphasizing proper hand-washing technique
- medication administration, dosage, and possible adverse effects.

Pancreatic cancer

DESCRIPTION

- Proliferation of cancer cells in the pancreas
- Fifth most lethal type of carcinoma
- Poor prognosis (most patients die within 1 year of diagnosis)
- Incidence highest in black men ages 35 to 70
- Three to four times more common in smokers than nonsmokers

PATHOPHYSIOLOGY

- Pancreatic cancer is almost always adenocarcinoma.
- Nearly two-thirds of tumors appear in the head of the pancreas; islet cell tumors are rare.
- A high-fat or excessive protein diet induces chronic hyperplasia of the pancreas, with increased cell turnover.
- Two main tissue types form fibrotic nodes. Cylinder cells arise in ducts and degenerate into cysts; large, fatty, granular cells arise in parenchyma.

CAUSES

- Possible link to inhalation or absorption of carcinogens (such as cigarette smoke, excessive fat and protein, food additives, and industrial chemicals), which the pancreas then excretes

ASSESSMENT FINDINGS

- Colicky, dull, or vague intermittent epigastric pain, which may radiate to the right upper quadrant or dorsolumbar area; unrelated to posture or activity and aggravated by meals
- Anorexia, nausea, and vomiting
- Rapid, profound weight loss
- Jaundice
- Large, palpable, well-defined mass in the subumbilical or left hypochondrial region
- Abdominal bruit or pulsation

TEST RESULTS

- Pancreatic enzymes are absent.
- Serum bilirubin level is increased.
- Serum lipase and amylase levels may be increased.
- Thrombin time is prolonged.
- Aspartate aminotransferase and alanine aminotransferase levels are elevated if liver cell necrosis is present.
- Alkaline phosphatase level is markedly elevated in biliary obstruction.
- Serum insulin is measurable if islet cell tumor is present.
- Hypoglycemia or hyperglycemia is present.
- Specific tumor markers for pancreatic cancer, including carcinoembryonic antigen, pancreatic oncofetal antigen, alpha-fetoprotein, and serum immunoreactive elastase I, are elevated.
- Barium swallow, retroperitoneal insufflation, cholangiography, and scintigraphy locate the neoplasm and detect changes in the duodenum or stomach.

- Ultrasonography and computed tomography scans identify masses.
- Magnetic resonance imaging scan disclose tumor location and size.
- Angiography reveal tumor vascularity.
- Endoscopic retrograde cholangiopancreatography allows tumor visualization and specimen biopsy.
- Percutaneous fine-needle aspiration biopsy may detect tumor cells.
- Laparotomy with biopsy allows definitive diagnosis.

TREATMENT

- Mainly palliative
- May involve radiation therapy as adjunct to fluorouracil chemotherapy
- Well-balanced diet, as tolerated
- Small, frequent meals
- Postoperative avoidance of lifting and contact sports
- After recovery, no activity restrictions
- Chemotherapy
- Antibiotics
- Anticholinergics
- Antacids
- Diuretics
- Insulin
- Analgesics
- Pancreatic enzymes
- Total pancreatectomy
- Cholecystojejunostomy, choledochoduodenostomy, and choledochojejunostomy
- Gastrojejunostomy
- Whipple's operation or radical pancreatoduodenectomy
- Biliary stent insertion

KEY PATIENT OUTCOMES

The patient will:
- maintain an adequate weight
- maintain normal fluid volume status
- maintain skin integrity
- verbalize increased comfort and pain relief
- avoid injury.

NURSING INTERVENTIONS

- Administer prescribed medications and blood transfusions.
- Provide small, frequent meals.

- Ensure adequate rest and sleep.
- Assist with range-of-motion and isometric exercises, as appropriate.
- Perform meticulous skin care.
- Apply antiembolism stockings.
- Encourage verbalization and provide emotional support.
- Monitor fluid balance and nutrition.
- Assess abdominal girth, metabolic state, and daily weight.
- Monitor blood glucose levels.
- Monitor complete blood count.
- Assess pain control and provide comfort measures.
- Observe for bleeding.
- Refer the patient to community resource and support services and hospice care, if indicated.

PATIENT TEACHING

Be sure to cover:
- the disorder, diagnosis, and treatment
- end-of-life issues
- medication administration, dosage, and possible adverse effects
- expected postoperative care
- information about diabetes, including signs and symptoms of hypo-glycemia and hyperglycemia
- adverse effects of radiation therapy and chemotherapy
- how to access the American Cancer Society.

Parkinson's disease

DESCRIPTION

- Brain disorder causing progressive deterioration, with muscle rigidity, akinesia, and involuntary tremors
- Usual cause of death: aspiration pneumonia
- One of the most common crippling diseases in the United States

PATHOPHYSIOLOGY

- Dopaminergic neurons degenerate, causing loss of available dopamine.
- Dopamine deficiency prevents affected brain cells from performing their normal inhibitory function.
- Excess excitatory acetylcholine occurs at synapses.
- Nondopaminergic receptors may contribute to depression and other non-motor symptoms.

FOCUS IN

NEUROTRANSMITTER ACTION IN PARKINSON'S DISEASE

Parkinson's disease is a degenerative process involving the dopaminergic neurons in the substantia nigra (the area of the basal ganglia that produces and stores the neurotransmitter dopamine). Dopamine deficiency prevents affected brain cells from performing their normal inhibitory function. Other nondopaminergic receptors may be affected, possibly contributing to depression and other nonmotor symptoms.

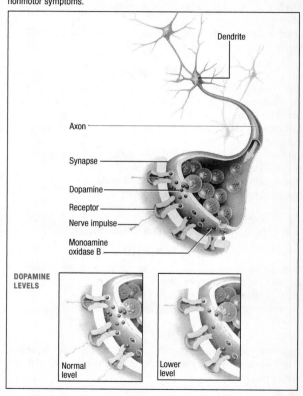

Dendrite

Axon

Synapse

Dopamine

Receptor

Nerve impulse

Monoamine oxidase B

DOPAMINE LEVELS

Normal level

Lower level

■ Motor neurons are depressed. (See *Neurotransmitter action in Parkinson's disease.*)

CAUSES

■ Usually unknown
■ Drug-induced (haloperidol [Haldol], methyldopa [Aldomet], reserpine)
■ Exposure to such toxins as manganese dust and carbon monoxide
■ Type A encephalitis

ASSESSMENT FINDINGS

■ Muscle rigidity
■ Akinesia
■ Insidious (unilateral pill-roll) tremor, which increases during stress or anxiety and decreases with purposeful movement and sleep
■ Dysphagia
■ Fatigue with activities of daily living (ADLs)
■ Muscle cramps of legs, neck, and trunk
■ Oily skin
■ Increased perspiration
■ Insomnia
■ Mood changes
■ Dysarthria
■ High-pitched, monotonous voice
■ Drooling
■ Masklike facial expression
■ Difficulty walking
■ Lack of parallel motion in gait
■ Loss of posture control with walking
■ Oculogyric crises (eyes fixed upward, with involuntary tonic movements)
■ Muscle rigidity causing resistance to passive muscle stretching
■ Difficulty pivoting
■ Loss of balance

TEST RESULTS

■ Computed tomography scan or magnetic resonance imaging rule out other disorders such as intracranial tumors.
■ Diagnosis is based primarily on neurologic examination.

TREATMENT

■ Small, frequent meals
■ High-bulk foods

- Physical therapy and occupational therapy
- Assistive devices to aid ambulation
- Dopamine replacement drugs
- Anticholinergics
- Antihistamines
- Antiviral agents
- Enzyme-inhibiting agents
- Tricyclic antidepressants
- Surgery used when drug therapy fails
- Stereotaxic neurosurgery
- Destruction of ventrolateral nucleus of thalamus

KEY PATIENT OUTCOMES

The patient will:
- perform ADLs
- avoid injury
- maintain adequate caloric intake
- express positive feelings about self
- develop adequate coping behaviors
- seek support resources.

NURSING INTERVENTIONS

- Take measures to prevent aspiration.
- Protect the patient from injury.
- Stress the importance of rest periods between activities.
- Ensure adequate nutrition.
- Provide frequent warm baths and massage.
- Provide emotional and psychological support.
- Encourage the patient to be independent.
- Assist with ambulation and range-of-motion exercises.
- Monitor vital signs.
- Measure and evaluate intake and output.
- Monitor response to drug therapy.
- Observe for adverse reactions to medications.
- Monitor ability to swallow.
- Postoperatively, observe for signs of hemorrhage and increased intracranial pressure.
- Refer the patient to a physical therapy program.
- Refer the patient to the National Parkinson foundation and Parkinson's Disease Foundation.

PATIENT TEACHING

Be sure to cover:
- the disorder, diagnosis, and treatment
- medication administration, dosage, and possible adverse effects
- measures to prevent pressure ulcers and contractures
- household safety measures
- importance of daily bathing
- methods to improve communication
- swallowing therapy regimen (aspiration precautions).

Polycythemia vera

DESCRIPTION

- Chronic, myeloproliferative disorder of increased red blood cell (RBC) mass, leukocytosis, thrombocytosis, and increased hemoglobin concentration
- Onset usually between ages 40 and 60
- Most common among Jewish men
- Also called *primary polycythemia*, *erythremia*, *polycythemia rubra vera*, *splenomegalic polycythemia*, and *Vaquez-Osler disease*

PATHOPHYSIOLOGY

- Uncontrolled and rapid cellular reproduction and maturation cause proliferation or hyperplasia of all bone marrow cells.
- Increased RBC mass makes the blood abnormally viscous and inhibits blood flow to the microcirculation.
- Diminished blood flow and thrombocytosis set the stage for intravascular thrombosis.

CAUSES

- Hyperplasia of all bone marrow cells (panmyelosis)

ASSESSMENT FINDINGS

- Vague feeling of fullness in the head or rushing in the ears
- Tinnitus
- Headache
- Dizziness, vertigo
- Epistaxis
- Night sweats
- Epigastric and joint pain

- Vision alterations, such as scotomas, double vision, and blurred vision
- Pruritus
- Abdominal fullness
- Congestion of the conjunctiva, retina, and retinal veins
- Oral mucous membrane congestion
- Hypertension
- Ruddy cyanosis (plethora)
- Ecchymosis
- Hepatosplenomegaly
- Joint pain

TEST RESULTS

- Uric acid level is increased.
- Increased RBC mass and normal arterial oxygen saturation confirm diagnosis with splenomegaly or two of the following:
  - Platelet count above 400,000/µl (thrombocytosis)
  - White blood cell count above 10,000/µl in adults
  - Elevated leukocyte alkaline phosphatase level
  - Elevated serum vitamin B_{12} levels or unbound B_{12}-binding capacity
- Bone marrow biopsy shows panmyelosis.
- Hematocrit greater than 55%.
- Ultrasonography reveals splenomegaly.

TREATMENT

- Phlebotomy
- Pheresis
- Myelosuppressive therapy using radioactive phosphorus or chemotherapeutic agents

KEY PATIENT OUTCOMES

The patient will:
- maintain strong peripheral pulses
- maintain normal skin color and temperature
- remain free from evidence of infection
- express feelings of increased comfort and decreased pain.

NURSING INTERVENTIONS

- Keep the patient active and ambulatory.
- If bed rest is necessary, elevate foot of bed to promote venous return and implement a daily program of active and passive range-of-motion exercises.

- Encourage additional fluid intake of at least 3,000 ml/day, if not contra-indicated.
- If the patient has symptomatic splenomegaly, suggest or provide small, frequent meals followed by a rest period.
- If the patient has pruritus, give prescribed medications.
- Encourage the patient to express concerns about the disease and its treatment.
- Monitor vital signs.
- Observe for adverse reactions to medications.
- Monitor complete blood count (CBC) and platelet count before and during therapy.
- Observe for the onset of complications.

> **ALERT** *Report acute abdominal pain immediately. It may signal splenic infarction, renal calculus formation, or abdominal organ thrombosis.*

- Observe for signs and symptoms of impending stroke.
- Monitor patient for hypertension.
- Observe for signs and symptoms of heart failure.
- Observe for signs and symptoms of bleeding.

During and after phlebotomy

- Make sure the patient is lying down comfortably. Stay alert for tachycardia, clamminess, and complaints of vertigo. If these effects occur, the procedure should be stopped.
- Immediately after phlebotomy, have the patient sit up for about 5 minutes before letting him walk. Give 24 oz (720 ml) of juice or water.

> **ALERT** *Elderly patients may require fluid replacement with normal saline solution after phlebotomy to decrease the risk of orthostatic hypertension.*

During myelosuppressive chemotherapy

- If nausea and vomiting occur, begin antiemetic therapy and adjust the patient's diet.
- During treatment with radioactive phosphorus, obtain a blood sample for CBC count and platelet count before starting treatment. (Personnel who administer radioactive phosphorus should take radiation precautions to prevent contamination.)
- Have the patient lie down during I.V. administration and for 15 to 20 minutes afterward.

PATIENT TEACHING

Be sure to cover:
- the disorder, diagnosis, and treatment
- importance of staying as active as possible
- use of an electric razor to prevent accidental cuts
- ways to minimize falls and contusions at home
- avoidance of high altitudes
- common bleeding sites, if the patient has thrombocytopenia
- importance of reporting abnormal bleeding promptly
- phlebotomy procedure (if scheduled) and its effects
- symptoms of iron deficiency to report
- possible adverse reactions to myelosuppressive therapy
- instructions about infection prevention for an outpatient who develops leukopenia (including avoiding crowds and watching for infection symptoms)
- radioactive phosphorus administration procedure (if scheduled) and the possible need for repeated phlebotomies
- dental care
- use of gloves when outdoors if temperature is below 50° F (10° C).

Pressure ulcers

DESCRIPTION

- Localized areas of ischemic tissue caused by pressure, shearing, or friction
- Most common over bony prominences, especially the sacrum, ischial tuberosities, greater trochanter, heels, malleoli, and elbows
- May be superficial, caused by localized skin irritation (with subsequent surface maceration), or deep, arising in underlying tissue (Deep lesions may go undetected until they penetrate the skin.)
- Also called *decubitus ulcers*, *pressure sores*, or *bedsores*

PATHOPHYSIOLOGY

- Impaired skin capillary pressure results in local tissue anoxia.
- Anoxia leads to edema and multiple capillary thromboses.
- An inflammatory reaction results in ulceration and necrosis of ischemic cells.

CAUSES

- Friction
- Local tissue compression
- Shearing force

ASSESSMENT FINDINGS

- Shiny, erythematous superficial lesion (early)
- Small blisters or erosions with progression of superficial erythema
- Possible necrosis and ulceration with deeper erosions and ulcerations
- Malodorous, purulent discharge (suggesting secondary bacterial infection)
- Black eschar around and over the lesion (see *Four stages of pressure ulcers*, page 220)

TEST RESULTS

- Wound culture and sensitivity testing of exudate identifies infecting organism.
- Total serum protein is decreased.

TREATMENT

- Measures to prevent pressure ulcers
- Relief of pressure on the affected area
- Meticulous skin care
- Devices such as pads, mattresses, and special beds
- Moist wound therapy dressings
- Whirlpool baths
- Diet high in protein, iron, and vitamin C (unless contraindicated)
- Activity, as tolerated
- Active and passive range-of-motion (ROM) exercises
- Frequent turning and repositioning
- Enzymatic ointments
- Healing ointments
- Antibiotics, if indicated
- Debridement of necrotic tissue
- Skin grafting (in severe cases)

▶ **COLLABORATION** *Consult a wound care specialist to help develop a treatment plan. The patient with advanced stages of a pressure ulcer may also benefit from hyperbaric therapy. Home care services and infusion therapy may also be required upon discharge from the hospital.*

FOUR STAGES OF PRESSURE ULCERS

The most widely used system for staging pressure ulcers is the classification system developed by the National Pressure Ulcer Advisory Panel. This staging system reflects the depth and extent of tissue involvement.

Stage I

An area of skin that develops observable, pressure-related changes that include persistent redness in patients with light skin or persistent red, blue, or purple in patients with darker skin. Other indicators include pain, itching, warmth, edema or hardness at the site.

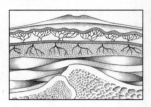

Stage II

Superficial partial-thickness wound that appears as an abrasion, blister, or shallow crater involving the epidermis, dermis, or both.

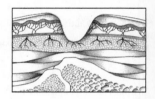

Stage III

Full-thickness wound with tissue damage or necrosis of subcutaneous tissue that can extend down to, but not through, underlying fasciae. The wound appears as a deep crater that may or may not undermine to neighboring tissue.

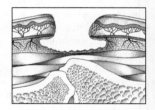

Stage IV

Full-thickness wound with extensive damage, tissue necrosis, or damage to muscle, bone, or structures, such as joints and tendons. The wound may undermine to neighboring tissues and develop sinus tracts.

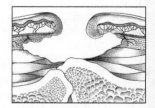

KEY PATIENT OUTCOMES

The patient will:
■ exhibit improved or healed lesions or wounds
■ maintain adequate daily caloric intake
■ maintain joint mobility and ROM
■ avoid infection and other complications.

NURSING INTERVENTIONS

■ Administer prescribed medications.
■ Apply dressings appropriate for the ulcer stage.
■ Encourage adequate food and fluid intake.
■ Reposition the bedridden patient at least every 2 hours.
■ Elevate the head of the bed 30 degrees or less.
■ Perform passive ROM exercises, and encourage active ROM exercises, if possible.
■ Use pressure-relief aids on the bed.
■ Provide meticulous skin care.
■ Assess for changes in skin color, turgor, temperature, sensation, and drainage.
■ Assess for a change in the ulcer stage.
■ Monitor laboratory results, especially serum protein, albumin, and electrolyte levels and white blood cell count
■ Observe for the onset of complications.
■ Monitor patient's response to treatment.
■ Record and evaluate intake and output.

PATIENT TEACHING

Be sure to cover:
■ the disorder, diagnosis, and treatment
■ techniques for changing positions
■ active and passive ROM exercises
■ avoidance of skin-damaging agents
■ debridement procedures
■ skin graft surgery, if required
■ signs and stages of healing
■ importance of a well-balanced diet and adequate fluid intake
■ medication administration, dosage, and possible adverse effects
■ importance of notifying the physician immediately of signs and symptoms of infection.

Prostate cancer

DESCRIPTION

- Proliferation of cancer cells that usually take the form of adenocarcinomas and typically originate in the posterior prostate gland
- May progress to widespread bone metastasis and death
- Leading cause of cancer death in men
- Most common neoplasm in men older than age 50

PATHOPHYSIOLOGY

- Slow-growing prostatic cancer seldom causes signs and symptoms until it's well advanced.
- Typically, when a primary prostatic lesion spreads beyond the prostate gland, it invades the prostatic capsule and spreads along ejaculatory ducts in the space between the seminal vesicles or perivesicular fascia. (See *How prostate cancer develops*.)
- Endocrine factors may play a role, leading researchers to suspect that androgens speed tumor growth.
- Malignant prostatic tumors seldom result from the benign hyperplastic enlargement that commonly develops around the prostatic urethra in older men.

CAUSES

- Unknown

ASSESSMENT FINDINGS

- Urinary problems, such as difficulty initiating a urinary stream, dribbling, painless hematuria, and urine retention
- Nonraised, firm, nodular mass with a sharp edge
- In advanced disease: edema of the scrotum or leg; a hard lump in the prostate region

TEST RESULTS

- Serum prostate-specific antigen (PSA) level is elevated, indicating possible cancer with or without metastases.
- Transrectal prostatic ultrasonography shows prostate size and presence of abnormal growths.
- Bone scan and excretory urography determine the extent of the disease.
- Magnetic resonance imaging and computed tomography scan define the extent of the tumor.

FOCUS IN
HOW PROSTATE CANCER DEVELOPS

Prostate cancer (commonly a form of adenocarcinoma) grows slowly. When primary lesions metastasize beyond the prostate, they invade the prostate capsule and spread along the ejaculatory ducts in the space between the seminal vesicles.

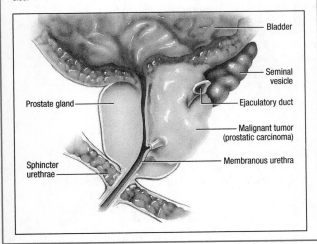

- Standard screening tests to identify prostate cancer include digital rectal examination and PSA test (recommended yearly by the American Cancer Society for men older than age 40).

TREATMENT

- Varies with cancer stage
- Radiation therapy or internal beam radiation
- Well-balanced diet
- Hormonal therapy
- Chemotherapy
- Prostatectomy
- Orchiectomy
- Radical prostatectomy
- Transurethral resection of prostate
- Cryosurgical ablation

KEY PATIENT OUTCOMES

The patient will:
- express feelings of increased comfort
- discuss the disease's impact on self and his family
- demonstrate effective coping mechanisms.

NURSING INTERVENTIONS

- Give prescribed medications.
- Encourage the patient to express his feelings.
- Provide emotional support.
- Monitor pain level and provide comfort measures.
- Assess wound site and provide wound care.
- Observe for postoperative complications.
- Monitor medication effects.

PATIENT TEACHING

Be sure to cover:
- the disorder, diagnosis, and treatment
- perineal exercises that decrease incontinence
- follow-up care
- medication administration, dosage, and possible adverse effects.

Psoriasis

DESCRIPTION

- Hereditary chronic skin disease marked by epidermal proliferation
- Causes lesions of erythematous papules and plaques covered with silvery scales that vary widely in severity and distribution
- Involves recurring remissions and exacerbations
- Exacerbations unpredictable, but usually controllable with therapy
- Affects about 2% of the U.S. population
- Two periods of onset: early (young adulthood) and late (middle adulthood)

PATHOPHYSIOLOGY

- Psoriatic skin cells have a shortened maturation time as they migrate from the basal membrane to the surface or stratum corneum.
- As a result, the stratum corneum develops thick, scaly plaques (the cardinal manifestation of psoriasis).

CAUSES

- Beta-hemolytic streptococci infection
- Genetic predisposition
- Physical trauma
- Possible autoimmune process

ASSESSMENT FINDINGS

- Family history of psoriasis
- Pruritus and burning
- Arthritic symptoms such as morning joint stiffness
- Remissions and exacerbations
- Erythematous, well-demarcated papules and plaques covered with silver scales, typically appearing on the scalp, chest, elbows, knees, back, and buttocks
- In mild psoriasis: plaques scattered over a small skin area
- In moderate psoriasis: plaques more numerous and larger (up to several centimeters in diameter)
- In severe psoriasis: plaques covering at least half the body
- Friable or adherent scales
- Fine bleeding points or Auspitz sign after attempts to remove scales
- Thin, erythematous guttate lesions, alone or with plaques, and with few scales (see *Identifying types of psoriasis*, page 226)
- Small indentations or pits, and yellow or brown discoloration of finger-nails or toenails

 ALERT *In severe cases of psoriasis, the nail may separate from the nail bed.*

TEST RESULTS

- Serum uric acid level is increased.
- In early-onset familial psoriasis, human leukocyte antigens Cw6, B13, and Bw-57 are present.
- Skin biopsy rules out other diseases.

TREATMENT

- Depends on the psoriasis type, extent, and effect on the patient's quality of life
- Lesion management
- Lukewarm baths
- Ultraviolet B light or natural sunlight
- Topical corticosteroid creams and ointments

IDENTIFYING TYPES OF PSORIASIS

Psoriasis occurs in various forms, ranging from one or two localized plaques that seldom require long-term medical attention to widespread lesions and crippling arthritis.

Erythrodermic psoriasis
This type is marked by extensive flushing all over the body, which may result in scaling. The rash may develop rapidly, signaling new psoriasis or gradually in chronic psoriasis. Sometimes the rash occurs as an adverse drug reaction.

Guttate psoriasis
This type typically affects children and young adults. Erupting in drop-sized plaques over the trunk, arms, legs and, sometimes, the scalp, this rash generalizes in several days. It's commonly associated with upper respiratory streptococcal infections.

Inverse psoriasis
Smooth, dry, bright red plaques characterize inverse psoriasis. Located in skin folds (armpits and groin, for example), the plaques fissure easily.

Psoriasis vulgaris
This psoriasis type is the most common. It begins with red, dotlike lesions that gradually enlarge and produce dry, silvery scales. The plaques usually appear symmetrically on the knees, elbows, extremities, genitalia, scalp, and nails.

Pustular psoriasis
This type features an eruption of local or extensive small, raised, pus-filled plaques. Possible triggers include emotional stress, sweating, infections, and adverse drug reactions.

- Antihistamines
- Analgesics
- Nonsteroidal anti-inflammatory drugs
- Occlusive ointment bases
- Urea or salicylic acid preparations
- Coal tar preparations
- Vitamin D analogs
- Emollients
- Keratolytics
- Methotrexate for severe, unresponsive psoriasis
- Potent retinoic acid derivative for resistant psoriasis
- Cyclosporine for severe, widespread psoriasis

■ Surgical nail removal to treat severely disfigured or damaged nails caused by psoriasis

KEY PATIENT OUTCOMES

The patient will:
■ exhibit improved or healed lesions
■ report feelings of increased comfort
■ verbalize feelings about changed body image
■ demonstrate understanding of proper skin care
■ express an understanding of the condition and its treatment.

NURSING INTERVENTIONS

■ Administer prescribed medications.
■ Apply topical medications using a downward motion.
■ Encourage the patient to verbalize his feelings.
■ Provide emotional support.
■ Involve family members in the treatment regimen.
■ Observe response to treatment.
■ Monitor lipid profile results.
■ Assess liver function tests.
■ Assess renal function.
■ Monitor blood pressure.
■ Observe for signs and symptoms of hepatic or bone marrow toxicity.

PATIENT TEACHING

Be sure to cover:
■ the disorder, diagnosis, and treatment
■ risk factors
■ incommunicability of psoriasis
■ likelihood of exacerbations and remissions
■ medication administration, dosage, and possible adverse effects
■ how to apply prescribed ointments, creams, and lotions
■ importance of avoiding scratching plaques
■ measures to relieve pruritus
■ importance of avoiding sun exposure
■ stress-reduction techniques
■ safety precautions
■ relationship between psoriasis and arthritis
■ when to notify the physician
■ how to access the National Psoriasis Foundation.

Radiation exposure

DESCRIPTION

- Results from exposure to excessive radiation that causes tissue damage
- Damage varies with amount of body area exposed, length of exposure, dosage absorbed, distance from the source, and presence of protective shielding
- Can result from cancer radiotherapy, working in a radiation facility, or other exposure to radioactive materials
- Can be acute or chronic

PATHOPHYSIOLOGY

- Ionization occurs in the molecules of living cells.
- Electrons are removed from atoms. Charged atoms or ions form and react with other atoms to cause cell damage.
- Rapidly dividing cells are the most susceptible to radiation damage. Highly differentiated cells are more resistant to radiation.

CAUSES

- Exposure to radiation through inhalation, ingestion, or direct contact

ASSESSMENT FINDINGS

Acute hematopoietic radiation toxicity

- Petechiae
- Pallor
- Weakness
- Oropharyngeal abscesses
- Bleeding from the skin, genitourinary tract, and GI tract
- Nosebleeds
- Hemorrhage
- Increased susceptibility to infection

GI radiation toxicity

- Mouth and throat ulcers and infection
- Intractable nausea, vomiting, and diarrhea
- Circulatory collapse and death

Cardiovascular radiation toxicity

- Hypotension, shock, and cardiac arrhythmias

Cerebral radiation toxicity
- Nausea, vomiting, and diarrhea
- Lethargy
- Tremors
- Seizures
- Confusion
- Coma and death

Generalized radiation exposure
- Signs of hypothyroidism
- Cataracts
- Skin dryness, erythema, pruritus, atrophy, and malignant lesions
- Alopecia
- Brittle nails

TEST RESULTS
- White blood cell, platelet, and lymphocyte counts are decreased.
- Serum potassium and chloride levels are decreased.
- X-rays may show bone necrosis.
- Bone marrow studies may reveal blood dyscrasia.
- Geiger counter determines if radioactive material was ingested or inhaled and evaluates the amount of radiation in open wounds.

TREATMENT
- Based on the type and extent of radiation injury
- Management of life-threatening injuries

  ALERT Hematologic, digestive, nervous, and integumentary systems are most affected after radiation exposure. Watch for signs of shock, infection, and respiratory difficulties.
- Symptomatic and supportive treatment
- High-protein, high-calorie diet
- Activity, as tolerated
- Chelating agents
- Potassium iodide (SSKI, Lugol's solution)
- Aluminum phosphate gel
- Barium sulfate

KEY PATIENT OUTCOMES
The patient will:
- maintain an acceptable weight
- maintain normal fluid volume

■ remain free from signs and symptoms of infection.

NURSING INTERVENTIONS

■ Implement all appropriate respiratory and cardiac support measures.
■ Give prescribed I.V. fluids and electrolytes.
■ For skin contamination, wash the patient's body thoroughly with mild soap and water.
■ Debride and irrigate open wounds, as ordered.
■ For ingested radioactive material, perform gastric lavage and whole-bowel irrigation, and administer activated charcoal, as ordered.
■ Dispose of contaminated clothing properly.
■ Dispose of contaminated excrement and body fluids according to facility policy.
■ Use strict sterile technique.
■ Measure and evaluate intake and output.
■ Monitor fluid and electrolyte balance.
■ Assess vital signs.
■ Observe for signs and symptoms of hemorrhage.
■ Assess nutritional status.

PATIENT TEACHING

Be sure to cover:
■ the injury process, diagnosis, and treatment
■ effects of radiation exposure
■ how to prevent a recurrence
■ skin care
■ wound care
■ need for follow-up care.

Renal failure, acute

DESCRIPTION

■ Results from sudden interruption of renal function resulting from obstruction, reduced circulation, or renal parenchymal disease
■ Classified as prerenal failure, intrarenal failure (also called *intrinsic* or *parenchymal failure*), or postrenal failure
■ Usually reversible with medical treatment
■ If not treated, may progress to end-stage renal disease, uremia, and death
■ Seen in 5% of hospitalized patients
■ Normally occurs in three distinct phases: oliguric, diuretic, and recovery

Oliguric phase

- This phase may last a few days or several weeks.
- A patient's urine output may drop below 400 ml/day.
- Fluid volume excess, azotemia, and electrolyte imbalance occur.
- Local mediators are released, causing intrarenal vasoconstriction.
- Medullary hypoxia causes cellular swelling and adherence of neutrophils to capillaries and venules.
- Hypoperfusion occurs in this phase.
- Cellular injury and necrosis occur.
- Reperfusion causes reactive oxygen species to form, leading to further cellular injury.

Diuretic phase

- Renal function is recovered.
- Urine output gradually increases.
- Glomerular filtration rate improves, although tubular transport systems remain abnormal.

Recovery phase

- This phase may last 3 to 12 months, or longer.
- The patient gradually returns to normal or near-normal renal function.

PATHOPHYSIOLOGY

Prerenal failure

- Prerenal failure is caused by impaired blood flow.
- Decrease in filtration pressure causes decline in glomerular filtration rate.
- Failure to restore blood volume or blood pressure may cause acute tubular necrosis (ATN) or acute cortical necrosis.

Intrarenal failure

- A severe episode of hypotension, commonly associated with hypovolemia, is often a significant contributing event.
- Cell swelling, injury, and necrosis — a form of reperfusion injury that may also be caused by nephrotoxins — results from ischemia-generated toxic oxygen-free radicals and anti-inflammatory mediators.

Postrenal failure

- Postrenal failure usually occurs with urinary tract obstruction that affects the kidneys bilaterally such as prostatic hyperplasia.

CAUSES

Prerenal failure
- Hemorrhagic blood loss
- Hypotension or hypoperfusion
- Hypovolemia
- Loss of plasma volume
- Water and electrolyte losses

Intrarenal failure
- ATN
- Coagulation defects
- Glomerulopathies
- Malignant hypertension

Postrenal failure
- Bladder neck obstruction
- Obstructive uropathies, usually bilateral
- Ureteral destruction

ASSESSMENT FINDINGS
- Oliguria or anuria, depending on renal failure phase
- Tachycardia
- Bibasilar crackles
- Irritability, drowsiness, or confusion
- Altered level of consciousness
- Bleeding abnormalities
- Dry, pruritic skin
- Dry mucous membranes
- Uremic breath odor

TEST RESULTS
- Blood urea nitrogen, serum creatinine, and potassium levels are elevated.
- Hematocrit and blood pH, bicarbonate, and hemoglobin levels are decreased.
- Urine casts and cellular debris are present, and specific gravity is decreased.
- In glomerular disease, proteinuria and urine osmolality are close to serum osmolality level.
- Urine sodium level is normal, decreased (below 20 mEq/L, caused by decreased perfusion in oliguria), or increased (above 40 mEq/L, caused by an intrarenal problem the oliguric phrase).

- Urine creatinine clearance measures glomerular filtration rate and estimates the number of remaining functioning nephrons.
- Kidney ultrasonography, kidney-ureter-bladder radiography, excretory urography renal scan, retrograde pyelography, computed tomography scan, and nephrotomography may reveal obstruction.
- Electrocardiography reveals tall, peaked T waves; a widening QRS complex; and disappearing P waves if hyperkalemia is present.

TREATMENT

- Hemodialysis or peritoneal dialysis (if appropriate)
- High-calorie, low-protein, low-sodium, and low-potassium diet
- Fluid restriction
- Rest periods when fatigued
- Supplemental vitamins
- Diuretics
- In hyperkalemia, hypertonic glucose-and-insulin infusions, sodium bicarbonate, sodium polystyrene sulfonate
- Creation of vascular access for hemodialysis

KEY PATIENT OUTCOMES

The patient will:
- avoid complications
- maintain fluid balance
- maintain hemodynamic stability
- verbalize risk factors for decreased tissue perfusion and modify lifestyle appropriately
- demonstrate the ability to manage urinary elimination problems
- verbalize diet and medication rationales and regimen.

NURSING INTERVENTIONS

- Administer prescribed medications.
- Encourage the patient to express his feelings.
- Provide emotional support.
- Identify patients who are at risk for ATN, and take appropriate preventative measures.
- Measure and evaluate intake and output.
- Monitor daily weight.
- Monitor appropriate renal function studies.
- Assess vital signs.
- Monitor the effects of excess fluid volume.
- Assess the dialysis access site for bruit and thrill.

PATIENT TEACHING

Be sure to cover:

- the disorder, diagnosis, and treatment
- medication administration, dosages, and possible adverse effects
- recommended fluid allowance
- compliance with diet and drug regimen
- importance of immediately reporting daily weight changes of 2 lb (0.9 kg) or more
- signs and symptoms of edema and importance of reporting them to the physician.

Respiratory acidosis

DESCRIPTION

- Acid-base disturbance characterized by reduced alveolar ventilation, as shown by hypercapnia (partial pressure of arterial carbon dioxide [$PaCO_2$] above 45 mm Hg)
- Varied prognosis, depending on severity of underlying disturbance and the patient's general clinical condition
- Can be acute or chronic

PATHOPHYSIOLOGY

- Depressed ventilation causes respiratory acidosis.
- Carbon dioxide is retained after acidosis occurs, and hydrogen ion concentration increases.

CAUSES

- Airway obstruction
- Asthma
- Central nervous system (CNS) trauma
- Chronic bronchitis
- Chronic metabolic alkalosis
- Chronic obstructive pulmonary disease
- CNS-depressant drugs
- Extensive pneumonia
- Large pneumothorax
- Neuromuscular disease
- Parenchymal lung disease
- Pulmonary edema
- Severe acute respiratory distress syndrome

ASSESSMENT FINDINGS

- Diaphoresis
- Bounding pulses
- Rapid, shallow respirations
- Tachycardia
- Hypotension
- Papilledema
- Mental status changes
- Asterixis (tremor)
- Depressed deep tendon reflexes

TEST RESULTS

- Arterial blood pH is below 7.35, and $PaCO_2$ is above 45 mm Hg (hypercapnia).

TREATMENT

- Correction of the condition causing alveolar hypoventilation
- Possible mechanical ventilation
- Possible dialysis
- I.V. fluid administration
- Possible need for parenteral nutrition
- Activity as tolerated
- Oxygen
- Bronchodilators
- Antibiotics
- Sodium bicarbonate
- Drug therapy for the underlying condition
- Bronchoscopy

KEY PATIENT OUTCOMES

The patient will:
- maintain a patent airway
- maintain adequate ventilation
- maintain fluid balance
- maintain adequate cardiac output
- demonstrate effective coping behaviors.

NURSING INTERVENTIONS

- Administer prescribed medications and oxygen.
- Provide adequate fluids.

- Maintain a patent airway.
- Perform tracheal suctioning, as needed.
- Assess vital signs.
- Measure and evaluate the patient's intake and output.
- Evaluate neurologic status.
- Evaluate respiratory status.
- Monitor arterial blood gas values.
- Monitor serum electrolyte values.
- Monitor mechanical ventilator settings.

ALERT *Be aware that pulse oximetry, used to monitor oxygen saturation, doesn't reveal increasing carbon dioxide levels.*

PATIENT TEACHING

Be sure to cover:
- the disorder, diagnosis, and treatment
- appropriate use and maintenance of supplemental oxygen
- prescribed drugs and possible adverse effects
- how to perform coughing and deep-breathing exercises
- signs and symptoms of acid-base imbalance and when to notify the physician.

Rhabdomyolysis

DESCRIPTION

- Breakdown of muscle tissue, causing myoglobinuria
- Usually follows major muscle trauma, especially a muscle crush injury
- Good prognosis if contributing causes are stopped or disease is checked before damage is irreversible

PATHOPHYSIOLOGY

- Muscle trauma that compresses tissue causes ischemia and necrosis.
- The ensuing local edema further increases compartment pressure and tamponade; pressure from severe swelling causes blood vessels to collapse, leading to tissue hypoxia, muscle infarction, neural damage in the area, and release of myoglobin from the necrotic muscle fibers into the circulation.

CAUSES

- Anesthetics that cause intraoperative rigidity
- Cardiac arrhythmias
- Electrolyte disturbances
- Excessive muscular activity associated with status epilepticus, electroconvulsive therapy, or high-voltage electrical shock
- Familial tendency
- Heat stroke
- Infection, especially severe infection
- Prescription and nonprescription drugs
- Strenuous exertion such as long-distance running
- Traumatic injury

ASSESSMENT FINDINGS

- Muscle trauma or breakdown
- Muscle pain
- Presence of any risk factors
- Dark, reddish-brown urine
- Tense, tender muscle compartment (compartment syndrome)

TEST RESULTS

- Urine myoglobin level exceeds 0.5 mg/dl (evident with only 200 g of muscle damage).
- Creatine kinase level is elevated (0.5 to 0.95 mg/dl) from muscle damage.
- Serum potassium, phosphate, creatinine, and creatine levels elevated.
- Hypocalcemia occurring in early stages; hypercalcemia, in later stages.
- Intracompartmental venous pressure measurements (using a wick catheter, needle, or slit catheter inserted into the muscle) are elevated.
- Computed tomography, magnetic resonance imaging, and bone scintigraphy detect muscle necrosis.

TREATMENT

- Treatment of potential underlying disorder
- Prevention of renal failure
- Bed rest
- Anti-inflammatory agents
- Corticosteroids (in extreme cases)
- Analgesics
- Immediate fasciotomy and debridement if compartment venous pressure exceeds 25 mm Hg

KEY PATIENT OUTCOMES

The patient will:
- maintain normal renal function
- express increased comfort and decreased pain
- verbalize understanding of the disorder and treatment.

NURSING INTERVENTIONS

- Give prescribed I.V. fluids and diuretics.
- Measure and evaluate intake and output accurately.
- Promote comfort measures.
- Monitor the patient's urine myoglobins.
- Monitor appropriate renal studies.
- Assess pain control.

PATIENT TEACHING

Be sure to cover:
- the disorder, diagnosis, and treatment
- need for prolonged, low-intensity training as opposed to short bursts of intense exercise.

Rheumatoid arthritis

DESCRIPTION

- Chronic, systemic, symmetrical inflammatory disease
- Primarily attacks peripheral joints and surrounding muscles, tendons, ligaments, and blood vessels
- Marked by spontaneous remissions and unpredictable exacerbations
- Potentially crippling
- Strikes three times as many women as men
- Can occur at any age; peak onset between ages 35 and 50

PATHOPHYSIOLOGY

- Cartilage damage resulting from inflammation triggers further immune responses, including complement activation.
- Complement, in turn, attracts polymorphonuclear leukocytes and stimulates release of inflammatory mediators, which exacerbates joint destruction. (See *Understanding rheumatoid arthritis*.)

FOCUS IN

UNDERSTANDING
RHEUMATOID ARTHRITIS

A potentially crippling disease, rheumatoid arthritis primarily attacks peripheral joints and surrounding tissues through chronic inflammation. If not arrested, the inflammatory process occurs in four stages:

- Synovitis develops from congestion and edema of the synovial membrane and joint capsule. Infiltration by lymphocytes, macrophages, and neutrophils continues the local inflammatory response. These cells, as well as fibroblast-like synovial cells, produce enzymes that help degrade bone and cartilage.
- Pannus (thickened layers of granulation tissue) covers and invades cartilage, eventually destroying the joint capsule and bone.
- Fibrous ankylosis (fibrous invasion of the pannus and scar formation) occludes the joint space. Bone atrophy and misalignment cause visible deformities and disrupt the articulation of opposing bones, resulting in muscle atrophy and imbalance and, possibly, partial dislocations (subluxations).
- Fibrous tissue calcifies, resulting in bony ankylosis and total immobility.

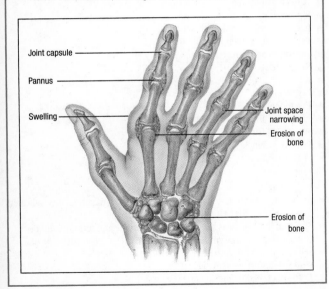

CAUSES

- Unknown
- Possible influence of infection (viral or bacterial), hormonal factors, and lifestyle

ASSESSMENT FINDINGS

- Insidious onset of nonspecific symptoms, including fatigue, malaise, anorexia, persistent low-grade fever, weight loss, and vague articular symptoms
- Later, more specific localized articular symptoms, commonly in the fingers
- Bilateral and symmetrical symptoms, which may extend to the wrists, elbows, knees, and ankles
- Stiff joints
- Numbness or tingling in the feet or weakness or loss of sensation in the fingers
- Pain on inspiration
- Shortness of breath
- Joint deformities and contractures
- Painful, red, swollen arms
- Foreshortened hands
- Boggy wrists
- Rheumatoid nodules
- Leg ulcers
- Eye redness
- Joints that are warm to the touch
- Pericardial friction rub
- Positive Babinski's sign
- Stiff, weak, or painful muscles

TEST RESULTS

- Rheumatoid factor test is positive in 75% to 80% of patients, as indicated by a titer of 1:160 or higher.
- Synovial fluid analysis shows increased volume and turbidity but decreased viscosity and complement (C3 and C4) levels, with white blood cell count possibly exceeding 10,000/µl.
- Serum globulin levels are elevated.
- Erythrocyte sedimentation rate is elevated.
- Complete blood count shows moderate anemia and slight leukocytosis. (See *Classifying rheumatoid arthritis*.)

CLASSIFYING RHEUMATOID ARTHRITIS

A patient who meets four of seven American College of Rheumatology criteria is classified as having rheumatoid arthritis. She must experience the first four criteria for at least 6 weeks, and a physician must observe the second through fifth criteria:

- Morning stiffness in and around the joints that lasts for 1 hour before full improvement
- Arthritis in three or more joint areas, with at least three joint areas (as observed by a physician) exhibiting soft-tissue swelling or joint effusions, not just bony overgrowth (the 14 possible areas involved include the right and left proximal interphalangeal, metacarpophalangeal, wrist, elbow, knee, ankle, and metatarsophalangeal joints)
- Arthritis of hand joints, including the wrist, the metacarpophalangeal joint, or the proximal interphalangeal joint
- Arthritis that involves the same joint areas on both sides of the body
- Subcutaneous rheumatoid nodules over bony prominences
- Demonstration of abnormal amounts of serum rheumatoid factor by any method that produces a positive result in less than 5% of patients without rheumatoid arthritis
- Radiographic changes, usually on posteroanterior hand and wrist radiographs, must show erosions or unequivocal bony decalcification localized in or most noticeable adjacent to the involved joints.

- In early stages, X-rays show bone demineralization and soft-tissue swelling. Later, they help determine the extent of cartilage and bone destruction, erosion, subluxations, and deformities and show the characteristic pattern of these abnormalities.
- Magnetic resonance imaging and computed tomography scan may provide information about the extent of damage.
- Synovial tissue biopsy shows inflammation.

TREATMENT

- Adequate sleep (8 to 10 hours every night)
- Splinting
- Range-of-motion (ROM) exercises and carefully individualized therapeutic exercises
- Moist heat application
- Frequent rest periods between activities
- Salicylates

- Nonsteroidal anti-inflammatory drugs
- Antimalarials (hydroxychloroquine)
- Gold salts
- Penicillamine
- Corticosteroids
- Antineoplastic agents
- Metatarsal head and distal ulnar resectional arthroplasty and insertion of silastic prosthesis between the metacarpophalangeal and proximal interphalangeal joints
- Arthrodesis (joint fusion)
- Synovectomy
- Osteotomy
- Repair of ruptured tendon
- In advanced disease, joint reconstruction or total joint arthroplasty

  COLLABORATION *Consult with physical and occupational therapists. A physical therapy program, including range-of-motion exercises and carefully individualized therapeutic exercises, forestalls loss of joint function. An occupational therapy program helps maintain independence.*

KEY PATIENT OUTCOMES

The patient will:

- express feelings of increased comfort and decreased pain
- attain the highest degree of mobility within the confines of the disease
- maintain skin integrity
- verbalize feelings about limitations
- express an increased sense of well-being.

NURSING INTERVENTIONS

- Administer prescribed analgesics, and watch for adverse reactions.
- Provide meticulous skin care.
- Supply adaptive devices, such as a zipper-pull, easy-to-open beverage cartons, lightweight cups, and unpackaged silverware.
- Assess joint mobility and pain level.
- Assess skin integrity.
- Assess vital signs and daily weight.
- Assess for sensory disturbances.
- Monitor serum electrolyte, hemoglobin, and hematocrit levels.
- Assess activity tolerance.
- Monitor for complications of corticosteroid therapy.

After total knee or hip arthroplasty

- Administer prescribed blood replacement products, antibiotics, and pain medication.
- Have the patient perform active dorsiflexion; immediately report inability to do so.
- Supervise isometric exercises every 2 hours.
- After total hip arthroplasty, check traction for pressure areas and keep the head of the bed raised 30 to 45 degrees.
- Change or reinforce dressings, as needed, using the aseptic technique.
- Have the patient turn, cough, and breathe deeply every 2 hours.
- After total knee arthroplasty, keep the leg extended and slightly elevated.
- After total hip arthroplasty, keep the hip in abduction. Watch for and immediately report any inability to rotate the hip or bear weight on it, increased pain, or a leg that appears shorter.
- Assist patient in activities, keeping the weight on the unaffected side.

PATIENT TEACHING

Be sure to cover:
- the disorder, diagnosis, and treatment
- chronic nature of rheumatoid arthritis and possible need for major lifestyle changes
- importance of a balanced diet and weight control
- importance of adequate sleep
- sexual concerns.

If the patient requires total knee or hip arthroplasty, be sure to cover:
- preoperative and surgical procedures
- postoperative exercises, with supervision
- deep-breathing and coughing exercises to perform after surgery
- performing frequent ROM leg exercises after surgery
- use of a constant-passive-motion device after total knee arthroplasty, or placement of an abduction pillow between the legs after total hip arthroplasty
- how to use a trapeze to move about in bed
- medication regimen and possible adverse effects
- information on the support and services offered by the Arthritis Foundation.

Severe acute respiratory syndrome

DESCRIPTION

- Severe viral infection (influenza-like disease) that may progress to pneumonia
- Believed to be less infectious than influenza
- Incubation period estimated to range from 2 to 7 days (average, 3 to 5 days)
- Not highly contagious when protective measures are used
- Also known as *SARS*

PATHOPHYSIOLOGY

- Coronaviruses cause diseases in pigs, birds, and other animals.
- A theory suggests that a coronavirus may have mutated, allowing transmission to and infection of humans.
- Cells in the respiratory tract are affected.

CAUSES

- A new type of coronavirus known as SARS-associated coronavirus (SARS-CoV)
- Ability of virus to live for a short time on contaminated surfaces and objects
- Ability of virus to spread by close direct contact with an infected person through aerosolized (exhaled) droplets and body secretions

ASSESSMENT FINDINGS

- Predisposing factors, such as contact with a person known to have SARS or travel to an endemic area
- Temperature over 100.4° F (38° C)
- Dry cough (within 2 to 7 days of infestation)
- Shortness of breath, hypoxia, or other respiratory difficulties
- Headache
- Muscular stiffness
- Loss of appetite
- Malaise
- Confusion
- Rash
- Sore throat

TEST RESULTS

- Serum antibodies to SARS-coronavirus (CoV) are detected.
- Sputum Gram stain and culture isolates coronavirus.
- Blood test reveals low platelet count.
- Changes in chest X-ray indicate pneumonia (infiltrates).
- SARS-specific polymerase chain reaction test detects SARS-CoV ribonucleic acid.
- Antibody testing via enzyme-linked immunosorbent assay and the immunofluorescent antibody test is in development for the diagnosis of SARS-CoV.

TREATMENT

- Treatment of symptoms
- Isolation of hospitalized patients
- Strict respiratory and mucosal barrier precautions
- Quarantine of exposed people to prevent spread
- Oxygen therapy as needed
- Diet as tolerated
- Activity as tolerated, with frequent rest periods
- Global surveillance and reporting of suspected cases to national health authorities
- Antivirals
- Combination of steroids and antimicrobials

KEY PATIENT OUTCOMES

The patient will:
- remain in isolation as recommended
- practice good hygiene to prevent further transmission
- maintain good nutritional status
- maintain a patent airway.

NURSING INTERVENTIONS

- Monitor the patient for complications, such as severe respiratory distress and thrombocytopenia (low platelet count) in later stages.
- Monitor vital signs.
- Administer prescribed medication.
- Encourage adequate nutritional intake.
- Observe, record, and report nature of rash.
- Maintain proper isolation technique.
- Collect laboratory specimens as needed.
- Monitor oxygen therapy as prescribed.

PATIENT TEACHING

Be sure to cover:
- the importance of frequent hand washing
- covering mouth and nose when coughing or sneezing
- avoiding close personal contact with friends and family
- the importance of not going to work, school, or other public places until 10 days after fever and respiratory symptoms resolve
- the wearing of a surgical mask by the patient or those in contact with him
- not sharing silverware, towels, or bedding until they've been washed in soap and hot water
- using disposable gloves and household disinfectant to clean any surface that might have been exposed to the patient's body fluids.

 Life-threatening disorder

Shock, cardiogenic

DESCRIPTION

- A condition of diminished cardiac output that severely impairs tissue perfusion (myocardial damage of more than 40% of the left ventricle most common)
- Failure of the heart to pump blood adequately to meet oxygenation needs of the body
- Most lethal form of shock

PATHOPHYSIOLOGY

- Left ventricular dysfunction initiates a series of compensatory mechanisms that attempt to increase cardiac output. (See *What happens in cardiogenic shock.*)
- As cardiac output decreases, aortic and carotid baroreceptors activate sympathetic nervous responses.
- Responses increase heart rate, left ventricular filling pressure, and peripheral resistance to flow to enhance venous return to the heart.
- This action initially stabilizes the patient but later causes deterioration with increasing oxygen demands on the already-compromised myocardium.
- These events consist of a cycle of low cardiac output, sympathetic compensation, myocardial ischemia, and even lower cardiac output.

FOCUS IN
WHAT HAPPENS IN CARDIOGENIC SHOCK

When the myocardium can't contract sufficiently to maintain adequate cardiac output, stroke volume decreases and the heart can't eject an adequate volume of blood with each contraction. The blood backs up behind the weakened left ventricle, increasing preload and causing pulmonary congestion. In addition, to compensate for the drop in stroke volume, the heart rate increases to maintain cardiac output. As a result of the diminished stroke volume, coronary artery perfusion and collateral blood flow decrease. All of these mechanisms increase the heart's workload and enhance left-sided heart failure. The result is myocardial hypoxia, further decreased cardiac output, and a triggering of compensatory mechanisms to prevent decompensation and death.

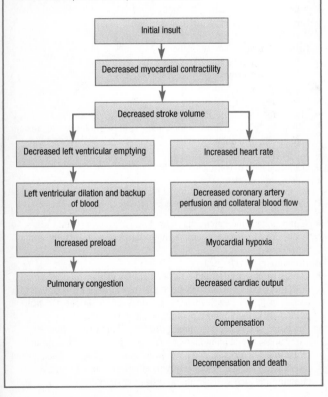

CAUSES

- Acute mitral or aortic insufficiency
- End-stage cardiomyopathy
- Myocardial infarction (MI); myocardial damage of more than 40% of the left ventricle most common
- Myocardial ischemia
- Myocarditis
- Papillary muscle dysfunction
- Ventricular aneurysm
- Ventricular septal defect

ASSESSMENT FINDINGS

- Determination of existing disorder, such as MI or cardiomyopathy that severely decreases left ventricular function
- Anginal pain
- Urine output less than 20 ml/hour
- Pale, cold, clammy skin
- Decreased sensorium
- Rapid, shallow respirations
- Rapid, thready pulse
- Mean arterial pressure of less than 60 mm Hg in adults
- Gallop rhythm, faint heart sounds, and, possibly, a holosystolic murmur
- Jugular vein distention
- Severe anxiety
- Decreased level of consciousness (LOC)
- Pulmonary crackles

TEST RESULTS

- Serum enzyme measurements show elevated levels of creatine kinase, lactate dehydrogenase, aspartate aminotransferase, and alanine aminotransferase.
- Troponin level is elevated.
- Cardiac catheterization and echocardiography may reveal other conditions that can lead to pump dysfunction and failure, such as cardiac tamponade, papillary muscle infarct or rupture, ventricular septal rupture, pulmonary emboli, venous pooling, and hypovolemia.
- Pulmonary artery pressure monitoring reveals increased pulmonary artery pressure and pulmonary artery wedge pressure, reflecting an increase in left ventricular end-diastolic pressure (preload) and heightened resistance to left ventricular emptying (afterload) caused by ineffective pumping and increased peripheral vascular resistance.

- Invasive arterial pressure monitoring shows systolic arterial pressure less than 80 mm Hg, caused by impaired ventricular ejection.
- Arterial blood gas (ABG) analysis may show metabolic and respiratory acidosis and hypoxia.
- Electrocardiography demonstrates possible evidence of acute MI, ischemia, or ventricular aneurysm.

TREATMENT

- Intra-aortic balloon pump (IABP)
- Vasopressors, inotropics, and vasoconstrictors

ALERT Monitor the patient closely when using vasoactive drugs, to maintain the balance between adequate perfusion pressure and reduced afterload. Report signs of hemodynamic decline promptly.

- Oxygen
- Osmotic diuretics
- Vasodilators
- Analgesics; sedatives
- Bed rest
- Possible parenteral nutrition or tube feedings
- Possible ventricular assist device
- Possible heart transplant

KEY PATIENT OUTCOMES

The patient will:
- maintain adequate cardiac output and hemodynamic stability
- develop no complications of fluid volume excess
- maintain adequate ventilation
- express feelings and develop adequate coping mechanisms.

NURSING INTERVENTIONS

- Administer prescribed oxygen.
- Follow IABP protocols and policies.

ALERT When a patient is receiving treatment with an IABP, move him as little as possible. Never place the patient in a sitting position higher than 45 degrees (including for chest X-rays) because the balloon may tear through the aorta and cause immediate death. Assess pedal pulses and skin temperature and color. Check the dressing on the insertion site frequently for bleeding, and change it according to facility protocol. Also check the site for hematomas or signs of infection, and culture drainage.

- Monitor the patient continuously for cardiac arrhythmias.
- Monitor ABG levels (acid-base balance) and pulse oximetry.
- Evaluate complete blood count and electrolyte levels.
- Obtain vital signs and peripheral pulses.
- Monitor hemodynamic parameters.
- Measure and record urine output every hour from indwelling catheter, and fluid intake.
- Monitor heart and breath sounds.
- Evaluate LOC.
- Be alert to adverse responses to drug therapy.
- Plan your care to allow frequent rest periods, and provide as much privacy as possible. Allow the patient's family to visit and comfort him as much as possible.
- Provide explanations and reassurance for the patient and his family as appropriate.
- Prepare the patient and his family for a possibly fatal outcome, and help them find effective coping strategies.
- Monitor the patient for possible multiple organ dysfunction.

PATIENT TEACHING

Be sure to cover:
- disorder, diagnosis, and treatment
- explanations and reassurance for patient and his family
- possible fatal outcome.

 Life-threatening disorder

Shock, hypovolemic

DESCRIPTION

- Reduced intravascular blood volume causing circulatory dysfunction and inadequate tissue perfusion resulting from loss of blood, plasma, or fluids
- Potentially life-threatening

PATHOPHYSIOLOGY

- When fluid is lost from the intravascular space, venous return to the heart is reduced.
- This decreases ventricular filling, which leads to a drop in stroke volume.
- Cardiac output falls, causing reduced perfusion to tissues and organs.
- Tissue anoxia prompts a shift in cellular metabolism from aerobic to anaerobic pathways.

■ This produces an accumulation of lactic acid, resulting in metabolic acidosis.

CAUSES

■ Acute blood loss (about one-fifth of total volume)
■ Acute pancreatitis
■ Ascites
■ Burns
■ Dehydration, as from excessive perspiration, severe diarrhea, protracted vomiting, diabetes insipidus, diuresis, or inadequate fluid intake
■ Diuretic abuse
■ High susceptibility to and low tolerance of reduced circulating blood volume in elderly patients
■ Internal hemorrhage
■ Intestinal obstruction
■ Peritonitis

ASSESSMENT FINDINGS

■ Preexisting disorders or conditions that reduced blood volume, such as GI hemorrhage, trauma, and severe diarrhea and vomiting
■ Some anginal pain in patients with cardiac disease, because of decreased myocardial perfusion and oxygenation
■ Physical symptoms consistent with reduced cardiac output due to reduced intravascular blood volume
  – Pale, cool, clammy skin
  – Decreased sensorium
  – Rapid, shallow respirations
  – Urine output usually less than 20 ml/hour
  – Rapid, thready pulse
  – Mean arterial pressure less than 60 mm Hg in adults (in chronic hypotension, mean pressure may fall below 50 mm Hg before signs of shock)
  – Orthostatic vital signs and tilt test results consistent with hypovolemic shock (see *Checking for early hypovolemic shock*, page 252)

TEST RESULTS

■ Hematocrit is low, and hemoglobin level and red blood cell and platelet counts are decreased.
■ Serum potassium, sodium, lactate dehydrogenase, creatinine, and blood urea nitrogen levels are elevated.
■ Urine specific gravity (greater than 1.020) and urine osmolality are increased.

CHECKING FOR EARLY HYPOVOLEMIC SHOCK

Orthostatic vital signs and tilt test results can help in assessing for the possibility
of impending hypovolemic shock.

Orthostatic vital signs
Measure the patient's blood pressure and pulse rate while he's lying in a supine
position, sitting, and standing. Wait at least 1 minute between each position
change. A systolic blood pressure decrease of 10 mm Hg or more between positions or a pulse rate increase of 10 beats/minute or more is a sign of volume
depletion and impending hypovolemic shock.

Tilt test
With the patient in a supine position, raise his legs above heart level. If his blood
pressure increases significantly, the test result is positive, indicating volume
depletion and impending hypovolemic shock.

- pH and partial pressure of arterial oxygen are decreased, and partial pres-
  sure of arterial carbon dioxide is increased.
- Aspiration of gastric contents through a nasogastric tube shows internal
  bleeding.
- Occult blood tests are positive.
- Coagulation studies show coagulopathy from disseminated intravascular
  coagulation.
- Chest or abdominal X-rays help to identify internal bleeding sites.
- Gastroscopy helps to identify internal bleeding sites.
- Invasive hemodynamic monitoring shows reduced central venous pres-
  sure, right atrial pressure, pulmonary artery pressure, pulmonary artery
  wedge pressure, and cardiac output.

TREATMENT

- In severe cases, an intra-aortic balloon pump, ventricular assist device, or
  pneumatic antishock garment (rare, only when unstable fractures in-
  volved)
- Oxygen administration
- Bleeding control by direct application of pressure and related measures
- Possible parenteral nutrition or tube feedings
- Bed rest
- Prompt and vigorous blood and fluid replacement
- Positive inotropes
- Possibly diuretics
- Possible surgery to correct underlying problem

KEY PATIENT OUTCOMES

The patient will:
- maintain adequate cardiac output
- maintain hemodynamic stability
- maintain adequate ventilation
- express feelings and develop adequate coping mechanisms
- regain adequate fluid volume.

NURSING INTERVENTIONS

- Check for a patent airway and adequate circulation. If blood pressure and heart rate are absent, start cardiopulmonary resuscitation.
- Obtain type and crossmatch as ordered.
- Administer prescribed I.V. solutions or blood products.
- Insert an indwelling urinary catheter.
- Administer prescribed oxygen.
- Provide emotional support to the patient and his family.
- Use modified Trendelenburg's position. (See *Positioning the patient*, page 254.)
- Monitor:
  - vital signs and peripheral pulses
  - cardiac rhythm
  - coagulation studies for signs of impending coagulopathy
  - complete blood count and electrolyte measurements
  - arterial blood gas levels
  - intake and output
  - hemodynamics.
- Monitor the patient for such complications as:
  - acute respiratory distress syndrome
  - acute tubular necrosis and renal failure
  - disseminated intravascular coagulation
  - multiple organ dysfunction.

PATIENT TEACHING

Be sure to cover:
- the disorder, diagnosis, and treatment
- procedures and their purpose
- risks associated with blood transfusions
- the purpose of all equipment such as mechanical ventilation
- dietary restrictions
- drugs and possible adverse effects.

POSITIONING THE PATIENT

This illustration shows proper positioning (modified Trendelenburg) for the patient who shows signs of shock. Elevate the legs to an angle of about 20 degrees and straighten the knees. Make sure the patient's trunk is horizontal and his head is slightly elevated.

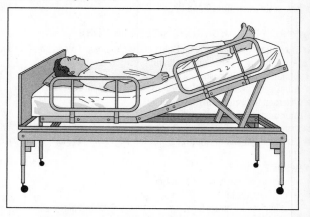

 Life-threatening disorder

Shock, septic

DESCRIPTION

■ Low systemic vascular resistance and elevated cardiac output
■ Occurs as a result of bacteria or their toxins circulating in the blood

PATHOPHYSIOLOGY

■ Initially, the body's defenses activate chemical mediators in response to the invading organisms.
■ The release of these mediators results in low systemic vascular resistance and increased cardiac output.
■ Blood flow is unevenly distributed in the microcirculation, and plasma leaking from capillaries causes functional hypovolemia.
■ Diffuse increase in capillary permeability occurs.

■ Eventually, cardiac output decreases, and poor tissue perfusion and hypotension cause multiple-organ-dysfunction syndrome and death.

CAUSES

■ Any pathogenic organism
■ Gram-negative bacteria, such as *Escherichia coli*, *Klebsiella pneumoniae*, *Serratia*, *Enterobacter*, and *Pseudomonas*, most common causes (up to 70% of cases)

 ALERT *Septic shock develops more easily in neonates and in patients who are elderly, debilitated, or immunocompromised.*

ASSESSMENT FINDINGS

Predisposing factors

■ Immunosuppression
■ Previous invasive tests
■ Chronic illness
■ Medication use
■ Malnutrition

Hyperdynamic, or warm, phase

■ Peripheral vasodilation
■ Skin possibly pink and flushed or warm and dry
■ Altered level of consciousness (LOC) reflected in agitation, anxiety, irritability, and shortened attention span
■ Respirations rapid and shallow
■ Urine output below normal
■ Rapid, full, bounding pulse
■ Blood pressure normal or slightly elevated

Hypodynamic, or cold, phase

■ Peripheral vasoconstriction and inadequate tissue perfusion
■ Pale skin and possible cyanosis
■ Decreased LOC; possible obtundation and coma
■ Respirations possibly rapid and shallow
■ Urine output possibly less than 25 ml/hour or absent
■ Rapid, weak, thready pulse
■ Irregular pulse if arrhythmias are present
■ Cold, clammy skin
■ Hypotension
■ Crackles or rhonchi if pulmonary congestion present

TEST RESULTS

- Blood cultures are positive for the causative organism.
- Complete blood count shows the presence or absence of anemia and leukopenia, severe or absent neutropenia, and usually the presence of thrombocytopenia.
- Blood urea nitrogen and creatinine levels are increased, and creatinine clearance is decreased.
- Prothrombin time and partial thromboplastin time are abnormal.
- Serum lactate dehydrogenase level is elevated, with metabolic acidosis.
- Urine studies show increased specific gravity (more than 1.02), increased osmolality, and decreased sodium level.
- Arterial blood gas (ABG) analysis demonstrates increased blood pH and partial pressure of arterial oxygen and decreased partial pressure of arterial carbon dioxide with respiratory alkalosis in early stages.
- Invasive hemodynamic monitoring shows:
  - increased cardiac output and decreased systemic vascular resistance in warm phase
  - decreased cardiac output and increased systemic vascular resistance in cold phase.

TREATMENT

- Removal of I.V., intra-arterial, or urinary drainage catheters whenever possible
- In patients immunosuppressed from drug therapy, drugs discontinued or dose reduced, if possible
- Mechanical ventilation if respiratory failure occurs
- Fluid volume replacement
- Possible parenteral nutrition or tube feedings
- Bed rest
- Granulocyte transfusions
- Colloid or crystalloid infusions
- Oxygen
- Antimicrobials
- Diuretics
- Vasopressors
- Antipyretics

KEY PATIENT OUTCOMES

The patient will:
- maintain adequate cardiac output
- maintain hemodynamic stability

- maintain adequate ventilation
- show no signs of infection
- express feelings and develop adequate coping mechanisms
- maintain adequate fluid volume.

NURSING INTERVENTIONS

- Remove potential routes of infection, such as I.V., intra-arterial, or urinary drainage catheters, and send them to the laboratory to culture for the presence of the causative organism.
- Administer prescribed I.V. fluids and blood products.

> **ALERT** *A progressive drop in blood pressure accompanied by a thready pulse usually signals inadequate cardiac output from reduced intravascular volume. Notify the physician immediately, and increase the I.V. infusion rate.*

- Administer appropriate antimicrobials and vasoactive I.V. drugs.
- Notify the physician if urine output is less than 30 ml/hour.
- Administer prescribed oxygen.
- Administer prescribed nutritional supplementation.
- Provide emotional support to the patient and his family.
- Document the occurrence of a nosocomial infection, and report it to the infection-control practitioner.
- Obtain specimens for culture (blood, urine, wound drainage, sputum).
- Use strict sterile technique for any invasive procedure.
- Monitor:
  - ABG levels and pulse oximetry
  - intake and output
  - vital signs and peripheral pulses
  - hemodynamics
  - heart and breath sounds
  - serum albumin levels.
- Monitor the patient for:
  - complications, such as disseminated intravascular coagulation, renal failure, heart failure, GI ulcers, and abnormal liver function
  - irregular cardiac rhythms when cardiac output, blood pressure, and pulse pressure decrease.

PATIENT TEACHING

Be sure to cover:
- the disorder, diagnosis, and treatment
- procedures and their purpose
- risks associated with blood transfusions

- all equipment and its purpose
- medications and possible adverse effects
- possible complications.

 Life-threatening disorder

Stroke

DESCRIPTION

- Sudden impairment of blood circulation to the brain
- Third most common cause of death in the United States
- Affects 500,000 people each year, causing death in 50% of these people
- Most common cause of neurologic disability
- About 50% of stroke survivors permanently disabled
- Recurrences possible within weeks, months, or years
- Also known as *cerebrovascular accident* or *brain attack*

PATHOPHYSIOLOGY

- The oxygen supply to the brain is interrupted or diminished.
- In ischemic (thrombotic or embolic) stroke, neurons die from lack of oxygen.
- In hemorrhagic stroke, impaired cerebral perfusion causes infarction.

CAUSES

- Cerebral embolism
  - After open-heart surgery
  - Cardiac arrhythmias
  - Carotid stenosis
  - Endocarditis
  - History of rheumatic heart disease
  - Posttraumatic valvular disease
- Cerebral hemorrhage
  - Arteriovenous malformation
  - Cerebral aneurysms
  - Chronic hypertension
- Cerebral thrombosis
  - Obstruction of a blood vessel in the extracerebral vessels
  - Site possibly intracerebral
- Other factors that can contribute to cause
  - Alcohol use
  - Diabetes mellitus

- Elevated cholesterol and triglyceride levels
- Family history of cerebrovascular disease
- Gout
- High red blood cell count
- History of transient ischemic attack
- Obesity
- Smoking
- Use of hormonal contraceptives, in those who smoke and have hypertension

ASSESSMENT FINDINGS

- Symptoms related to artery affected, extent of injury, extent of collateral circulation, and contributing factors
- Sudden onset of hemiparesis or hemiplegia
- Gradual onset of dizziness, mental disturbances, or seizures
- Loss of consciousness or sudden aphasia (expressive, receptive, or global)
- Sudden severe headache (not always present)
- Signs and symptoms on right side with stroke in left hemisphere
- Signs and symptoms on left side with stroke in right hemisphere
- Signs and symptoms on the affected side with stroke that causes cranial nerve damage
- Dysphagia
- Urinary incontinence
- Decreased deep tendon reflexes
- Hemianopsia on the affected side of the body
- With right-sided hemiplegia, problems with visuospatial relations
- Sensory losses
- Cognitive and emotional deficits

TEST RESULTS

- Laboratory tests — including anticardiolipin antibodies, antiphospholipid, factor V (Leiden) mutation (the most common hereditary contributor to hypercoagulability), antithrombin III, protein S, and protein C — show increased thrombotic risk.
- Magnetic resonance imaging and magnetic resonance angiography show the location and size of the lesion.
- Cerebral angiography details the disruption of cerebral circulation and is the test of choice for examining the entire cerebral blood flow.
- Computed tomography scan detects structural abnormalities.
- Positron emission tomography provides data on cerebral metabolism and on cerebral blood flow changes.

- Other tests include:
  - transcranial Doppler studies to evaluate the velocity of blood flow
  - carotid Doppler to measure blood flow through the carotid arteries
  - two-dimensional echocardiogram to evaluate the heart for dysfunction
  - cerebral blood flow studies to measure blood flow to the brain
  - EEG to evaluate electrical activity in an area of cortical infarction.

TREATMENT

- Careful blood pressure management
- Pureed dysphagia diet or tube feedings, if indicated
- Physical, speech, and occupational rehabilitation
- Helping patient adapt to specific deficits
- Tissue plasminogen activator when the cause isn't hemorrhagic (emergency care within 3 hours of onset of the symptoms)
- Anticonvulsants
- Stool softeners
- Anticoagulants
- Analgesics
- Antidepressants
- Antiplatelets
- Antilipemics
- Antihypertensives
- Surgery, if indicated, which may include craniotomy, endarterectomy, extracranial-intracranial bypass, ventricular shunts

▶ *COLLABORATION* *An interdisciplinary approach involving a stroke team, including the physician, nurse, physical therapist, occupational therapist, speech therapist, dietitian, social worker, and vocational counselor, is vital to helping the stroke survivor regain lost skills and function.*

KEY PATIENT OUTCOMES

The patient will:

- maintain adequate ventilation
- remain free from injury
- achieve maximal independence
- maintain joint mobility and range of motion.

NURSING INTERVENTIONS

- Maintain a patent airway and oxygenation.
- Offer the urinal or bedpan every 2 hours.
- Insert an indwelling urinary catheter if necessary.

PREVENTING STROKE

To decrease the risk of another stroke, teach the patient and family members about the need to correct risk factors. For example, if the patient smokes, refer him to a smoking-cessation program. Teach the importance of maintaining an ideal weight and controlling diabetes and hypertension. Teach all patients to follow a low-cholesterol, low-salt diet; perform regular physical exercise; avoid prolonged bed rest; and minimize stress. Early recognition of signs and symptoms of complications or impending stroke is imperative, as is seeking prompt treatment.

- Ensure adequate fluid, electrolyte, and nutritional intake.
- Provide careful mouth and eye care.
- Follow the physical therapy program, and assist the patient with exercise.
- Establish and maintain patient communication.
- Provide psychological support for patient and family members.
- Set realistic short-term goals.
- Protect the patient from injury and complications.
- Provide careful positioning to prevent aspiration and contractures.
- Administer prescribed medications.
- Monitor patient for complications related to immobility.
- Refer the patient to home care and outpatient services, as needed.

PATIENT TEACHING

Be sure to cover:
- the disorder, diagnosis, and treatment
- occupational and speech therapy programs
- dietary and drug regimens
- adverse drug reactions
- stroke prevention. (See *Preventing stroke.*)

Life-threatening disorder

Syndrome of inappropriate antidiuretic hormone

DESCRIPTION

- Disease of the posterior pituitary, marked by excessive release of antidiuretic hormone (ADH or vasopressin)

- Potentially life-threatening
- Prognosis dependent on underlying disorder and response to treatment
- Also known as *SIADH*

PATHOPHYSIOLOGY

- Excessive ADH secretion occurs without normal physiologic stimuli for its release.
- Excessive water reabsorption from the distal convoluted tubule and collecting ducts results in hyponatremia and normal to slightly increased extracellular fluid volume. (See *Understanding SIADH.*)

CAUSES

- Central nervous system disorders
- Drugs
- Miscellaneous conditions, such as myxedema and psychosis
- Neoplastic diseases
- Oat cell carcinoma of the lung
- Pulmonary disorders

ASSESSMENT FINDINGS

- Determination of possible underlying causes
  - Cerebrovascular disease
  - Cancer
  - Pulmonary disease
  - Recent head injury
- Anorexia, nausea, vomiting
- Weight gain
- Lethargy, headaches, emotional and behavioral changes
- Tachycardia
- Disorientation
- Seizures and coma
- Sluggish deep tendon reflexes
- Muscle weakness
- Fluid and electrolyte imbalance
- Hyponatremia

TEST RESULTS

- Serum osmolality level is less than 280 mOsm/kg.
- Serum sodium level is less than 123 mEq/L.
- Urine sodium level is more than 20 mEq/L without diuretics.
- Renal function test result is normal.

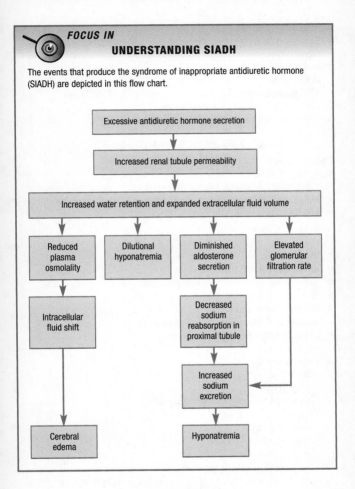

FOCUS IN

UNDERSTANDING SIADH

The events that produce the syndrome of inappropriate antidiuretic hormone (SIADH) are depicted in this flow chart.

Excessive antidiuretic hormone secretion

↓

Increased renal tubule permeability

↓

Increased water retention and expanded extracellular fluid volume

↓

- Reduced plasma osmolality
- Dilutional hyponatremia
- Diminished aldosterone secretion
- Elevated glomerular filtration rate

Reduced plasma osmolality → Intracellular fluid shift → Cerebral edema

Diminished aldosterone secretion → Decreased sodium reabsorption in proximal tubule → Increased sodium excretion → Hyponatremia

Elevated glomerular filtration rate → Increased sodium excretion

TREATMENT

- Based primarily on symptoms
- Correction of the underlying cause
- Restricted water intake (500 to 1,000 ml/day)
- High-salt, high-protein diet or urea supplements to enhance water excretion

- Activity as tolerated
- Demeclocycline (Declomycin) or lithium (Eskalith) for long-term treatment
- Loop diuretics if fluid overload, history of heart failure, or resistance to treatment
- 3% sodium chloride solution if serum sodium level is less than 120 mmol/L or if the patient is seizing
- Surgery to treat underlying cause such as cancer

KEY PATIENT OUTCOMES

The patient will:
- develop no complications
- remain alert and oriented to the environment
- verbalize an understanding of the disorder and treatment regimen
- maintain adequate fluid balance.

NURSING INTERVENTIONS

- Restrict fluids.
- Provide comfort measures for thirst.
- Reduce unnecessary environmental stimuli.
- Orient as needed.
- Provide a safe environment.
- Institute seizure precautions as needed.
- Administer prescribed medication.
- Monitor:
  - intake and output
  - vital signs
  - daily weight
  - serum electrolytes, especially sodium
  - response to treatment
  - breath sounds
  - heart sounds
  - neurologic checks
  - for changes in level of consciousness
  - for complications, such as cerebral edema, water intoxication, severe hyponatremia, coma.

ALERT *Watch closely for signs and symptoms of heart failure, which may occur because of fluid overload.*

PATIENT TEACHING

Be sure to cover:
- the disorder, diagnosis, and treatment
- fluid restriction
- methods to decrease discomfort from thirst
- medications and possible adverse effects
- self-monitoring techniques for fluid retention such as daily weight
- signs and symptoms that require immediate medical intervention.

Systemic lupus erythematosus

DESCRIPTION

- A chronic inflammatory autoimmune disorder that affects connective tissues
- Two forms: discoid lupus erythematosus (DLE) and systemic lupus erythematosus (SLE)
- Only the skin affected by DLE
- Recurrent seasonal remissions and exacerbations, especially during spring and summer

PATHOPHYSIOLOGY

- The body produces antibodies, such as antinuclear antibodies (ANAs), against its own cells.
- The formed antigen-antibody complexes suppress the body's normal immunity and damage tissues.
- Patients with SLE produce antibodies against many different tissue components, such as red blood cells (RBCs), neutrophils, platelets, lymphocytes, and almost any organ or tissue in the body.

CAUSES

- Unknown
- Predisposing factors
  - Abnormal estrogen metabolism
  - Emotional upsets
  - Exhaustion
  - Exposure to sunlight or ultraviolet light
  - Gender: Affects women between ages 15 and 40 at a rate 8 to 10 times greater than men; onset most common during childbearing years
  - Immunization, pregnancy
  - Injury

- Race: Most prevalent in Asians and Blacks
- Streptococcal or viral infections
- Stress
- Surgery

ASSESSMENT FINDINGS

- Onset acute or insidious; no characteristic clinical pattern
- Possible fever, anorexia, weight loss, malaise, fatigue, abdominal pain, nausea, vomiting, diarrhea, constipation, rash, and polyarthralgia
- Possible drug history with 1 of 25 drugs that can cause SLE-like reaction
- Irregular menstruation or amenorrhea, particularly during flare-ups
- Chest pain and dyspnea
- Emotional instability, psychosis, organic brain syndrome, headaches, irritability, and depression
- Oliguria, urinary frequency, dysuria, and bladder spasms
- Joint involvement that resembles rheumatoid arthritis
- Raynaud's phenomenon
- Skin eruptions aggravated by sunlight or ultraviolet light
- Tachycardia, central cyanosis, and hypotension
- Altered level of consciousness, weakness of the arms and legs, and speech disturbances
- Skin lesions
- Butterfly rash over nose and cheeks
- Patchy alopecia
- Vasculitis
- Lymph node enlargement
- Pericardial friction rub

TEST RESULTS

- Complete blood count with differential shows anemia and a reduced white blood cell (WBC) count, decreased platelet count, and elevated erythrocyte sedimentation rate; serum electrophoresis shows hypergamma-globulinemia.
- ANA, anti-deoxyribonucleic acid, and lupus erythematosus cell test findings are usually positive.
- Urine studies show RBCs, WBCs, urine casts, sediment, and significant protein loss (more than 3.5 g in 24 hours).
- Blood studies demonstrate decreased serum complement (C3 and C4) levels, indicating active disease.
- C-reactive protein level is increased.
- Rheumatoid factor is positive in 30% to 40% of patients.

- Chest X-rays may disclose pleurisy or lupus pneumonitis.
- EEG results are abnormal in about 70% of patients because of central nervous system (CNS) involvement.
- Results of brain and magnetic resonance imaging scans may be normal despite CNS involvement.
- Electrocardiography may show a conduction defect with cardiac involvement or pericarditis.
- Renal biopsy shows progression of SLE and the extent of renal involvement.
- Skin biopsy shows immunoglobulin and complement deposition in the dermal-epidermal junction in 90% of patients.

TREATMENT

- Use of sunscreen with sun protection factor of at least 15
- No dietary restrictions unless renal failure occurs
- Regular exercise program
- Nonsteroidal anti-inflammatory drugs
- Topical corticosteroids
- Fluorinated steroids
- Antimalarials
- Corticosteroids
- Cytotoxic drugs
- Antihypertensives
- Possible joint replacement

KEY PATIENT OUTCOMES

The patient will:
- express feelings of increased comfort and decreased pain
- express feelings of increased energy
- maintain joint mobility and range of motion (ROM)
- maintain skin integrity
- maintain fluid balance.

NURSING INTERVENTIONS

- Provide a balanced diet.
- Provide bland, cool foods if the patient has a sore mouth.
- Provide a mouth rinse of normal saline solution after meals to assist healing of oral lesions.
- Apply heat packs to relieve joint pain and stiffness.
- Encourage regular exercise to maintain full ROM.

- Explain the expected benefit of prescribed medication, and watch for adverse effects.
- Institute seizure precautions if you suspect CNS involvement.
- Warm and protect the patient's hands and feet if he has Raynaud's phenomenon.
- Support the patient's self-image and emotional well-being.
- Encourage verbalization of fears and anxieties.
- Monitor:
  - signs and symptoms of organ involvement
  - blood in urine, stools, and GI secretions
  - hair loss on scalp and petechiae, bleeding, ulceration, pallor, and bruising of skin or mucous membranes
  - response to treatment
  - respiratory, cardiac, renal, and neurologic complications
  - nutritional status
  - joint mobility
  - seizure activity.
- Refer the patient to a rheumatology specialist if she becomes pregnant.

> **COLLABORATION** *Arrange for a physical therapy and occupational therapy consultation if musculoskeletal involvement compromises mobility.*

PATIENT TEACHING

Be sure to cover:
- the disorder, diagnosis, and treatment
- ROM exercises and body alignment and postural techniques
- ways to avoid infection, such as avoiding crowds and people with known infections
- need to notify a physician if fever, cough, or rash occurs or if chest, abdominal, muscle, or joint pain worsens
- importance of eating a balanced diet and the restrictions associated with prescribed medication
- importance of good skin care
- benefits of exercise
- importance of keeping regular follow-up appointments and contacting a physician if flare-ups occur
- need to wear protective clothing and use a sunscreen
- how to perform meticulous mouth care
- signs and symptoms of abnormal estrogen metabolism, particularly during flare-ups.

Thrombophlebitis

DESCRIPTION

- Development of a thrombus that may cause vessel occlusion or embolization
- Acute condition characterized by inflammation and thrombus formation
- May occur in deep or superficial veins (see *Major venous pathways of the leg*)

MAJOR VENOUS PATHWAYS OF THE LEG

Thrombophlebitis can occur in any leg vein. It most commonly occurs at valve sites.

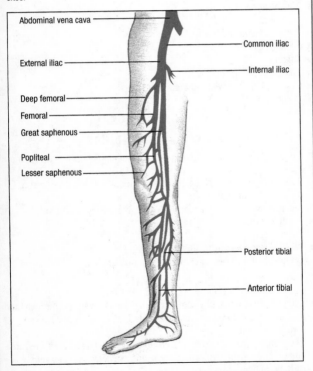

- Abdominal vena cava
- Common iliac
- External iliac
- Internal iliac
- Deep femoral
- Femoral
- Great saphenous
- Popliteal
- Lesser saphenous
- Posterior tibial
- Anterior tibial

- Typically occurs at the valve cusps because venous stasis encourages accumulation and adherence of platelet and fibrin

PATHOPHYSIOLOGY

- Changes in epithelial lining cause platelet aggregation and fibrin entrapment of red blood cells, white blood cells, and additional platelets.
- The thrombus starts a chemical inflammatory process in the vessel epithelium, leading to fibrosis, which may occlude the vessel lumen or embolize.

CAUSES

- Fracture of the spine, pelvis, femur, or tibia
- Hormonal contraceptives such as estrogens
- May be idiopathic
- Neoplasms
- Pregnancy and childbirth
- Prolonged bed rest
- Surgery
- Trauma
- Use of subclavian vein catheters
- Venous stasis
- Venulitis

ASSESSMENT FINDINGS

- Up to 50% of patients with deep vein thrombophlebitis may be asymptomatic
- Possible tenderness, aching, or severe pain in the affected leg or arm; fever, chills, and malaise
- Redness, swelling, and tenderness of the affected leg or arm
- Possible positive Homans' sign
- Positive cuff sign
- Possible warm feeling in affected leg or arm
- Lymphadenitis in case of extensive vein involvement

TEST RESULTS

- Doppler ultrasonography shows reduced blood flow to specific areas and any obstruction to venous flow, particularly in iliofemoral deep vein thrombophlebitis.
- Plethysmography shows decreased circulation distal to the affected area and is more sensitive than ultrasonography in detecting deep vein thrombophlebitis.

■ Phlebography confirms the diagnosis and shows filling defects and diverted blood flow.

TREATMENT

■ Application of warm, moist compresses to the affected area
■ Antiembolism stockings
■ Bed rest, with elevation of the affected extremity
■ Anticoagulants
■ Thrombolytics
■ Analgesics
■ Surgery, possibly including simple ligation to vein plication, embolectomy, caval interruption with transvenous placement of a vena cava filter

KEY PATIENT OUTCOMES

The patient will:
■ maintain collateral circulation
■ express feelings of increased comfort and decreased pain
■ maintain tissue perfusion and cellular oxygenation
■ develop no signs or symptoms of infection.

NURSING INTERVENTIONS

■ Enforce bed rest and elevate the patient's affected arm or leg, but avoid compressing the popliteal space.
■ Apply warm compresses or a covered aquathermia pad.
■ Administer prescribed analgesics.
■ Mark, measure, and record the circumference of the affected arm or leg daily, and compare this measurement with that of the other arm or leg.
■ Administer prescribed anticoagulants.
■ Perform or encourage range-of-motion exercises.
■ Use pneumatic compression devices.
■ Apply antiembolism stockings.
■ Encourage early ambulation.
■ Monitor:
  – response to treatment
  – vital signs
  – partial thromboplastin time for patient receiving heparin (Calciparin)
  – prothrombin time for patient receiving warfarin (Coumadin)
  – for signs and symptoms of bleeding
  – for signs and symptoms of heparin-induced thrombocytopenia
  – for signs and symptoms of pulmonary embolism.

PATIENT TEACHING

Be sure to cover:
- the disorder, diagnosis, and treatment
- importance of follow-up blood studies to monitor anticoagulant therapy
- how to give injections (if the patient is being discharged on subcutaneous anticoagulation therapy)
- need to avoid prolonged sitting or standing to help prevent a recurrence
- proper application and use of antiembolism stockings
- importance of adequate hydration
- use of an electric razor
- avoidance of aspirin-containing products.

Thyroid cancer

DESCRIPTION

- Proliferation of cancer cells in the thyroid gland
- Most common endocrine malignancy
- Papillary cancer: 50% of all cases
- Medullary cancer: may be linked to pheochromocytoma; curable when detected before it causes symptoms

PATHOPHYSIOLOGY

- Papillary cancer is usually multifocal and bilateral. It metastasizes slowly into regional nodes of the neck, mediastinum, lungs, and other distant organs. It's the least virulent form of thyroid cancer.
- Follicular cancer is less common but is more likely to recur and metastasize to the regional lymph nodes and spread through blood vessels into the bones, liver, and lungs.
- Medullary, or solid, cancer originates in the parafollicular cells derived from the last branchial pouch and contains amyloid and calcium deposits. It can produce calcitonin, histaminase, corticotropin, and prostaglandin E_2 and F_3. Untreated medullary cancer grows rapidly, commonly metastasizing to bones, liver, and kidneys.
- Anaplastic cancer, or giant and spindly cell cancer, resists radiation and is almost never curable by resection. This cancer metastasizes rapidly, causing death by invading the trachea and compressing adjacent structures.

CAUSES

- Chronic goiter
- Familial predisposition, possibly inherited as an autosomal dominant trait

- Previous exposure to radiation treatment in the neck area
- Prolonged secretion of thyroid-stimulating hormone

ASSESSMENT FINDINGS

- Possible history of:
  - Sensitivity to cold and mental apathy (hypothyroidism)
  - Sensitivity to heat, restlessness, and overactivity (hyperthyroidism)
  - Diarrhea
  - Dysphagia
  - Anorexia
  - Irritability
  - Ear pain
- Hard, painless nodule in an enlarged thyroid gland or palpable lymph nodes with thyroid enlargement
- Hoarseness and vocal stridor
- Disfiguring thyroid mass
- Bruits

TEST RESULTS

- Elevated fasting calcitonin level and an abnormal response to calcium stimulation identify "silent" medullary carcinoma.
- Thyroid scan differentiates functional nodes, which are rarely malignant, from hypofunctional nodes, which are usually malignant.
- Ultrasonography shows changes in the size of thyroid nodules after thyroxine suppression therapy and detects recurrent disease.
- Magnetic resonance imaging and computed tomography scans show the extent of disease in the thyroid and surrounding structures.
- Fine-needle aspiration biopsy differentiates benign from malignant thyroid nodules.
- Histologic analysis stages the disease and thereby guides treatment plans.

TREATMENT

- Radioisotope, or ^{131}I, therapy with external radiation or alone
- Soft diet with small, frequent meals if dysphagia occurs
- Suppressive thyroid hormone therapy
- Chemotherapy
- Total or subtotal thyroidectomy with modified node dissection, either bilateral or unilateral, on the side of the primary cancer in the case of papillary or follicular cancer
- Total thyroidectomy and radical neck excision in the case of medullary or anaplastic cancer

KEY PATIENT OUTCOMES

The patient will:
- not aspirate
- maintain current weight without further loss
- express positive feelings about self
- express feelings of increased comfort and decreased pain.

NURSING INTERVENTIONS

- Encourage verbalization and provide support.
- Before surgery:
  - Prepare the patient for scheduled surgery.
  - Establish a way to communicate postoperatively.
- After surgery:
  - Keep the patient in semi-Fowler's position, with adequate neck support.
  - Keep a tracheotomy set and oxygen equipment nearby in case of respiratory obstruction.
  - Monitor the patient's vital signs, wound site, pain control, serum calcium levels, hydration and nutritional status and for complications
- Refer the patient to available resource and support services, including the American Cancer Society.

PATIENT TEACHING

Be sure to cover:
- the disorder, diagnosis, and treatment
- before surgery, the operation and postoperative procedures and positioning
- treatments and home care
- medication administration, dosage, and possible adverse effects.

Toxoplasmosis

DESCRIPTION

- One of the most common parasitic infectious diseases
- Usually causes localized infection
- May produce significant generalized infection, especially in an immuno-deficient patient
- Once infected, organism carried for life and acute infection can reactivate
- Congenital type characterized by lesions in the central nervous system (CNS); may result in stillbirth or serious birth defects

OCULAR TOXOPLASMOSIS

Ocular toxoplasmosis (active chorioretinitis) is characterized by focal necrotizing retinitis. It accounts for about 25% of all cases of granulomatous uveitis. Although usually the result of a congenital infection, it may not appear until adolescence or young adulthood, when infection is reactivated.

Symptoms include blurred vision, scotoma, pain, photophobia, and impairment or loss of central vision. Vision improves as inflammation subsides, but usually without recovery of lost visual acuity. Ocular toxoplasmosis may subside after treatment with prednisone (Deltasone).

PATHOPHYSIOLOGY

- After ingestion, parasites are released from latent cysts by the digestive process; they then invade the GI tract and multiply.
- Parasites disseminate to various organs, especially lymphatic tissue, skeletal muscle, myocardium, retina, placenta, and the CNS. (See *Ocular toxoplasmosis*.)
- The parasite infects host cells, replicates, and then invades adjoining cells, resulting in cell death and focal necrosis surrounded by an acute inflammatory response.

CAUSES

- Congenital toxoplasmosis from transplacental transmission
- The protozoan *Toxoplasma gondii*, which exists in trophozoite forms in the acute stages of infection and in cystic forms in latent stages
- Transmitted by ingestion of tissue cysts in raw or undercooked meat or by fecal-oral contamination from infected cats

ASSESSMENT FINDINGS

- Predisposing factors, such as immunocompromised state, exposure to cat feces, and ingestion of poorly cooked meat
- Assess patient for history of symptoms, such as headache, fatigue, malaise, myalgia, sore throat, and vomiting
- Fever (if generalized, possibly 106.7° F [41.5° C])
- Cough
- Dyspnea
- Cyanosis
- Coarse crackles
- Delirium, seizures
- Diffuse maculopapular rash (except on the palms, soles, and scalp)

- In an infant with congenital toxoplasmosis:
  - Hydrocephalus or microcephalus
  - Jaundice, purpura, rash
  - Strabismus, blindness
  - Epilepsy, mental retardation
  - Lymphadenopathy, splenomegaly, and hepatomegaly

TEST RESULTS

- Specimens, such as bronchoalveolar lavage material from immunocompromised patients or lymph node biopsy, contain parasites.
- Intraperitoneal inoculation with blood or other body fluids into mice or tissue cultures show isolation of parasites.
- Polymerase chain reaction detects parasite's genetic material.

TREATMENT

- No treatment in otherwise healthy patient who isn't pregnant
- Rest periods when fatigued
- Seizure precautions
- Pyrimethamine (Daraprim) plus sulfadiazine with leucovorin (Wellcovorin)

 COLLABORATION *A neurologist or infectious disease specialist may be consulted.*

KEY PATIENT OUTCOMES

The patient will:
- have normal vital signs
- have an adequate fluid volume
- report an increased energy level
- develop no complications
- maintain respiratory rate within 5 breaths/minute of baseline.

NURSING INTERVENTIONS

- Administer tepid sponge baths to decrease fever.
- Administer drug therapy.
- Provide chest physiotherapy and administer oxygen, as needed. Assist ventilations if needed.
- Institute seizure precautions.

ALERT *Don't palpate the patient's abdomen vigorously; this could lead to a ruptured spleen. For the same reason, discourage vigorous activity.*

- Report all cases of toxoplasmosis to the local public health department.
- Monitor the patient's neurologic status and response to treatment.
- Monitor the patient for potential complications, including seizure disorder, vision loss, mental retardation, deafness, generalized infection, still-birth, and congenital toxoplasmosis.

PATIENT TEACHING

Be sure to cover:
- the disorder, diagnosis, and treatment
- necessary drugs, including the need for frequent blood tests
- importance of regularly scheduled follow-up care
- ways to prevent the spread of toxoplasmosis, including washing hands after working with soil, cooking meat thoroughly and freezing promptly, covering children's sandboxes, and keeping flies away from food
- need for pregnant women to avoid cleaning and handling cat litter boxes, or to wear gloves when doing so.

Tuberculosis

DESCRIPTION

- Acute or chronic lung infection characterized by pulmonary infiltrates and the formation of granulomas with caseation, fibrosis, and cavitation
- Can occur in other organs, bone, or lymph nodes
- Prognosis excellent with proper treatment and compliance except in cases of multidrug-resistant tuberculosis (MDR-TB)
- Also known as *TB*

PATHOPHYSIOLOGY

- Multiplication of the bacillus *Mycobacterium tuberculosis* causes an inflammatory process where deposited.
- A cell-mediated immune response follows, usually containing the infection within 4 to 6 weeks.
- The T-cell response causes granulomas to form around the bacilli, making them go dormant. This confers immunity to subsequent infection.
- Bacilli within granulomas may remain viable for many years, causing a positive result for the purified protein derivative or other skin test for TB.
- Active disease develops in 5% to 15% of those infected.
- Transmission occurs when an infected person coughs, sneezes, shouts, or sings.

CAUSES

- Exposure to *M. tuberculosis*
- Exposure to other strains of mycobacteria (sometimes)

ASSESSMENT FINDINGS

- Patients at high risk:
  - Those having close contact with newly diagnosed TB patient
  - Those with a history of TB exposure
  - Those with multiple sexual partners
  - Recent immigrants from Africa, Asia, Mexico, or South America
  - Those who have had a gastrectomy
  - Those with a history of silicosis, diabetes, malnutrition, cancer, Hodgkin's disease, or leukemia
  - Those with drug or alcohol abuse problems
  - Residents in nursing home, mental health facility, or prison
  - Immunosuppressed patients and those who use corticosteroids
  - Homeless patients
  - Those in crowded, poorly ventilated, unsanitary living conditions
  - Health care workers
- Signs and symptoms of primary infection:
  - May be asymptomatic after a 4- to 8-week incubation period
  - Weakness and fatigue
  - Anorexia, weight loss
  - Low-grade fever
  - Night sweats
- Signs and symptoms of reactivated infection:
  - Chest pain
  - Productive cough for blood, or mucopurulent or blood-tinged sputum
  - Low-grade fever
- Other possible signs and symptoms:
  - Dullness over the affected area
  - Crepitant crackles
  - Bronchial breath sounds
  - Wheezes
  - Whispered pectoriloquy

TEST RESULTS

- Tuberculin skin test result is positive for induration in both active and inactive tuberculosis.
- Stains and cultures of sputum, cerebrospinal fluid, urine, abscess drainage, or pleural fluid show heat-sensitive, nonmotile, aerobic, acid-fast bacilli.

- Chest X-rays show nodular lesions, patchy infiltrates, cavity formation, scar tissue, and calcium deposits.
- Computed tomography or magnetic resonance imaging shows presence and extent of lung damage.
- Bronchoscopy specimens show heat-sensitive, nonmotile, aerobic, acid-fast bacilli in specimens.

TREATMENT

- Well-balanced, high-calorie diet
- Rest, initially; then, activity as tolerated
- Antitubercular therapy for at least 6 months, with a prescribed schedule of oral doses of four of these drugs initially:
  – ethambutol (EMB), until drug sensitivity tests show no drug resistance (about 2 weeks)
  – isoniazid (INH)
  – pyrazinamide (PZA)
  – rifampin (Rifadin, RIF)
  – rifapentine (Priftin)
  – rifabutin (Mycobutin)
- Second-line drugs for MDR-TB:
  – amikacin (Amikin)
  – capreomycin (Capastat)
  – cycloserine (Seromycin)
  – ethionamide (Ethomid)
  – gatifloxacin (Tequin)
  – levofloxacin (Levaquin, Quixin)
  – moxifloxacin (Avelox)
  – para-aminosalicylic acid (Paser)
  – streptomycin
- Possible surgery for certain complications

KEY PATIENT OUTCOMES

The patient will:
- express an understanding of the illness
- maintain adequate ventilation
- use support systems to assist with coping
- identify measures to prevent or reduce fatigue
- comply with treatment regimen
- resume normal activities after 2- to 4-week infectious period, while continuing to take medication.

PREVENTING TUBERCULOSIS

Explain respiratory and standard precautions to a hospitalized patient with tuberculosis (TB). Before discharge, tell him that he must take precautions to prevent spreading the disease, such as wearing a mask around others, until his physician tells him he's no longer contagious. He should tell all health care providers he sees, including his dentist and optometrist, that he has TB so that they can institute infection-control precautions.

Teach the patient other specific precautions to avoid spreading the infection. Tell him to cough and sneeze into tissues and to dispose of the tissues properly. Stress the importance of washing his hands thoroughly in hot, soapy water after handling his own secretions. Also instruct him to wash his eating utensils separately in hot, soapy water.

NURSING INTERVENTIONS

- Administer drug therapy.
- Isolate the patient in a quiet, properly ventilated room, and maintain tuberculosis precautions. (See *Preventing tuberculosis*.)
- Provide diversional activities.
- Properly dispose of secretions.
- Provide adequate rest periods.
- Provide small, frequent, well-balanced, high-calorie meals.
- Consult with dietitian if oral supplements are needed.
- Perform chest physiotherapy.
- Provide supportive care.
- Include the patient in care decisions.
- Monitor the patient's vital signs, intake and output, and daily weight.
- Monitor the patient for potential complications including massive pulmonary tissue damage, respiratory failure, bronchopleural fistulas, pneumothorax, pleural effusion, pneumonia, infection of other body organs by small mycobacterial foci, liver involvement, and disease caused by drug therapy.
- Observe the patient for adverse reactions to drugs; monitor his visual acuity if he's taking ethambutol.
- Monitor the results of liver and kidney function tests.
- Assist in notification of local and state public health officials as required.
- Explain how to access support services such as the American Lung Association and the local Public Health Department.
- Provide information on smoking-cessation programs, if indicated.
- Refer anyone exposed to an infected patient for testing and follow-up.

PATIENT TEACHING

Be sure to cover:
- the disorder, diagnosis, and treatment
- medication and potential adverse effects
- where to obtain free medication locally
- when to notify the physician
- need for isolation
- postural drainage and chest percussion
- coughing and deep-breathing exercises
- regular follow-up examinations
- signs and symptoms of recurring TB
- possible decreased hormonal contraceptive effectiveness during rifampin therapy
- need for a high-calorie, high-protein, balanced diet.

West Nile encephalitis

DESCRIPTION

- An infectious disease, part of a family of vector-borne diseases that also includes malaria, yellow fever, and Lyme disease
- Mortality from 3% to 15%; higher in elderly patients
- Ticks infected with the virus found in Africa and Asia only; role of ticks in transmission and maintenance of the virus uncertain
- Also called *West Nile virus*

PATHOPHYSIOLOGY

- The incubation period is 5 to 15 days after exposure.
- Mosquitoes become infected by feeding on birds contaminated with the virus. (See *Transmission routes of West Nile encephalitis,* page 282.)
- The virus is transmitted to a human by the bite of an infected mosquito (mostly the *Culex* species).
- Disease primarily causes encephalitis.

CAUSES

- A flavivirus commonly found in humans, birds, and other vertebrates in Africa, West Asia, and the Middle East
- Greatest risk in those older than age 50 and those with compromised immune systems

TRANSMISSION ROUTES OF WEST NILE ENCEPHALITIS

Birds harbor the virus that causes West Nile encephalitis, but they can't spread it. Mosquitoes serve as the vectors, spreading it from bird to bird and from bird to human. Humans are thought to be "dead-end hosts" because the virus can live and cause illness in humans, but a feeding mosquito can't acquire the virus from an infected person.

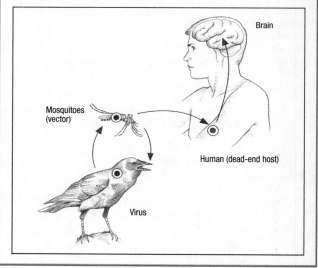

ASSESSMENT FINDINGS

- History of recent exposure to bodies of water, dead birds, or mosquitoes
- Symptoms:
  - Headache
  - Myalgia
  - Neck stiffness
  - Decreased appetite
  - Nausea and vomiting
  - Diarrhea
- Signs:
  - Fever
  - Rash
  - Swollen lymph glands

- Stupor and disorientation
- Decreased neck motion
- Change in mental status

TEST RESULTS

■ White blood cell (WBC) count is normal or increased.
■ Enzyme-linked immunosorbent assay (ELISA) indicates a recent infection, thus allowing for a rapid and definitive diagnosis.
■ Accurate diagnosis is possible only when serum or cerebrospinal fluid specimens are obtained while the patient is hospitalized with acute illness and they show elevated WBC count and protein levels.
■ Magnetic resonance imaging may show inflammation.

TREATMENT

■ No specific treatment
■ Respiratory support
■ Increased fluid intake
■ Rest periods when fatigued
■ Antipyretics

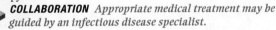 **COLLABORATION** *Appropriate medical treatment may be guided by an infectious disease specialist.*

KEY PATIENT OUTCOMES

The patient will:
■ maintain collateral circulation
■ maintain hemodynamic stability
■ have adequate cardiac output
■ remain afebrile
■ have an adequate fluid volume.

NURSING INTERVENTIONS

■ Maintain adequate hydration with I.V. fluids.
■ Administer prescribed medications.
■ Provide respiratory support measures when needed.
■ Follow standard precautions when handling blood or other body fluids.
■ Report any suspected cases of West Nile encephalitis to the state department of health.
■ Monitor:
  - fluid and electrolyte status
  - neurologic status
  - vital signs.

PREVENTING WEST NILE ENCEPHALITIS

To reduce the risk of infection with West Nile encephalitis, advise patients to do the following:

- Stay indoors at dawn and dusk and in early evening when mosquitoes are biting.
- Wear long-sleeved shirts and long pants when outdoors.
- Apply insect repellent sparingly to exposed skin. Effective repellents contain 20% to 30% N,N-diethyltoluamide (deet). In concentrations greater than 30%, deet can cause adverse effects, particularly in children, and should be avoided; adults should apply repellent with no more than 10% deet on children.
- Avoid applying repellent under clothing.
- Avoid applying repellent over cuts, wounds, sunburn, or irritated skin.
- Wash repellent off daily and reapply as needed.

PATIENT TEACHING

Be sure to cover:
- the disorder, diagnosis, and treatment
- proper use of insect repellants, which can irritate the eyes and mouth, and to avoid applying repellant to the hands of children (shouldn't be applied to children younger than age 3) (see *Preventing West Nile encephalitis*)
- expected course and outcomes of the illness
- need to drink fluids to avoid dehydration
- how to stop mosquitoes from breeding by:
  - cleaning out birdbaths and wading pools at least once per week
  - cleaning roof gutters and downspout screens
  - eliminating any standing water
  - not allowing water to collect in trash cans
  - turning over or removing containers in yards where rainwater collects, such as toys and old tires.

Part two

Treatments

Adrenalectomy

DESCRIPTION

- Surgical resection or removal of one or both of the adrenal glands

PURPOSE

- To resolve adrenal hyperfunction or hyperaldosteronism
- To remove a benign or malignant adrenal tumor
- Secondary treatment of neoplasms
- Secondary treatment of corticotropin oversecretion

PATIENT PREPARATION

- Explain the treatment and preparation to the patient and his family.
- Make sure the patient has signed an appropriate consent form.
- Give drugs to control hypertension, edema, diabetes, cardiovascular symptoms, and increased infection risk, as needed and ordered.
- Administer aldosterone antagonists for blood pressure control as ordered.
- Administer glucocorticoids on the morning of surgery as ordered.
- Draw blood samples for laboratory tests as ordered.
- Administer potassium supplements as ordered.
- Provide a low-sodium, high-potassium diet as ordered.
- Administer catecholamine-syntheses blockers and medications to control hypertension and tachycardia as ordered, 1 to 2 weeks before surgery for patients with pheochromocytoma.
- Monitor the patient for arrhythmias, palpitations, severe headache, hypertension, hyperglycemia, nausea, vomiting, diaphoresis, and vision disturbances.

PROCEDURE

- After the patient is anesthetized, an anterior (transperitoneal) or a posterior (lumbar) approach is used.
- The adrenal gland is identified and dissected free from the upper pole of the kidney.
- The wound is closed.
- If the procedure was done because of a tumor, the adrenal gland is explored first; then the tumor is resected or one or both of the glands is removed.
- In pheochromocytoma, the affected adrenal gland is excised, and the abdominal organs are palpated for other tumors.

POSTPROCEDURE CARE

- Administer I.V. vasopressors; titrate the dosage to the patient's blood pressure response as ordered.
- Increase the I.V. infusion rate as ordered.
- Administer glucocorticoids I.V. as ordered.
- Administer analgesics as ordered.
- Maintain asepsis.
- Keep the room cool.
- Monitor the patient's vital signs, intake and output, invasive arterial pressure, serum electrolyte levels, and surgical wound and dressings.
- Assess the patient for hemorrhage and shock, adrenal hypofunction, acute adrenal crisis, hypoglycemia, abdominal distention, and return of bowel sounds.
- Refer the patient to a local support group.
- Be sure to teach the patient about:
  - medications and possible adverse reactions
  - avoidance of sudden steroid withdrawal
  - potential complications, including acute life-threatening adrenal crisis, hemorrhage, poor wound healing, hypoglycemia, electrolyte disturbances, pancreatic injury, hypotension, and possible hypertension
  - when to notify the physician
  - follow-up medical care
  - adjustment of steroid dosage during stress or illness
  - signs and symptoms of adrenal insufficiency
  - reversal of physical disease signs within a few months in cases of adrenal hyperfunction
  - wound care instructions
  - signs and symptoms of infection
  - stress-reduction techniques, if appropriate
  - importance of wearing medical identification.

Amputation

DESCRIPTION

- Surgical removal of an extremity
- Closed technique: skin flaps are used to cover the residual bone
- Open (guillotine) amputation: tissue and bone are cut flush, and the wound is left open to be repaired in a second operation

PURPOSE

- To preserve function in a remaining part

- To prevent death caused by:
  - cancer
  - gangrene
  - thermal injury
  - vascular disease
- To correct a congenital deformity

PATIENT PREPARATION

- Explain the treatment and preparation to the patient and his family.
- Make sure that the patient has signed an appropriate consent form.
- Provide emotional support.
- Arrange for the patient to meet with a patient who has adjusted well to the procedure, if possible.
- Demonstrate prescribed exercises.

PROCEDURE

- The patient receives general or local anesthesia.

Closed technique

- All involved tissue is incised to the bone, leaving sufficient skin to cover the limb end.
- Bleeding is controlled by tying off the bleeding vessels above the amputation site.
- The bone (or joint) is sawed and filed, with the periosteum removed about $^1/_4$" (0.6 cm) from the bone end.
- All vessels are ligated and nerves divided.
- Opposing muscles are sutured over the bone end and periosteum.
- Skin flaps are closed and an incisional drain is placed.
- Soft dressings are applied; rigid dressings may be used in below-the-knee amputation.

Emergency or guillotine amputation

- A perpendicular incision is made through the bone and all tissue.
- The wound isn't sutured closed.
- A large, bulky dressing is applied.

POSTPROCEDURE CARE

- Elevate the affected limb as ordered.
- Provide analgesics as ordered.
- Keep the residual limb wrapped properly with elastic compression bandages or a limb shrinker as ordered.

- Provide cast care if a rigid plaster dressing has been applied.
- Maintain the patient in proper body alignment.
- Provide regular physical therapy to prevent contractures.
- Encourage frequent ambulation.
- Encourage active or passive range-of-motion exercises.
- Help the patient with turning and positioning without propping the limb on a pillow.
- Monitor the patient's vital signs, intake and output, surgical wound and dressings, bleeding, drain patency and drainage, pain, and skin breakdown.

 COLLABORATION *Arrange for a consultation with a psychologist or social services, as indicated.*

- Be sure to teach the patient about:
  - medications and possible adverse reactions
  - postoperative care and rehabilitation
  - the prosthesis and its care
  - phantom limb sensation
  - daily examination of the distal limb
  - daily limb care and dressings
  - signs and symptoms of infection
  - complications, such as signs and symptoms of infection, contractures, skin breakdown, and phantom pain
  - when to notify the physician
  - the use of elastic bandages or a limb shrinker
  - proper crutch use as appropriate
  - activities to toughen the residual limb
  - follow-up care.

Appendectomy

DESCRIPTION

- Surgical removal of an inflamed vermiform appendix
- May involve laparoscopy for diagnosis and appendix removal

PURPOSE

- To prevent imminent rupture or perforation of the appendix

PATIENT PREPARATION

- Explain the treatment and preparation to the patient and his family.
- Make sure the patient has signed an appropriate consent form.

- Administer preventive antibiotics as ordered.
- Administer I.V. fluids as ordered.
- Insert a nasogastric (NG) tube as ordered.
- Place the patient in Fowler's position.
- Avoid giving analgesics, cathartics, or enemas or applying heat to the abdomen.

PROCEDURE

- The patient receives general anesthesia.
- The surgeon makes an incision in the right lower abdominal quadrant to expose the appendix.
- In laparoscopic appendectomy, three to four small abdominal incisions are made.
- The base of the appendix is ligated.
- A purse-string suture is placed in the cecum.
- Excessive fluid or tissue debris is removed from the abdominal cavity.
- If perforation occurs, one or more Penrose drains or abdominal sump tubes, or both, are placed before the incision is closed.
- The incision is closed.

POSTPROCEDURE CARE

- After anesthesia wears off, place the patient in Fowler's position.
- Ensure the patency of drainage catheters and tubes.
- Encourage the patient to ambulate as soon as possible.
- Encourage coughing, deep breathing, and frequent position changes.
- After NG tube removal, gradually resume oral intake.
- Assist with emergency treatment of peritonitis if needed.
- Monitor the patient's vital signs, intake and output, bowel sounds, surgical wounds and dressings, peritonitis, drainage, and complications related to infection, paralytic ileus, and peritonitis.
- Be sure to teach the patient about:
  - medications and possible adverse reactions
  - signs and symptoms of infection
  - signs and symptoms of intestinal obstruction
  - complications
  - when to notify the physician
  - wound care
  - activity restrictions
  - follow-up care.

Bowel resection with ostomy

DESCRIPTION

- Excision of diseased bowel and creation of a stoma on the outer abdominal wall to allow feces elimination
- Laparoscopic approach possible for both standard colostomy and end-ileostomy

PURPOSE

- To treat inflammatory bowel disease
- To treat familial adenomatous polyposis
- To treat diverticulitis
- To treat advanced colorectal cancer

PATIENT PREPARATION

- Make sure the patient has signed an appropriate consent form.
- Provide total parenteral nutrition as ordered.
- Administer antibiotics and other medications as ordered.
- Monitor the patient's vital signs, nutritional status, fluid and electrolyte status, intake and output, and daily weight.

PROCEDURE

- After the patient receives a general anesthetic, the surgeon makes an incision in the abdominal wall near the bowel area to be resected.
- The diseased bowel segment is resected, possibly along with several more inches of bowel.
- The surgeon creates a stoma.

Abdominoperineal resection

- A low abdominal incision is made, and the sigmoid colon is divided.
- The proximal end of the colon is brought out through another, smaller abdominal incision to create an end stoma.
- A wide perineal incision is made, and the anus, rectum, and distal portion of the sigmoid colon are resected.
- The abdominal wound is closed, and abdominal drains are placed.
- The perineal wound may be left open, packed with gauze, or closed; several Penrose drains are placed.

Ileostomy

- The surgeon resects all or part of the colon and rectum.

- A permanent ileostomy is created by bringing the end of the ileum out through a small abdominal incision in the right lower quadrant.

Ileoanal reservoir

- A colectomy is made, and a loop or an end stoma is created for a temporary ileostomy.
- The rectal mucosa is stripped, and an internal pouch is made with a portion of the ileum.
- A pouch-anal anastomosis is performed.
- A temporary ileostomy is made; usually, it's closed after 3 or 4 months.

Kock ileostomy

- The surgeon removes the colon, rectum, and anus and closes the anus.
- A reservoir is constructed from a loop of the terminal ileum.
- A portion of the ileum is intussuscepted to form a nipple valve.
- The upper part of the sutured and cut ileum is pulled down and sutured to form a pouch.
- The nipple valve is used to create a stoma by pulling it through the abdominal wall and suturing it flush with the skin.

POSTPROCEDURE CARE

- Provide meticulous wound care.
- Administer analgesics as ordered.
- After an abdominoperineal resection, irrigate the perineal area as ordered.
- If the patient has a Kock pouch with a catheter inserted in the stoma:
  - Connect the catheter to low intermittent suction or to straight drainage as ordered.
  - Check catheter patency regularly, and irrigate with 20 to 30 ml of normal saline solution as ordered.
  - Assess pouch drainage, and advance the patient's diet as ordered.
  - Clamp and unclamp the pouch catheter to increase its capacity as ordered.
- Encourage the patient to express feelings and concerns.

   ▶ **COLLABORATION** *Arrange for a consultation with an enterostomal therapist if possible. Arrange for the patient to meet with a patient who has adjusted well to an ostomy, if possible.*

- Monitor the patient's vital signs, intake and output, fluid and electrolyte imbalance, stoma drainage, and stoma appearance.
- Assess the patient for such potential complications as infection, peritonitis, ileus, sepsis, skin irritation and excoriation, pelvic abscess, incompetent nipple valve, and psychological problems.

ALERT *Immediately report excessive blood or mucus drain-ing from the stoma, which could indicate hemorrhage or in-fection.*

■ Refer the patient to appropriate community resources and support ser-vices, such as home care and ostomy product suppliers.
■ Be sure to teach the patient about:
  – what to expect for fecal drainage and bowel movement control
  – medications and possible adverse reactions
  – ostomy type and function
  – ostomy appliances
  – resumption of sexual intercourse
  – stoma and skin care
  – dietary restrictions
  – importance of a high fluid intake
  – avoidance of alcohol, laxatives, and diuretics
  – bowel retraining
  – sitz baths, after abdominoperineal resection
  – signs and symptoms of inflammation and infection
  – complications
  – when to notify the physician
  – follow-up care.

Cancer care

DESCRIPTION

■ Required for patients who have cancer

PURPOSE

■ To care for patients receiving cancer therapy

PATIENT PREPARATION

■ Explain the treatment and preparation to the patient and his family.
■ Make sure that the patient has signed an appropriate consent form.
■ Provide emotional support to the patient and his family.
■ Obtain a medical history.
■ Perform a physical assessment.
■ Review the diagnostic test results.
■ Assess the patient's nutritional status.
■ Assess the patient's rehabilitation needs and self-care ability.
■ Develop a care plan for managing symptoms.

IMMUNOTHERAPIES

Immunotherapies offer promise in treating cancer. Specific immunotherapies that have proved useful are discussed below.

■ *Nonspecific immunostimulation* uses biological agents, such as bacille Calmette-Guérin vaccine and *Corynebacterium parvum,* to stimulate the reticuloendothelial system. This therapy augments the patient's immune system and combats the immunosuppressive effects of cancer and its treatment.

■ *Intralesional stimulation* involves injecting a biological agent directly into the tumor. This initiates specific and nonspecific responses that trigger local cancer cell destruction.

■ *Active specific immunostimulation* uses specific tumor antigen vaccines that stimulate the immune system to control or reject malignant cells by producing antibodies and lymphocytes.

■ *Adoptive transfer of immunity* involves transferring immunologically active cells from a donor with established immunity to stimulate active immunity in the patient.

■ Identify the patient's long-term and short-term needs.
■ Administer pretreatment medications as ordered.

PROCEDURE

■ Treatment options depend on tumor type, stage, localization, and responsiveness and may include:
  – surgery
  – radiation
  – chemotherapy
  – hormone therapy
  – immunotherapy or biotherapy. (See *Immunotherapies.*)

POSTPROCEDURE CARE

■ Consult a dietitian.
■ Provide a diet high in protein, carbohydrates, and calories.
■ As indicated and ordered, provide total parenteral nutrition or deliver nutrition by nasogastric tube.
■ Provide adequate fluids.
■ Administer analgesics as ordered.
■ Implement noninvasive pain-relief techniques.
■ Explain palliative treatments if indicated.

- Assist the patient in developing effective coping strategies.
- Monitor the patient's vital signs, intake and output, daily weight, and ability to cope effectively.
- If radiation treatment was used, monitor the patient for complications such as weakness, fatigue, anorexia, anemia, nausea, vomiting, and diarrhea.
- If an antineoplastic was used, monitor the patient for complications such as bone marrow depression, GI epithelial cell irritation, destruction of hair follicles and skin cells, venous sclerosis, and deep cutaneous necrosis.
- If a biotherapeutic agent was used, monitor the patient for complications such as fever, flulike symptoms, fatigue, central nervous system effects, and capillary leakage syndrome.
- Refer the patient to the American Cancer Society, home care, or palliative or hospice care, as indicated.
- Be sure to teach the patient about:
  - medications and possible adverse reactions
  - complications
  - the prescribed diet
  - feeding tube care as indicated
  - parenteral nutrition as indicated
  - adverse effects of chemotherapy if indicated
  - noninvasive pain-relief techniques
  - cancer signs and symptoms (see *CAUTION: Cancer signs and symptoms*)
  - when to notify the physician
  - follow-up care.

CAUTION: CANCER SIGNS AND SYMPTOMS

Use *CAUTION*, the American Cancer Society's mnemonic device, to assess your patient for signs and symptoms of cancer.

- **C**hange in bowel or bladder habits
- **A** sore that doesn't heal
- **U**nusual bleeding or discharge
- **T**hickening or lump in the breast or elsewhere
- **I**ndigestion or difficulty swallowing
- **O**bvious change in a wart or mole
- **N**agging cough or hoarseness

Cholecystectomy

DESCRIPTION

- Surgical removal of the gallbladder
- May be performed as an open abdominal surgical procedure or as a laparoscopic procedure

PURPOSE

- To resolve gallbladder or biliary duct disease refractory to drug therapy, dietary changes, and other supportive treatments

PATIENT PREPARATION

- Explain the treatment and preparation to the patient and his family.
- Make sure the patient has signed an appropriate consent form.
- Withhold oral intake as ordered.
- Administer preoperative medications as ordered.

PROCEDURE

- Patients having either the open abdominal or the laparoscopic approach undergo general anesthesia.

Abdominal cholecystectomy

- A right subcostal or paramedial incision is made.
- The surgeon surveys the abdomen.
- Laparotomy packs are used to isolate the gallbladder from the surrounding organs.
- After biliary tract structures are identified, cholangiography or ultrasonography may be used to identify gallstones.
- The bile ducts are visualized using a choledoscope.
- The ducts are cleared of stones after insertion of a Fogarty balloon-tip catheter.
- The surgeon ligates and divides the cystic duct and artery and removes the entire gallbladder.
- A choledochotomy may be performed, with a T tube inserted into the common bile duct.
- A Penrose drain may be placed into the ducts.
- The incision is closed and a dressing is applied.

Laparoscopic cholecystectomy

- A small incision is made just above the umbilicus.
- Carbon dioxide or nitrous oxide is injected into the abdominal cavity.

- A trocar, connected to an insufflator, is inserted through the incision.
- A laparoscope is passed through the trocar to view the intra-abdominal contents.
- The patient is placed in a 30-degree reverse Trendelenburg position and tilted slightly to the left.
- With laparoscopic guidance, the surgeon makes three incisions in the right upper quadrant: one below the xiphoid process in the midline; one below the right costal margin in the midclavicular line; and one in the anterior axillary line at the umbilical level.
- Using the laparoscope, the surgeon passes instruments through the three incisions to clamp and tie off the cystic duct and excise the gallbladder.
- The gallbladder is removed through the umbilical opening.
- The surgeon sutures all four incisions and places a dressing over each.

POSTPROCEDURE CARE

- Administer medications as ordered.
- Place the patient in low Fowler's position.
- Attach the nasogastric (NG) tube to low intermittent suction as ordered.
- Report drainage greater than 500 ml after 48 hours.
- Provide meticulous skin care, especially around drainage tube insertion sites.
- After NG tube removal, introduce foods as ordered.
- Clamp the T tube before and after each meal as ordered.
- After laparoscopic cholecystectomy, start clear liquids as ordered when the patient has fully recovered from anesthesia.
- Assist with early ambulation.
- Encourage coughing and deep-breathing exercises.
- Encourage incentive spirometry use.
- Provide analgesics as ordered.
- Monitor the patient's vital signs, intake and output, respiratory status, amount and characteristics of drainage, surgical dressings, and position and patency of drainage tubes.
- Monitor the patient for complications such as peritonitis, postcholecystectomy syndrome, atelectasis, bile duct injury, small bowel injury, wound infection, ileus, urine retention, and retained gallstones.
- Be sure to teach the patient about:
  - medications and possible adverse reactions
  - coughing and deep-breathing exercises
  - tube home care if applicable
  - signs and symptoms of biliary obstruction
  - signs and symptoms of infection
  - complications

- when to notify the physician
- follow-up care.

■ If the abdominal approach is used, be sure to teach the patient that:
  - an NG tube will be in place for 1 to 2 days and an abdominal drain will be in place for 3 to 5 days after surgery
  - a T tube may remain in place for up to 2 weeks
  - the patient may be discharged with the T tube in place.

■ If the laparoscopic approach is used, be sure to teach the patient that:
  - an indwelling urinary catheter will be inserted into the bladder
  - an NG tube will be placed in the stomach
  - tubes are usually removed in the postanesthesia room
  - three small incisions will be covered with a small sterile dressing
  - discharge may occur on the day of surgery or 1 day after.

Conization

DESCRIPTION

■ Removal of a cone of tissue; most commonly referring to excision of the entire transformation zone and endocervical canal

PURPOSE

■ To diagnose or treat microinvasive cervical cancer
■ To investigate an abnormal Papanicolaou test result and remove abnormal cervical tissue

PATIENT PREPARATION

■ Explain the treatment and preparation to the patient and her family.
■ Make sure the patient has signed an appropriate consent form.
■ Provide emotional support.
■ Obtain results of diagnostic studies, medical history, and physical examination; notify the physician of any abnormalities.
■ Make sure the patient has fasted and used an enema preoperatively.
■ Administer I.V. fluids as ordered.

PROCEDURE

■ The patient receives a general or local anesthetic.
■ The surgeon uses carbon dioxide, a large hot loop, a scalpel, or a laser to cut a circular incision around the external os of the cervix.
■ A cone-shaped piece of tissue is removed.
■ Biopsies are taken at the apex of the cone.

- The cervix is sutured.
- Dilatation and curettage may be performed.

POSTPROCEDURE CARE

- Administer analgesics as ordered.
- Administer fluids as ordered.
- Provide the ordered diet as tolerated.

> **ALERT** *Be sure to report continuous, sharp abdominal pain that doesn't respond to analgesics, which may be a symptom of uterine perforation, a potentially life-threatening complication.*

- Monitor the patient's vital signs, intake and output, and vaginal drainage.
- Monitor the patient for complications such as uterine perforation, bleeding, infection, cervical stenosis, infertility, decreased cervical mucus, and cervical incompetence.
- Be sure to teach the patient about:
  - medications and possible adverse reactions
  - the possibility of postoperative abdominal cramping and pain in the pelvis and lower back
  - postoperative vaginal drainage
  - abnormal bleeding
  - signs and symptoms of infection
  - complications
  - when to notify the physician
  - follow-up care
  - the possibility of heavier-than-normal menses for the first two or three menstrual cycles after the procedure
  - avoidance of tampons, douches, or sexual intercourse until the physician permits it.

Gastric surgery

DESCRIPTION

- Surgery involving the stomach, the specific procedure depending on the location and extent of the disorder
- *Partial gastrectomy:* excision of part of the stomach
- *Bilateral vagotomy:* transection of the right and left vagus nerves, typically done to relieve ulcer symptoms and eliminate vagal nerve stimulation of gastric secretions
- *Pyloroplasty:* incision of the pylorus and reconstruction of the pyloric channel, typically done to relieve pyloric obstruction or speed gastric emptying after vagotomy

PURPOSE

- To treat chronic ulcer disease
- To treat cancer
- To treat pyloric obstruction
- To treat GI hemorrhage
- To treat perforated ulcer

PATIENT PREPARATION

- With emergency surgery, preparation may be limited.
- Explain the treatment and preparation to the patient and his family.
- Make sure the patient has signed an appropriate consent form.
- Stabilize the patient's fluid and electrolyte status as ordered.
- Obtain serum samples for hematologic studies.
- Begin I.V. fluid replacement and total parenteral nutrition (TPN).
- Prepare the patient for abdominal X-rays as ordered.
- Explain postoperative care and equipment.
- Monitor the patient's vital signs, intake and output, nutritional status, and appropriate laboratory test results.

PROCEDURE

- After the patient is anesthetized, an upper abdominal incision is performed.
- The stomach and part of the intestine are exposed.
- Total gastrectomy or removal of the entire stomach requires a more extensive incision.
- The rest of the procedure varies with the type of surgery.
- To complete the operation, the surgeon inserts abdominal drains and closes the incision.

POSTPROCEDURE CARE

- Administer medications as ordered.
- Place the patient in low or semi-Fowler's position.

  ALERT *Watch for hypotension, bradycardia, and respiratory changes. These findings may signal hemorrhage and shock.*

- Administer tube feedings or TPN as ordered.
- Administer I.V. fluid and electrolyte replacement therapy as ordered.
- Encourage coughing, deep breathing, use of incentive spirometry, and position changes.
- Monitor the patient's vital signs, intake and output, nutritional status, laboratory test results, surgical wound site and dressings, fluid and electrolyte imbalance, bowel sounds, and respiratory status.

■ Monitor the patient for complications such as hemorrhage, obstruction, dumping syndrome, paralytic ileus, perforation, vitamin B_{12} deficiency, anemia, and atelectasis.

ALERT *Watch for and report weakness, nausea, flatulence, and palpitations occurring within 30 minutes after a meal. These findings suggest that the patient has dumping syndrome.*

■ Be sure to teach the patient about:
  – medications and possible adverse reactions
  – abnormal bleeding
  – signs and symptoms of infection
  – signs and symptoms of obstruction or perforation
  – complications
  – when to notify the physician
  – coughing and deep-breathing exercises
  – splinting of the incision
  – surgical wound care
  – dumping syndrome and its prevention
  – dietary restrictions
  – tube feedings procedure and treatment, if appropriate
  – stress-management techniques
  – smoking cessation, if indicated.

Hernia repair

DESCRIPTION

■ May involve herniorrhaphy, which returns the protruding intestine to the abdominal cavity and repairs an abdominal wall defect
■ May involve hernioplasty, which reinforces the weakened area around the repair with plastic, steel or tantalum mesh, or wire
■ Laparoscopic repair typical for uncomplicated hernias
■ Usually done on an elective basis, but emergency surgery necessary for a strangulated or incarcerated hernia

PURPOSE

■ To treat groin hernias and hernias of the anterior abdominal wall

PATIENT PREPARATION

■ Explain the treatment and preparation to the patient and his family.
■ Make sure the patient has signed an appropriate consent form.
■ Explain postoperative care.
■ Shave the surgical site as ordered.

- Administer an enema as ordered.
- Administer a sedative as ordered.

PROCEDURE

- General or spinal anesthesia is used.
- The surgeon makes an incision over the herniated area.
- The herniated tissue is manipulated back to its proper position.
- The defect in the muscle or fascia is repaired.
- If necessary, the defect is reinforced with wire, mesh, or another material.
- The incision is closed and a dressing applied.

POSTPROCEDURE CARE

- Administer medications as ordered.
- Reduce pressure on the incision site.
- Take measures to prevent constipation.
- Encourage early ambulation.
- Make sure the patient voids within 12 hours after surgery; if necessary, insert a urinary catheter or assist with insertion.
- Provide comfort measures.
- Apply an ice bag to the scrotum if appropriate.
- Apply a scrotal bridge or truss if appropriate.
- Monitor the patient's vital signs, intake and output, surgical wound and dressings, and drainage.
- Monitor the patient for complications, such as infection and bleeding.
- Refer the patient to a weight reduction program if indicated.
- Refer the patient to a smoking-cessation program if indicated.
- Be sure to teach the patient about:
  - medications and possible adverse reactions
  - activity restrictions
  - incision care
  - signs and symptoms of infection
  - complications of hernia recurrence and transient voiding problems
  - when to notify the physician
  - follow-up care
  - possible need for a job change if the patient regularly does heavy lifting or other strenuous activities
  - signs and symptoms of hernia recurrence
  - hernia prevention
  - use of scrotal support or ice packs in males
  - a high-fiber diet
  - adequate oral fluid intake.

Hysterectomy

DESCRIPTION

- Surgical removal of the uterus
- May be performed abdominally, vaginally, or through a laparoscope
- When done laparoscopically, allows the surgeon to perform preparatory steps before removing the uterus through the vagina
- *Subtotal hysterectomy:* removal of the entire uterus except the cervix
- *Total hysterectomy:* removal of both the uterus and cervix
- *Panhysterectomy:* removal of the entire uterus, ovaries, and fallopian tubes
- *Radical hysterectomy:* removal of the uterus, ovaries, fallopian tubes, adjoining ligaments and lymph nodes, upper one-third of the vagina, and surrounding tissues

PURPOSE

- To treat malignant or benign tumor of the uterus, cervix, or adnexa
- To treat uterine bleeding and hemorrhage
- To treat uterine rupture or perforation
- To treat life-threatening pelvic infection
- To treat endometriosis unresponsive to conservative treatment
- To treat pelvic floor relaxation or prolapse

PATIENT PREPARATION

- Explain the treatment and preparation to the patient and her family.
- Make sure the patient has signed an appropriate consent form.
- Administer an enema the evening before surgery.
- Administer prophylactic antibiotics as ordered.
- Make sure laboratory tests have been performed, including a pregnancy test if indicated; report abnormal results.
- Institute deep vein thrombosis prophylaxis as ordered.
- Teach the patient what to expect. If the patient will have an abdominal hysterectomy, explain that an indwelling catheter or suprapubic tube as well as a nasogastric or rectal tube, may be inserted.

PROCEDURE

- The patient receives general anesthesia.

Abdominal approach

- A midline vertical incision is made from the umbilicus to the symphysis pubis or a horizontal incision is made in the lower abdomen.
- The uterus and accompanying structures are excised and removed.
- The incision is closed, and a dressing and perineal pad are applied.

Vaginal approach

- An incision is made above the vagina near the cervix.
- The uterus is excised and removed through the vaginal canal.
- The opening is closed to the peritoneal cavity with sutures.
- A perineal pad is applied.

Laparoscopic approach

- An incision is made in the umbilicus.
- Nitrous oxide or carbon dioxide is infused into the abdominal cavity.
- The patient is placed in Trendelenburg's position.
- The laparoscope is inserted.
- Several other small abdominal incisions are made to pass instruments.
- The uterus is excised vaginally, along with other accompanying structures as necessary.
- The incision is closed, and a dressing and perineal pad are applied.

POSTPROCEDURE CARE

- Administer medications as ordered.
- Provide indwelling urinary catheter or suprapubic catheter care if appropriate.
- Provide perineal care.
- Notify the physician if the patient saturates more than one pad every 4 hours.
- Encourage the patient to cough, breathe deeply, and turn at least every 2 hours.
- Administer I.V. fluids as ordered.
- Withhold oral intake status until peristalsis returns.
- Keep the patient in a supine position, low Fowler's, or semi-Fowler's position as ordered.
- Assist with early ambulation.
- Encourage the patient to perform prescribed exercises.
- Monitor the patient's vital signs, intake and output, vaginal drainage, surgical wound and dressings, abnormal bleeding, bowel sounds, respiratory status, and pain management.
- Monitor the patient for complications such as wound infection, urine retention, abdominal distention, thromboembolism, atelectasis, pneumo-

nia, hemorrhage, ureteral or bowel injury, wound dehiscence, pulmonary embolism, paralytic ileus, and psychological problems.

■ Be sure to teach the patient about:
  – medications and possible adverse reactions
  – coughing and deep-breathing exercises
  – use of incentive spirometry
  – signs and symptoms of infection
  – complications
  – when to notify the physician
  – activity restrictions, including sexual activity
  – early ambulation
  – avoidance of tub baths, douching, and sexual activity until after the 6-week checkup
  – importance of a high-protein, high-residue diet
  – increased oral fluid intake (3,000 ml/day) as ordered
  – follow-up care
  – wound care
  – pain management
  – potential abdominal cramping and expected drainage
  – estrogen replacement therapy, if indicated.

Implantable cardioverter-defibrillator

DESCRIPTION

■ An implantable electronic device that monitors the heart for bradycardia, ventricular tachycardia, and fibrillation and delivers shocks or paced beats when indicated
■ Stores information and electrocardiograms (ECGs) and tracks treatments and their outcome
■ Allows information retrieval to evaluate the device's function and battery status and to adjust the settings
■ Depending on the model, may deliver bradycardia pacing, antitachycardia pacing, cardioversion, and defibrillation
■ Also called an *ICD*

PURPOSE

■ To treat cardiac arrhythmias such as atrial fibrillation that are refractory to drug therapy, surgery, or catheter ablation

PATIENT PREPARATION

■ Explain the preparation, treatment, and postoperative care.

- Make sure the patient has signed an appropriate consent form.
- Obtain baseline vital signs and a 12-lead ECG.
- Evaluate the patient's radial and pedal pulses.
- Assess the patient's mental status.
- Restrict food and fluids before the procedure as ordered.
- If the patient is monitored, document and report any arrhythmias.
- Administer medications as ordered, and prepare to assist with medical procedures, such as defibrillation, if indicated.

PROCEDURE

- The following methods may be used:
  - transvenous route with fluoroscopy
  - thoracotomy approach, for patients who have mediastinal adhesions from previous sternal surgery
  - subxiphoid approach
  - median sternotomy, for patients who need other cardiac surgery such as revascularization.
- One or more leadwires are attached to the epicardium.
- A programmable pulse generator is inserted into a pocket made under the right or left clavicle.
- The device is programmed and checked for proper functioning.

POSTPROCEDURE CARE

- Obtain a printed status report verifying the ICD type and model, status, detection rates, and therapies to be delivered, such as pacing, antitachycardia pacing, cardioversion, and defibrillation.
- Don't remove the occlusive dressing for the first 24 hours without a physician's order.
- After the first 24 hours, begin passive range-of-motion exercises if ordered, and progress as tolerated.
- If the patient experiences cardiac arrest, initiate cardiopulmonary resuscitation and advanced cardiac life support.

ALERT *For external defibrillation, use anteroposterior paddle placement; don't place paddles directly over the pulse generator.*

- Monitor the patient's vital signs, intake and output, heart rate and rhythm, surgical incision and dressings, and drainage.
- Monitor the patient for complications such as infection, venous thrombosis and embolism, pneumothorax, pectoral or diaphragmatic muscle stimulation, arrhythmias, cardiac tamponade, heart failure, lead dislodgment,

and ICD malfunction resulting in untreated ventricular fibrillation and cardiac arrest.

ALERT *Monitor the patient for signs and symptoms of a per- forated ventricle with resultant cardiac tamponade. Find- ings may include persistent hiccups, distant heart sounds, pulsus paradoxus, hypotension accompanied by narrow pulse pressure, in- creased venous pressure, jugular vein distention, cyanosis, de- creased urine output, restlessness, and complaints of fullness in the chest. Notify the physician immediately, and prepare the patient for emergency surgery.*

■ Be sure to teach the patient about:
  – medications and possible adverse reactions
  – signs and symptoms of infection
  – complications
  – when to notify the physician
  – importance of wearing medical alert identification that indicates ICD placement and of carrying ICD information at all times
  – what to do in an emergency, such as calling 911 and having a family member perform cardiopulmonary resuscitation if the ICD fails
  – avoidance of placing excessive pressure over the insertion site or mov- ing or jerking the area, until the physician approves
  – prescribed activity restrictions
  – what to expect when the ICD discharges
  – notifying the physician when the ICD discharges
  – importance of informing airline personnel and health care workers who perform diagnostic tests (such as computed tomography scans and magnetic resonance imaging) of ICD presence
  – possible disruption of the ICD by electrical or electronic devices
  – follow-up care.

Joint replacement

DESCRIPTION

■ Total or partial replacement of a joint with a synthetic prosthesis
■ Restores joint mobility and stability and relieves pain
■ May involve any joint except a spinal joint
■ Most commonly involves the hip, knee, and shoulder (see *Arthroplasty variations*, page 308)
■ Also called *arthroplasty*

ARTHROPLASTY VARIATIONS

Arthroplasty, the surgical reconstruction or replacement of a joint, is done to restore mobility of the joint and function to the muscles and ligaments. Other than total joint replacement, types of arthroplastic surgery include joint resection and interpositional reconstruction.

Joint resection involves removing a portion of the bone from a stiffened joint, creating a gap between the bone and the socket, to improve the range of motion. Scar tissue eventually fills this gap. Although pain is relieved and motion is restored, the joint is less stable.

Interpositional reconstruction involves reshaping the joint and placing a prosthetic disk between the reshaped bony ends forming the joint. The prosthesis may be made of metal, plastic, skin, or body tissue such as fascia. However, with repeated injury and surgical reshaping, the patient eventually may need total joint replacement.

In recent years, joint replacement has become the operation of choice for most knee and hip problems. Elbow, shoulder, ankle, and finger joints are more likely to be treated with joint resection or interpositional reconstruction.

PURPOSE

■ To treat severe chronic arthritis
■ To treat degenerative joint disorders
■ To treat extensive joint trauma

PATIENT PREPARATION

■ Make sure the patient has signed an appropriate consent form.
■ Reassure the patient that analgesics will be available as needed.
■ Provide emotional support.

PROCEDURE

The procedure varies slightly depending on the joint and its condition.

■ The patient is placed in the appropriate position and receives a regional or general anesthetic.
■ An incision is made to expose the affected joint.
■ The joint capsule is incised or excised as indicated.
■ The joint is dislocated to expose all parts of the affected joint as indicated.
■ The intact bone of one side of the joint is shaped and reamed to accept the prosthetic part.
■ The device is secured in place by cement, press fit, or bone ingrowth.
■ Polymethylmethacrylate adhesive is used to secure the device in place if the prosthesis is cemented.

- The process is repeated for the other side of the joint.
- After the prosthetic parts are in place, the surgeon fits them together to restore the joint.
- The incision is closed in layers and a dressing is applied.

POSTPROCEDURE CARE

- Administer medications as ordered.
- Maintain bed rest for the prescribed period.
- Maintain the affected joint in proper alignment.
- Assess the patient's pain level and provide analgesics as ordered.
- Change dressings as ordered.
- Reposition the patient frequently.
- Encourage frequent coughing and deep breathing.
- Encourage adequate fluid intake.
- Exercise the affected joint as ordered.
- If joint displacement occurs, notify the physician.
- If traction is used to correct joint displacement, periodically check weights and other equipment.
- Monitor the patient's vital signs, intake and output, surgical wound and dressings, drainage, abnormal bleeding, respiratory status, and neurovascular status of the affected extremity.
- Monitor for complications such as infection, hypovolemic shock, fat embolism, thromboembolism, pulmonary embolism (PE), nerve compromise, prosthesis dislocation or loosening, heterotrophic ossification, avascular necrosis, atelectasis, pneumonia, and deep vein thrombosis (DVT).
- Be sure to teach the patient about:
  - medications and possible adverse reactions
  - signs and symptoms of infection
  - signs and symptoms of joint dislodgment
  - complications
  - when to notify the physician
  - incision care
  - follow-up care
  - signs and symptoms of DVT and PE
  - the need to follow a prescribed exercise regimen as directed by a physical therapist
  - prescribed activity restrictions
  - range-of-motion exercises and use of a continuous passive motion device as appropriate
  - infective endocarditis prophylaxis.
- After hip replacement, be sure to teach the patient about:
  - importance of maintaining hip abduction

- avoidance of crossing legs when sitting
- avoidance of flexing hips more than 90 degrees when rising from a bed or chair
- using a chair with high arms and a firm seat
- importance of sleeping on a firm mattress
- the proper use of crutches or a cane.
■ After shoulder joint replacement, be sure to teach the patient about:
- importance of keeping the affected arm in a sling until postoperative swelling subsides.

Laminectomy and spinal fusion

DESCRIPTION

■ *Laminectomy:* removal of one or more of the bony laminae that cover the vertebrae; typically done to relieve pressure on the spinal cord or spinal nerve roots
■ *Spinal fusion:* grafting of bone chips between the vertebral spaces to stabilize the spine; it follows laminectomy
■ Spinal fusion used when more conservative treatments, such as prolonged bed rest, traction, and use of a back brace, prove ineffective
■ *Percutaneous diskectomy:* alternative to laminectomy for decompressing and repairing damaged lumbar disks (see *Laminectomy alternative*)

PURPOSE

■ To treat herniated disk
■ To treat compression fracture
■ To treat vertebral dislocation
■ To treat spinal cord tumor
■ To treat vertebrae seriously weakened by trauma or disease

PATIENT PREPARATION

■ Make sure the patient has signed an appropriate consent form.
■ Perform a baseline assessment of motor function and sensation.
■ Show the patient how to perform the logrolling method of turning, and explain that he'll use this technique later to get in and out of bed by himself.

PROCEDURE

■ The patient receives a general anesthetic and is placed in a prone position.

LAMINECTOMY ALTERNATIVE

Percutaneous (endoscopic) diskectomy is an alternative to traditional surgery for a herniated disk. In this technique, the physician uses arthroscopy with suction and X-ray visualization to insert a small instrument to remove only the disk portion that's causing pain.

Typically used for smaller, less-severe disk abnormalities, percutaneous automated diskectomy, a slightly different method in which a needle is placed instead of the small instrument, has only a 50% success rate, perhaps because the operative site isn't visualized directly. One report indicates a high incidence of postoperative diskitis.

Nursing care after diskectomy resembles postlaminectomy care. Typically, the patient is allowed out of bed in 24 to 48 hours and is encouraged to walk without assistance as soon as possible.

Laminectomy
■ A midline vertical incision is made.
■ The fascia and muscles are stripped off the bony laminae.
■ One or more sections of laminae are removed to expose the spinal defect.

Herniated disk
■ Part or all of the disk is removed.

Spinal cord tumor
■ The dura is incised, and the cord is explored for metastasis.
■ The tumor is dissected and removed, using suction, forceps, or dissecting scissors.

Spinal fusion
■ The surgeon exposes the affected vertebrae.
■ Bone chips from the iliac crest, bone bank, or both are inserted.
■ Wire, spinal plates, rods, or screws are used to secure bone grafts into several vertebrae surrounding the unstable area.
■ The incision is closed and a dressing is applied.
■ External traction, such as a halo device, may be applied if surgery involved the cervical spine.

POSTPROCEDURE CARE
■ Administer medications as ordered.
■ Keep the head of the bed flat or elevated no more than 45 degrees for at least 24 hours after surgery.

- Urge the patient to remain in a supine position for the prescribed period.
- When the patient can lie on his side, make sure the spine is straight, with his knees flexed and drawn up toward his chest.
- Insert a pillow between the patient's knees.
- Assist the surgeon with the initial dressing change.
- If the patient doesn't void within 8 to 12 hours after surgery, notify the physician, and prepare to insert a urinary catheter (or assist with insertion).
- If the patient can void normally, provide assistance in getting on and off the bedpan while maintaining proper body alignment.
- Monitor the patient's vital signs, intake and output, surgical wound and dressings, drainage, abnormal bleeding, cerebrospinal fluid leakage, motor and neurologic function, peripheral vascular status, bowel sounds, and respiratory status.
- Be sure to teach the patient about:
  - medications and possible adverse reactions
  - incision care
  - signs and symptoms of infection
  - complications related to herniation relapse, arachnoiditis, chronic neuritis, nerve or muscle damage
  - when to notify the physician
  - showering with his back facing away from the stream of water
  - prescribed activity restrictions
  - prescribed exercises
  - proper body mechanics
  - avoidance of lying on his stomach or on his back with legs flat
  - sitting up straight with his feet on a low stool
  - using a firm, straight-backed chair
  - alternating placing each foot on a low stool
  - sleeping only on a firm mattress or inserting a bed board between the mattress and box spring
  - postoperative and follow-up care
  - pain relief, after chronic nerve irritation and swelling subside
  - availability of analgesics and muscle relaxants

Laparoscopy and laparotomy

DESCRIPTION

- *Laparoscopy,* also called *pelvic peritoneoscopy:* insertion of a laparoscope through the abdominal wall near the umbilicus
- *Laparotomy:* a general term for any surgical incision made into the ab-

dominal wall; called an *exploratory laparotomy* when the extent of abdominal injury or disease is unknown

PURPOSE

■ To examine the pelvic cavity and repair or remove diseased or injured structures

Laparoscopy
■ To allow for certain abdominal surgical procedures, such as:
    – cholecystectomy
    – tubal ligation
    – ovarian cyst aspiration
    – ovarian biopsy
    – graafian follicle aspiration
    – cauterization of endometrial implants
    – oophorectomy
    – salpingectomy
■ To resolve lysis of adhesions
■ To detect abnormalities, such as cysts, adhesions, fibroids, and infection
■ To identify the cause of pelvic pain
■ To diagnose endometriosis, ectopic pregnancy, or pelvic inflammatory disease
■ To evaluate pelvic masses
■ To examine the fallopian tubes in an infertile patient

Laparotomy
■ To allow extensive surgical repair
■ To treat pelvic conditions untreatable by laparoscopy
■ To resect ovarian cysts containing endometrial tissue

PATIENT PREPARATION

■ Make sure the patient has signed an appropriate consent form.
■ Restrict food and fluids as ordered.
■ Obtain laboratory results and report abnormal findings to the physician.

PROCEDURE

Laparoscopy
■ The patient receives regional or general anesthesia.
■ The patient is placed in the lithotomy position.
■ A needle is inserted below the umbilicus, and carbon dioxide is infused into the pelvic cavity.
■ An infra-umbilical incision is made, and a trocar and cannula are inserted.

- The trocar is removed, and the laparoscope is inserted through the cannula.
- The pelvic cavity is visualized, and additional instruments are inserted through a second small incision close to the infra-umbilical incision, or they may be passed through the laparoscope.
- Carbon dioxide is removed.
- The incision is sutured and a dressing is applied.

Laparotomy
- The patient receives general anesthesia.
- An abdominal incision is made, and the abdominal cavity is explored.
- Necessary repairs or excisions are made.
- The incision is sutured, and a sterile dressing is applied.

POSTPROCEDURE CARE
- Administer medications as ordered.
- Assess for abdominal pain and, if the patient had a laparoscopy, for abdominal cramps or shoulder pain.
- Provide comfort measures.
- Explain that bloating or abdominal fullness from laparoscopy will subside as gas is absorbed.
- Monitor the patient's vital signs, intake and output, surgical wound and dressings, drainage, and signs of infection as well as for such complications as infection and hemorrhage.
- Be sure to teach the patient about:
  - medications and possible adverse reactions
  - coughing and deep-breathing exercises
  - use of incentive spirometry
  - incision care
  - signs and symptoms of infection
  - complications
  - when to notify the physician
  - prescribed activity restrictions
  - follow-up care.

Mastectomy

DESCRIPTION
- Breast excision done primarily to remove malignant breast tissue and regional lymphatic metastasis
- May involve one of various procedures (see *Types of mastectomy*)

TYPES OF MASTECTOMY

The type of mastectomy performed depends on the extent of tissue and lymph node involvement.

- A *lumpectomy (partial mastectomy)* or a *total (simple) mastectomy* may be done if the tumor is confined to breast tissue and no lymph node involvement is detected. A total mastectomy also may be used palliatively for advanced, ulcerative cancer and to treat extensive benign disease.
- *Modified radical mastectomy*—the standard surgery for stages I and II breast cancer—removes small, localized tumors. It has replaced radical mastectomy as the most widely used breast cancer surgery. Besides causing less disfigurement than radical mastectomy, it reduces postoperative arm edema and shoulder problems.
- *Radical mastectomy* controls the spread of larger, metastatic lesions. Later, breast reconstruction may be performed using a portion of the latissimus dorsi.
- *Extended radical mastectomy* is used to treat cancer in the medial quadrant of the breast or in subareolar tissue. This rare procedure may prevent metastasis to the internal mammary lymph nodes.

- May be combined with radiation and chemotherapy

PURPOSE

- To treat breast cancer

PATIENT PREPARATION

- Make sure the patient has signed an appropriate consent form.
- Take baseline arm measurements on both sides.
- Provide emotional support.

PROCEDURE

Total mastectomy

- The entire breast is removed without dissecting the lymph nodes.
- A skin graft may be applied if necessary.

Modified radical mastectomy

- Axillary lymph nodes are resected while the pectoralis major is left intact.
- The pectoralis minor may be removed.
- If the patient has small lesions and no metastasis, breast reconstruction may follow immediately or a few days later.

Radical mastectomy

- The entire breast, axillary lymph nodes, underlying pectoral muscles, and adjacent tissues are removed.
- Skin flaps and exposed tissue are covered with moist packs.
- The chest wall and axilla are irrigated before closure.

Extended radical mastectomy

- The breast, underlying pectoral muscles, axillary contents, and upper internal mammary (mediastinal) lymph node chain are removed.
- After closure of the mastectomy site, a drain or catheter may be inserted.
- Large pressure dressings may be applied if a drain isn't inserted.

POSTPROCEDURE CARE

- Administer medications as ordered.
- Elevate the patient's affected arm on a pillow.
- Regularly check the suction tubing to ensure proper functioning.
- Initiate flexion and extension arm exercises as ordered.
- Place a sign in the patient's room indicating that no blood pressure readings, injections, or venipunctures should be performed on the affected arm.
- Gently encourage the patient to look at the operative site.
- Encourage her to express her feelings.
- Arrange a fitting for a temporary breast pad after 2 to 3 days.
- Monitor the patient's vital signs, intake and output, surgical wound and dressings, drainage, and emotional response.
- Monitor the patient for complications such as infection, delayed healing, lymphedema, and change in self-concept.
- Refer the patient to the American Cancer Society and Reach to Recovery.
- Be sure to teach the patient about:
  - medications and possible adverse reactions
  - signs and symptoms of infection
  - complications
  - when to notify the physician
  - ways to prevent infection
  - importance of using the affected arm as much as possible
  - range-of-motion exercises and other postoperative exercises
  - temporary breast prosthesis as needed
  - avoidance of blood pressure readings, injections, and venipunctures on the affected arm
  - avoidance of keeping the affected arm in a dependent position for a prolonged period

- protecting the affected arm from injury
- adequate rest periods
- monthly breast self-examinations
- follow-up care, including chemotherapy, hormonal therapy, or relaxation therapy
- permanent prosthesis, which can be fitted 3 to 4 weeks after surgery.

Prostatectomy

DESCRIPTION

- Surgical removal of the prostate
- *Transurethral resection of the prostate:* prostate removal via insertion of a resectoscope into the urethra
- May be performed by an open surgical approach, such as suprapubic prostatectomy, retropubic prostatectomy, or perineal prostatectomy

PURPOSE

- To treat prostate cancer
- To treat obstructive benign prostatic hyperplasia

PATIENT PREPARATION

- Make sure the patient has signed an appropriate consent form.
- Administer an enema.
- Restrict foods and fluids as ordered.

PROCEDURE

Transurethral resection of the prostate

- The patient is placed in a lithotomy position and anesthetized.
- The surgeon introduces a resectoscope into the urethra and advances it to the prostate.
- A clear irrigating solution is instilled, and the obstruction is visualized.
- The resectoscope's cutting loop is used to resect prostatic tissue and restore the urethral opening.

Suprapubic prostatectomy

- The patient is placed in a supine position and anesthetized.
- A horizontal incision is made just above the pubic symphysis.
- Fluid is instilled into the bladder.
- A small incision is made in the bladder wall to expose the prostate.
- The surgeon shells out prostatic tissue with a finger.

- The obstruction is cleared and bleeding points are ligated.
- A suprapubic drainage tube and Penrose drain are inserted.

Retropubic prostatectomy

- The patient is placed in a supine position and anesthetized.
- A horizontal suprapubic incision is made.
- The prostate is approached from between the bladder and pubic arch.
- Another incision is made in the prostatic capsule, and the obstructing tissue is removed.
- Bleeding is controlled.
- A suprapubic tube and Penrose drain are inserted.

Perineal prostatectomy

- The patient is placed in an exaggerated lithotomy position and anesthetized.
- The surgeon makes an inverted U-shaped incision in the perineum.
- The entire prostate is removed, along with the seminal vesicles.
- The urethra is anastomosed to the bladder.
- The incision is closed, leaving a Penrose drain in place.

POSTPROCEDURE CARE

- Administer medications as ordered.

   ALERT *Never administer medication rectally in a patient who has had a total prostatectomy.*

- Maintain urinary catheter and suprapubic tube patency as ordered.
- Keep the urine collection container below the bladder level.
- Administer antispasmodics and analgesics as ordered.
- Offer sitz baths.

    COLLABORATION *Arrange for psychological and sexual counseling as needed.*

   ALERT *Watch for and report signs and symptoms of dilutional hyponatremia, such as altered mental status, muscle twitching, and seizures.*

- Monitor the patient's vital signs, intake and output, urine characteristics, surgical wound and dressings, drainage, and fluid and electrolyte status.
- Monitor the patient for such complications as hemorrhage, infection, urine retention, urinary incontinence, and impotence.

   ALERT *Watch for and report signs and symptoms of epididymitis, including fever, chills, groin pain, and a swollen, tender epididymis.*

- Be sure to teach the patient about:

- medications and possible adverse reactions
- incision care
- signs and symptoms of infection and abnormal bleeding
- complications
- when to notify the physician
- importance of drinking ten 8-oz glasses of water daily and urinating at least every 2 hours
- likelihood of experiencing transient urinary frequency and dribbling after catheter removal
- how to perform Kegel exercises
- avoidance of caffeine-containing beverages
- prescribed activity restrictions
- sitz baths
- follow-up care
- annual prostate-specific antigen testing.

Thoracotomy

DESCRIPTION

- Surgical incision into the thoracic cavity, most commonly performed to remove part or all of a lung and thus spare healthy lung tissue from disease
- May involve pneumonectomy, lobectomy, segmental resection, or wedge resection
- *Exploratory thoracotomy:* done to evaluate the chest and pleural space for chest trauma and tumors
- *Decortication:* removal or stripping of the fibrous membrane covering the visceral pleura; helps reexpand the lung in empyema
- *Thoracoplasty:* removes part or all of one rib to reduce chest cavity size, decreasing the risk of mediastinal shift; may be done when tuberculosis has reduced lung volume

PURPOSE

- To locate and examine thoracic abnormalities
- To perform a biopsy
- To remove diseased lung tissue

PATIENT PREPARATION

- Make sure the patient has signed an appropriate consent form.
- Arrange for laboratory studies and tests; report abnormal results.
- Withhold food and fluids as ordered.

PROCEDURE

- The patient is anesthetized.
- In a *posterolateral thoracotomy*, the incision starts in the submammary fold of the anterior chest, is drawn below the scapular tip and along the ribs, and then curves posteriorly and up to the scapular spine.
- In an *anterolateral thoracotomy*, the incision begins below the breast and above the costal margins, extending from the anterior axillary line and then turning downward to avoid the axillary apex.
- In a *median sternotomy*, a straight incision is made from the suprasternal notch to below the xiphoid process; the sternum must be transected with an electric or air-driven saw.
- Once the incision is made, the surgeon removes tissue for a biopsy.
- Bleeding sources are tied off.
- Injuries within the thoracic cavity are located and repaired.
- The ribs may be spread and the lung exposed for excision.

Pneumonectomy
- The surgeon ligates and severs the pulmonary arteries.
- The mainstem bronchus leading to the affected lung is clamped.
- The bronchus is divided and closed with nonabsorbable sutures or staples.
- The lung is removed.
- To ensure airtight closure, a pleural flap is placed over the bronchus and closed.
- The phrenic nerve is severed on the affected side.
- After air pressure in the pleural cavity stabilizes, the chest is closed.

Lobectomy
- The surgeon resects the affected lobe.
- Appropriate arteries, veins, and bronchial passages are ligated and severed.
- One or two chest tubes are inserted for drainage and lung reexpansion.

Segmental resection
- The surgeon removes the affected lung segment.
- The appropriate artery, vein, and bronchus are ligated and severed.
- Two chest tubes are inserted to aid lung reexpansion.

Wedge resection
- The affected area is clamped, excised, and sutured.
- The surgeon inserts two chest tubes to aid lung reexpansion.

■ After completing the procedure requiring the thoracotomy, the surgeon closes the chest cavity and applies a dressing.

POSTPROCEDURE CARE

■ Administer medications as ordered.
■ After pneumonectomy, make sure the patient lies only on the operative side or his back until stabilized.
■ Make sure chest tubes are patent and functioning.
■ Provide comfort measures.
■ Encourage coughing, deep breathing, and incentive spirometry use.
■ Have the patient splint the incision as needed.
■ Perform passive range-of-motion (ROM) exercises, progressing to active ROM exercises.
■ Perform incision care and dressing changes as ordered.
■ Monitor the patient's vital signs, intake and output, respiratory status, breath sounds, surgical wound and dressings, and drainage.
■ Monitor patient for complications such as hemorrhage, infection, tension pneumothorax, bronchopleural fistula, empyema, and persistent air space that the remaining lung tissue doesn't expand to fill.

ALERT *Watch for and immediately report dyspnea, chest pain, hypotension, irritating cough, vertigo, syncope, anxiety, subcutaneous emphysema, or tracheal deviation from the midline. These findings indicate tension pneumothorax.*

■ Refer the patient to home health care as needed.
■ Refer the patient to a smoking-cessation program, if needed.
■ Be sure to teach the patient about:
  – medications and possible adverse reactions
  – coughing and deep-breathing techniques
  – incentive spirometry
  – incision care and dressing changes
  – signs and symptoms of infection
  – complications
  – when to notify the physician
  – monitoring of sputum characteristics
  – ROM exercises
  – prescribed physical activity restrictions
  – ways to prevent infection
  – wound care and dressing change care
  – postoperative and follow-up care.

Thrombolytic therapy

DESCRIPTION

- Administration of a thrombolytic, such as streptokinase (Streptase), alteplase (Activase), anistreplase (Eminase), or reteplase (Retavase), to rapidly correct acute and extensive thrombotic disorders
- Involves conversion of plasminogen to plasmin by thrombolytics, which leads to lysis of thrombi, fibrinogen, and other plasma proteins

PURPOSE

- To treat thromboembolic disorders
- To treat deep vein thrombosis
- To treat peripheral arterial occlusion
- To treat acute myocardial infarction
- To treat acute pulmonary emboli
- To treat failing or failed atrioventricular fistulas

PATIENT PREPARATION

- Make sure the patient has signed an appropriate consent form.
- Obtain samples for blood typing and crossmatching and for coagulation studies.
- Obtain a baseline electrocardiogram and serum electrolyte, arterial blood gas, blood urea nitrogen, creatinine, and cardiac enzyme levels as ordered.

PROCEDURE

- The thrombolytic is usually given by I.V. bolus, with I.V. infusion given at a specific rate in a separate I.V. line.
- Some thrombolytics are given by intracoronary infusion.
- The thrombolytic can also be given locally or directly into the thrombus.

POSTPROCEDURE CARE

- Administer medications as ordered.
- Minimize invasive procedures and venipunctures.
- Administer anticoagulants as ordered.
- Provide comfort measures.
- Provide supplemental oxygen as ordered.
- Restrict physical activity as ordered.
- Monitor patient's vital signs, intake and output, hypersensitivity reactions, heart rate and rhythm, peripheral pulses, motor and sensory function, and respiratory status.

- Monitor the patient for complications, such as bleeding, adverse reactions to the thrombolytic, streptokinase resistance, and arrhythmias.
- Be sure to teach the patient about:
  - medications and possible adverse reactions
  - abnormal bleeding
  - signs and symptoms of thrombus formation and thromboembolic events
  - complications
  - when to notify the physician
  - prevention of thrombotic events
  - smoking cessation, if indicated
  - postoperative and follow-up care.

Thyroidectomy

DESCRIPTION

- Surgical removal of all or part of the thyroid gland

PURPOSE

- To resolve hyperthyroidism or respiratory obstruction caused by goiter
- To treat thyroid cancer

PATIENT PREPARATION

- Make sure the patient has signed an appropriate consent form.
- Make sure the patient has followed the preoperative drug regimen as ordered.
- Collect blood samples for serum thyroid hormone measurement.
- Obtain a 12-lead electrocardiogram.

PROCEDURE

- The patient is anesthetized.
- The surgeon extends the patient's neck fully and determines the incision line by measuring bilaterally from each clavicle.
- The surgeon cuts through the skin, fascia, and muscle and raises skin flaps from the strap muscles.
- The muscles are separated at midline, revealing the isthmus of the thyroid.
- The thyroid artery and veins are ligated to help prevent bleeding.
- The surgeon locates and visualizes the laryngeal nerves and parathyroid glands.

■ Thyroid tissue is dissected and removed.
■ A Penrose drain or a closed wound drainage device is inserted, and the wound is closed.

POSTPROCEDURE CARE

■ Administer medications as ordered.
■ Keep the patient in high Fowler's position.
■ Evaluate the patient's speech for signs of laryngeal nerve damage.
■ Keep a tracheotomy tray at the bedside for 24 hours after surgery.
■ Provide surgical wound care and dressing changes as ordered.
■ Provide comfort measures.
■ Maintain patency of drains.
■ Monitor the patient's vital signs, intake and output, surgical wound and dressings, drainage, and respiratory status.
■ Monitor the patient for complications, such as hypocalcemia, thyroid storm, hemorrhage, parathyroid damage, tetany, laryngeal nerve damage, and vocal cord paralysis.
■ Inform the patient that some hoarseness and a sore throat will occur after surgery.
■ Be sure to teach the patient about:
   – medications and possible adverse reactions
   – signs and symptoms of respiratory distress
   – signs and symptoms of hypothyroidism and hyperthyroidism
   – signs and symptoms of infection
   – signs and symptoms of hypocalcemia
   – abnormal bleeding
   – complications
   – when to notify the physician
   – prescribed thyroid hormone replacement therapy
   – calcium supplements as indicated
   – incision care and dressing changes
   – follow-up care.

Urinary diversion surgery

DESCRIPTION

■ Provides an alternative route for urine excretion when disease impedes normal urine flow through the bladder
■ *Incontinent diversion:* used when urine flow is constant and the patient requires an external collection device permanently; types include ileal conduit, ureterosigmoidostomy, and nephrostomy

■ *Continent diversion:* used when an external collection bag isn't needed; types include the Kock pouch, Indiana pouch, Mainz pouch, and Camey procedure in men

PURPOSE

■ To treat cystectomy
■ To treat congenital urinary tract defect
■ To treat severe, unmanageable urinary tract infection that threatens renal function
■ To treat chronic cystitis
■ To treat injury to the ureters, bladder, or urethra
■ To treat obstructive malignancy
■ To treat neurogenic bladder

PATIENT PREPARATION

■ Make sure the patient has signed an appropriate consent form.
■ Initiate referrals if the patient needs assistance with stoma management.
■ Prepare the bowel as ordered.

PROCEDURE

■ The patient receives a general anesthetic.
■ The surgeon makes a midline or paramedial abdominal incision.

To construct an ileal conduit

■ The surgeon excises a segment of the ileum measuring 6″ to 8″ (15 to 20.5 cm).
■ The remaining ileal ends are anastomosed to maintain intestinal integrity.
■ The ureters are dissected from the bladder and implanted in the ileal segment.
■ The surgeon sutures one end of the ileal segment closed.
■ The other end of the segment is brought through the abdominal wall to form a stoma.

To create a nephrostomy

■ The surgeon inserts a catheter into the renal pelvis percutaneously or through a flank incision.
■ This procedure is usually palliative because it carries a high risk of infection and renal calculus formation.

To create a continent internal ileal reservoir (such as the Kock pouch)

■ Segments of the small bowel and colon are used.

- For a Kock pouch, the surgeon excises 24″ to 32″ (61 to 81 cm) of ileum and anastomoses the remaining ileal ends.
- The isolated ileum segment is shaped into a pocket to serve as a bladder.
- The Kock pouch is connected to the urethra, or an intussuscepted nipple valve is used to connect the pouch to the external skin of the anterior abdominal wall.
- A second nipple valve is constructed at the other end of the pouch.
- The ureters are implanted at the site of the second nipple valve, along with ureteral stents.
- Ureteral stents originate in the pelvis of the kidneys and extend through the ureter into the reservoir and out through the abdominal opening or separate stab wounds.
- Stents may be attached to dependent drainage or may be contained with a pouching system.
- One or two drainage tubes are inserted into the reservoir and remain there until healing has occurred and pouch integrity is confirmed.

Camey procedure (orthotopic bladder replacement)

- The surgeon creates a pouch from both the small and large bowels and connects it to the urethral stump.
- An indwelling catheter is inserted and remains in place for about 3 weeks.
- After the catheter is removed, the patient voids through the urethra by means of abdominal straining.

POSTPROCEDURE CARE

- Administer medications as ordered.
- Provide comfort measures.
- Observe urine drainage for pus and blood; report these findings.
- Maintain patency of drainage catheters as ordered and report urine leakage from the drain or suture line.

  ALERT *Report signs and symptoms of peritonitis—fever, abdominal distention, and pain.*

- Perform surgical wound care and dressing changes as ordered.
- Continue I.V. replacement therapy and total parenteral nutrition.
- Provide emotional support.
- Monitor the patient's vital signs, intake and output, surgical wound and dressings, stoma and peristomal skin, drainage, urine characteristics, and bowel sounds.
- Monitor the patient for complications, such as abnormal bleeding, skin breakdown, infection, urinary extravasation, ureteral obstruction, small-

bowel obstruction, peritonitis, hydronephrosis, stomal stenosis, pyelonephritis, renal calculi, and psychological problems.
■ Refer the patient to sexual counseling as needed.
■ Refer the patient to support groups.
■ Be sure to teach the patient about:
  – medications and adverse reactions
  – signs and symptoms of infection
  – complications
  – when to notify the physician
  – stoma care and abnormal changes
  – pouch drainage tube care until it's removed (with a continent internal ileal reservoir)
  – prescribed activity restrictions
  – follow-up care.

Vascular repair

DESCRIPTION

■ Treatment of choice for damaged vessels
■ May involve aneurysm resection, bypass grafting, embolectomy, or vein stripping

PURPOSE

■ To repair a vessel damaged by an arteriosclerotic or thromboembolic disorder
■ To treat aortic aneurysm
■ To treat arterial occlusive disease
■ To treat limb-threatening acute arterial occlusion
■ To resolve vessel trauma, infection, or congenital defect
■ To treat vascular disease that doesn't respond to drug therapy or nonsurgical revascularization

PATIENT PREPARATION

■ Make sure the patient has signed an appropriate consent form.
■ Perform a complete vascular assessment.
■ Obtain baseline vital signs.
■ Evaluate pulses, noting bruits.
■ Restrict food and fluids as ordered.
■ Administer sedation as ordered.

> **ALERT** *If the patient is waiting for aortic aneurysm repair surgery, be sure to watch for and immediately report the classic triad of shock, pulsatile mass, and abdominal or back pain, which highly suggests rupture.*

PROCEDURE

- Typically, the patient receives general anesthesia.
- The procedure varies with the vessel affected and the specific repair needed.

POSTPROCEDURE CARE

- Administer medications as ordered.
- Position the patient as ordered.
- Explain recommended activity levels during the early recovery stage.
- Provide comfort measures.
- Use Doppler ultrasonography if peripheral pulses aren't palpable.
- As the patient's condition improves assist with weaning from the mechanical ventilator.
- Encourage frequent coughing, turning, and deep breathing.
- Assist with range-of-motion exercises.
- Provide incision care.
- Change dressings as ordered.
- Monitor the patient's vital signs, intake and output, neurovascular status, heart rate and rhythm, hemodynamic values, surgical wound and dressings, and drainage.
- Monitor the patient for complications, such as vessel trauma; thrombus formation; embolism; hemorrhage; infection; and graft occlusion, narrowing, dilation, or rupture involved with bypass grafting.
- Be sure to teach the patient about:
  - medications and possible adverse reactions
  - palpation and monitoring of peripheral pulses
  - monitoring of extremities for changes in temperature, sensation, and motor ability
  - incision care
  - signs and symptoms of infection
  - complications
  - when to notify the physician
  - follow-up care
  - smoking cessation, if indicated
  - risk factor modification.

Procedures

Part three

Bladder irrigation, continuous

DESCRIPTION

- Helps prevent urinary tract obstruction by flushing out small blood clots that form after prostate or bladder surgery
- Can be used to treat an irritated, inflamed, or infected bladder lining
- Continuous flow of irrigating solution through the bladder to create a mild tamponade that may help prevent venous hemorrhage
- Catheter usually inserted during prostate or bladder surgery but possibly inserted at bedside for a nonsurgical patient

EQUIPMENT

One 4,000-ml container or two 2,000-ml containers of irrigating solution or prescribed amount of medicated solution ♦ Y-type tubing made specifically for bladder irrigation ♦ alcohol or povidone-iodine pad (see *Setup for continuous bladder irrigation*)

ESSENTIAL STEPS

- Wash your hands.
- Use large volumes of irrigating solution, if necessary, during the first 24 to 48 hours after surgery.
- Double-check the irrigating solution against the physician's order before starting.
- Check the patient's chart to make sure he isn't allergic to any antibiotics in the solution.
- Assemble all equipment at the patient's bedside.
- Explain the procedure and provide privacy.
- Keep the patient on bed rest throughout continuous bladder irrigation, unless specified otherwise.
- Insert the spike of the Y-type tubing into the container of irrigating solution.
- Insert one spike into each container if you are using a two-container system.
- Squeeze the drip chamber on the spike of the tubing.
- Open the flow clamp and flush the tubing to remove air that could cause bladder distention.
- Close the clamp.
- Hang the bag of irrigating solution on the I.V. pole.
- Clean the opening to the inflow lumen of the catheter with the alcohol or povidone-iodine pad.

SETUP FOR CONTINUOUS BLADDER IRRIGATION

In continuous bladder irrigation, a triple-lumen catheter allows irrigating solution to flow into the bladder through one lumen and flow out through another, as shown in the inset. The third lumen is used to inflate the balloon that holds the catheter in place.

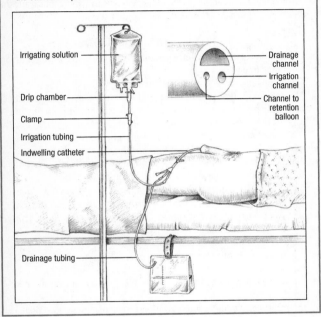

- Insert the distal end of the Y-type tubing securely into the third port of the catheter.
- Make sure the catheter's outflow lumen is securely attached to the drainage bag tubing.
- Open the flow clamp under the container of irrigating solution and set the drip rate as ordered.
- Replace the primary container before it empties completely, in order to prevent air from entering the system.
- Close the flow clamp under the nearly empty container and open the flow clamp under the reserve container simultaneously if you have a two-

container system. This prevents reflux of irrigating solution from the re-
serve container into the nearly empty one.
- Hang a new reserve container on the I.V. pole and insert the tubing, main-
taining asepsis.
- Empty the drainage bag about every 4 hours or as often as needed.
- Use sterile technique to avoid risk of contamination.
- Monitor vital signs at least every 4 hours during irrigation, increasing the
frequency if the patient becomes unstable.

NURSING CONSIDERATIONS

- Check inflow and outflow lines periodically for kinks to ensure solution
is running freely.
- Check the lines frequently if solution flows rapidly.
- Measure the outflow volume accurately. The outflow should be the same
or slightly more than the inflow volume, allowing for urine production.

*ALERT Postoperative inflow volume exceeding outflow vol-
ume may indicate bladder rupture at the suture lines or renal
damage; notify the physician immediately.*

- Assess outflow for changes in appearance and for blood clots, especially if
irrigation is being done postoperatively to control bleeding.

*ALERT If drainage is bright red, irrigating solution should
be infused rapidly with the clamp wide open until drainage
clears. Notify the physician immediately if you suspect hemorrhage.*

- Administer the solution at a rate of 40 to 60 drops/minute if the
drainage is clear.
- Administer antibiotic solutions at a rate usually specified by the physi-
cian.
- Encourage oral fluid intake of 2 to 3 qt (2 to 3 L)/day unless contraindi-
cated.
- Interruptions in a continuous irrigation system may cause infection.
- Obstruction in the catheter's outflow lumen may cause bladder disten-
tion.
- Record the date, time, and amount of fluids on the intake and output
record each time a container of solution is finished.
- Record the time and amount of fluid each time you empty the drainage
bag.
- Note the appearance of the drainage and patient complaints.
- Instruct the patient to report bladder distention or spasms.

Bone growth stimulation, electrical

DESCRIPTION

- Initiates or accelerates healing in patients with a fractured bone that fails to heal (about 1 in 20 fractures), by imitating the body's natural electrical forces
- Failure to heal possibly resulting from infection, insufficient reduction or fixation, pseudarthrosis, or severe tissue trauma around the fracture
- The stimulating effects of electrical currents first used on osteogenesis, which led to its use to promote healing
- May also be used for treating spinal fusions
- Three techniques: fully implantable direct-current stimulation, semi-invasive percutaneous stimulation, and noninvasive electromagnetic coil stimulation (see *Methods of electrical bone growth stimulation*, page 334)
- Choice of technique dependent on the fracture type and location, the physician's preference, and the patient's ability and willingness to comply
- Fully implantable device requiring little or no patient management
- Semi-invasive and noninvasive techniques requiring the patient to manage his own treatment schedule and maintain the equipment
- Treatment time: averages 3 to 6 months
- Electromagnetic coils contraindicated for pregnant patients, patients with tumors, and patients with arm fractures who also have a pacemaker
- Percutaneous electrical bone stimulation contraindicated if the patient has any kind of inflammatory process

ALERT Use caution in patients who are sensitive to nickel or chromium because both are present in the electrical bone stimulation system.

EQUIPMENT

All equipment comes with instructions provided by the manufacturer. Follow the instructions carefully. Make sure all parts are included and sterilized according to facility policy and procedure.

Direct-current stimulation
Small generator ◆ leadwires that connect to titanium cathode wire to be surgically implanted into nonunited bone site

Percutaneous stimulation
External anode skin pad with a leadwire ◆ lithium battery pack ◆ 1 to 4 Teflon-coated stainless steel cathode wires to be surgically implanted

METHODS OF ELECTRICAL BONE GROWTH STIMULATION

Electrical bone growth stimulation may be invasive or noninvasive.

Invasive system

An invasive system involves placing a spiral cathode inside the bone at the fracture site. A wire leads from the cathode to a battery-powered generator, also implanted in local tissues. The patient's body completes the circuit.

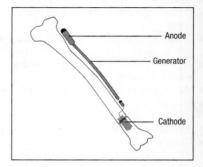

Noninvasive system

A noninvasive system may include a cufflike transducer or fitted ring that wraps around the patient's limb at the level of the injury. Electric current penetrates the limb.

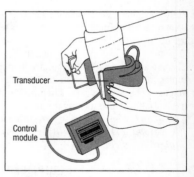

Electromagnetic stimulation

Generator that plugs into a standard 110-volt outlet ◆ two strong electromagnetic coils to be placed on either side of injured area, incorporated into a cast, cuff, or orthotic device

ESSENTIAL STEPS

■ Discuss the use of anesthetics with the patient.
■ Note the type of electrical bone stimulation equipment provided.
■ Note the date, time, and location, as appropriate.

- Record the patient's skin condition and tolerance of procedure.
- Document instructions given to the patient and his family.

Direct-current stimulation

- Implantation is performed with the patient under general anesthesia.
- The physician may apply a cast or external fixator to immobilize the limb.
- The patient is usually hospitalized for 2 to 3 days after implantation.
- Weight bearing may be ordered as tolerated.
- After the bone fragments join, the generator and leadwire can be removed under local anesthesia.
- The titanium cathode remains implanted.

Percutaneous stimulation

- Remove excessive hair from the injury site before applying the anode pad.
- Avoid stressing or pulling on the anode wire.
- Tell the patient to change the anode pad every 48 hours.
- Tell the patient to report local pain to his physician and not to bear weight on the limb for the duration of treatment.

Electromagnetic stimulation

- Show the patient where to place the coils and tell him to apply them for 3 to 10 hours each day, or as ordered.
- Many patients find it most convenient to perform the procedure at night.
- Advise the patient to not interrupt the treatments for more than 10 minutes at a time.
- Teach the patient how to use and care for the generator.
- Restate the physician's instructions for weight bearing. The physician will usually advise against bearing weight until evidence of healing appears on X-rays.

NURSING CONSIDERATIONS

- A patient with a direct-current electrical bone stimulation shouldn't undergo electrocauterization, diathermy, or magnetic resonance imaging (MRI).
  - Electrocautery may "short" the system.
  - Diathermy may potentiate the electrical current, possibly causing tissue damage.
  - MRI will interfere with or stop the current.
- Increased risk of infection exists with direct-current electrical bone stimulation equipment.

- Local irritation or skin ulceration may occur around cathode pin sites with percutaneous devices.
- No known complications are associated with electromagnetic coils.
- Teach the patient how to care for his cast or external fixation devices.
- Tell the patient how to care for the electrical generator.
- Urge the patient to follow treatment instructions.

Burn care

DESCRIPTION

- Competent care immediately after a burn to dramatically improve the success of overall treatment
- Goals: To maintain the patient's physiologic stability, repair skin integrity, prevent infection, and maximize functionality and psychosocial health
- Burn severity determined by the depth and extent of the burn, age, complications (such as infection, pulmonary problems), and coexisting illness (see *Evaluating burn severity*)
- Initial step: aggressive wound debridement, followed by maintenance of a clean wound bed until the wound heals or is covered with a skin graft
- Full-thickness burns and some deep partial-thickness burns debrided and grafted in the operating room; surgery as soon as possible after fluid resuscitation
- Most wounds managed with twice-daily dressing changes using topical antibiotics
- Dressings to bar germ entry and remove exudate, eschar, and other debris that host infection, encouraging healing

EQUIPMENT

A sterile field is required, and all equipment and supplies used in the dressing should be sterile.

Normal saline solution ◆ sterile bowl ◆ scissors ◆ tissue forceps ◆ ordered topical medication ◆ burn gauze ◆ roller gauze ◆ elastic netting or tape ◆ fine-mesh gauze ◆ elastic gauze ◆ cotton-tipped applicators or sterile tongue depressor ◆ ordered pain medication ◆ three pairs of sterile gloves ◆ sterile gown ◆ mask ◆ surgical cap ◆ heat lamps ◆ impervious plastic trash bag ◆ cotton bath blanket ◆ 4″ × 4″ gauze pads

FOCUS IN
EVALUATING BURN SEVERITY

To judge a burn's severity, assess its depth and extent as well as presence of other factors.

Superficial partial-thickness (first-degree) burn

Does the burned area appear pink or red with minimal edema? Is the area sensitive to touch and temperature changes? If so, your patient probably has a superficial partial-thickness, or first-degree, burn (shown here) affecting only the epidermal skin layer.

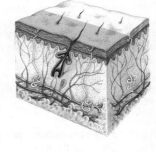

Deep partial-thickness (second-degree) burn

Does the burned area look pink or red, and have a mottled appearance? Do red areas blanch when you touch them? Does the skin have large, thick-walled blisters with subcutaneous edema? Does touching the burn cause severe pain? Is hair still present? If so, your patient probably has a deep partial-thickness, or second-degree, burn (shown here) affecting the epidermal and dermal layers.

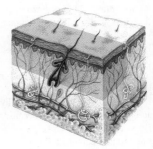

Full-thickness (third-degree) burn

Does the burned area appear red, waxy white, brown, or black? Does red skin remain red with no blanching when you touch it? Is the skin leathery with extensive subcutaneous edema? Is the skin insensitive to touch? Does the hair fall out easily? If so, your patient probably has a full-thickness, or third-degree, burn (shown here) that affects all skin layers.

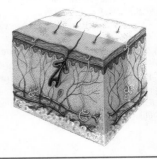

ESSENTIAL STEPS

- Give the ordered analgesic about 20 minutes before beginning wound care to maximize patient comfort and cooperation.
- Explain the procedure and provide privacy.
- Open equipment packages using sterile technique.
- Arrange supplies on a sterile field in order of use.
- Dress the cleanest areas first and the dirtiest or most contaminated areas last to prevent cross-contamination.
- Dress in stages if necessary to avoid exposing all wounds at the same time to help prevent excessive pain or cross-contamination.
- Turn on overhead heat lamps to keep the patient warm. Make sure they don't overheat him.
- Pour warmed normal saline solution into the sterile bowl in the sterile field.
- Wash your hands.

Removing a dressing without hydrotherapy

- Put on a gown, a mask, and sterile gloves.
- Remove dressing layers down to the innermost layer by cutting the outer dressings with sterile blunt scissors.
- Lay open these dressings.
- If the inner layer appears dry, soak it with warm normal saline solution to ease removal.
- Remove the inner dressing with sterile tissue forceps or your sterile gloved hand.
- Dispose of soiled dressings carefully in an impervious plastic trash bag according to facility policy, because these dressings harbor infection.
- Dispose of gloves and wash your hands.
- Put on a new pair of sterile gloves.
- Using gauze pads moistened with normal saline solution, gently remove exudate and old topical drug.
- Carefully remove all loose eschar with sterile forceps and scissors, if ordered.
- Assess the wound condition. It should appear clean, with no debris, loose tissue, purulence, inflammation, or darkened margins.
- Before applying a new dressing, remove your surgical cap, gown, gloves, and mask.
- Discard them properly; put on a clean mask, a cap, a gown, and sterile gloves.

Applying a wet dressing

■ Soak fine-mesh gauze and the elastic gauze dressing in a large sterile basin containing the ordered solution.

■ Wring out the fine-mesh gauze until it's moist but not dripping, and apply it to the wound.

■ Warn the patient he may feel transient pain when you apply the dressing.

■ Wring out the elastic gauze dressing and position it to hold the fine-mesh gauze in place.

■ Roll an elastic gauze dressing over the fine-mesh dressing to keep it intact.

■ Cover the patient with a cotton bath blanket to prevent chills.

■ Change the blanket if it becomes damp.

■ Use an overhead heat lamp, if necessary.

■ Change the dressings frequently, as ordered, to keep the wound moist, especially if you're using silver nitrate.

■ If the dressings become dry, silver nitrate becomes ineffective and the silver ions may damage tissue.

■ To maintain moist dressings, some protocols call for irrigating the dressing with solution at least every 4 hours through small slits cut into the outer dressing.

Applying a dry dressing with a topical drug

■ Remove old dressings and clean the wound.

■ Apply the drug to the wound in a thin layer — about 2 to 4 mm thick — with your sterile gloved hand or a sterile tongue blade.

■ Apply several layers of burn gauze over the wound to contain the drug but allow exudate to escape.

■ Cut the dressing to fit only the wound areas.

■ Don't cover unburned areas.

■ Cover the entire dressing with roller gauze and secure it with elastic netting or tape.

Providing arm and leg care

■ Apply the dressings from the distal to the proximal area to stimulate circulation and prevent constriction.

■ Wrap the burn gauze once around the arm or leg so the edges overlap slightly.

■ Continue wrapping until the gauze covers the wound.

■ Apply a dry roller gauze dressing to hold bottom layers in place.

■ Secure with elastic netting or tape.

Providing hand and foot care

■ Wrap each finger separately with a single 4″ × 4″ gauze pad to allow the patient to use his hands and to prevent webbing contractures.
■ Place the hand in a functional position, and secure using a dressing.
■ Apply splints if ordered.
■ Put gauze between each toe as appropriate to prevent webbing contractures.

Providing chest, abdomen, and back care

■ Apply the ordered drug to the wound in a thin layer.
■ Cover the entire burned area with sheets of burn gauze.
■ Wrap with roller gauze or apply a specialty vest dressing to hold the burn gauze in place.
■ Secure the dressing with elastic netting or tape.
■ Make sure the dressing doesn't restrict respiratory motion, especially in very young or elderly patients, or in those with circumferential injuries.

Providing facial care

■ If the patient has scalp burns, clip or shave the hair around the burn, as ordered.
■ Clip other hair until it's about 2″ (5 cm) long to prevent contamination of burned scalp areas.
■ Shave facial hair if it comes in contact with burned areas.
■ Typically, facial burns are managed with milder topical agents, such as triple antibiotic ointment, and are left open to air.
■ If dressings are required, make sure they don't cover the eyes, nostrils, or mouth.

Providing ear care

■ Clip or shave hair around the affected ear.
■ Remove exudate and crusts with cotton-tipped applicators dipped in normal saline solution.
■ Place a layer of 4″ × 4″ gauze behind the auricle to prevent webbing.
■ Apply the ordered topical drug to 4″ × 4″ gauze pads and place them over the burned area.
■ Before securing the dressing with a roller bandage, position the patient's ears normally to avoid damaging the auricular cartilage.
■ Assess the patient's hearing ability.

Providing eye care

■ Clean the area around the patient's eyes and eyelids with a cotton-tipped applicator and normal saline solution every 4 to 6 hours, or as needed, to remove crust and drainage.

- Give ordered eye ointments or drops.
- If the patient's eyes can't be closed, apply lubricating ointments or drops, as ordered.
- Be sure to close his eyes before applying eye pads to prevent corneal abrasion.
- Don't apply topical ointments near his eyes without a physician's order.

Providing nasal care

- Check the patient's nostrils for inhalation injury, such as the presence of inflamed mucosa, singed vibrissae, and soot.
- Clean the patient's nostrils with cotton-tipped applicators dipped in normal saline solution.
- Remove crust.
- Apply the ordered ointments.
- If the patient has a nasogastric tube, use tracheostomy ties to secure the tube.
- Be sure to check tracheostomy ties frequently for tightness caused by swelling facial tissue.
- Clean the area around the tube every 4 to 6 hours.

NURSING CONSIDERATIONS

- Thorough assessment and documentation of the wound's appearance are essential to detect infection and other complications.

> **ALERT** *A purulent wound or wound with green-gray exudate indicates infection, an overly dry wound suggests dehydration, and a wound with a swollen red edge suggests cellulitis. Suspect a fungal infection if the wound is white and powdery.*

- Healthy granulation tissue appears clean, pinkish, faintly shiny, and free of exudate.
- Blisters protect underlying tissue; leave them intact unless they impede joint motion, become infected, or cause discomfort.
- Be certain to meet the increased nutritional needs of the patient with healing burns; extra protein and carbohydrates are required to accommodate an almost doubled basal metabolism.
- If you must manage a burn with topical drugs, exposure to air, and no dressing, watch for such problems as wound adherence to bed linens, poor drainage control, and partial loss of topical drugs.
- Watch for complications such as infection, sepsis, allergic reactions to ointments or dressings, renal failure, and multisystem organ dysfunction.
- Record the dates and times for all care provided.
- Describe wound condition.

(Text continues on page 344.)

POSITIONING THE BURN PATIENT TO PREVENT DEFORMITY

For each of the potential deformities listed below, you can use the corresponding positioning and interventions to help prevent the deformity.

Burned area	Potential deformity
Neck	■ Flexion contraction of neck ■ Extensor contraction of neck
Axilla	■ Adduction and internal rotation ■ Adduction and external rotation
Pectoral region	■ Shoulder protraction
Chest or abdomen	■ Kyphosis
Lateral trunk	■ Scoliosis
Elbow	■ Flexion and pronation
Wrist	■ Flexion ■ Extension
Fingers	■ Adhesions of the extensor tendons; loss of palmar grip
Hip	■ Internal rotation, flexion, and adduction; possibly, joint subluxation if contracture is severe
Knee	■ Flexion
Ankle	■ Plantar flexion if foot muscles are weak or their tendons are divided

Preventive positioning	Nursing interventions
■ Extension ■ Prone with head slightly raised	■ Remove pillows from the bed. ■ Place a pillow or rolled towel under upper chest to flex cervical spine, or apply cervical collar.
■ Shoulder joint in external rotation and 100- to 130-degree abduction ■ Shoulder joint in forward flexion and 100- to 130-degree abduction	■ Use an I.V. pole, bedside table, or sling to suspend arm. ■ Use an I.V. pole, bedside table, or sling to suspend arm.
■ Shoulders abducted and externally rotated	■ Remove pillow from bed.
■ Same as for pectoral region, with hips neutral (not flexed)	■ Use no pillow under head or legs.
■ Supine; affected arm abducted	■ Put pillows or blanket rolls at sides.
■ Arm extended and supinated	■ Use an elbow splint, arm board, or bedside table.
■ Splint in 15-degree extension ■ Splint in 15-degree flexion	■ Apply a hand splint. ■ Apply a hand splint.
■ Metacarpophalangeal joints in maximum flexion; interphalangeal joints in slight flexion; thumb in maximum abduction	■ Apply a hand splint; wrap fingers separately.
■ Neutral rotation and abduction; maintain extension by prone position	■ Put a pillow under buttocks (if supine) or use trochanter rolls or knee or long leg splints.
■ Maintain extension	■ Use a knee splint with no pillows under legs.
■ 90-degree dorsiflexion	■ Use a footboard or ankle splint.

- Report special dressing-change techniques.
- List topical drugs given.
- Note positioning of the burned area.
- Describe the patient's tolerance of the procedure.
- Monitor the patient's respiratory status carefully in order to promote stability, especially if he suffered smoke inhalation.
- A patient with burns involving more than 20% of his total body surface area usually needs fluid resuscitation to support his body's compensatory mechanisms without overwhelming them.
- Give fluids, such as lactated Ringer's solution, to keep the patient's urine output at 30 to 50 ml/hour; monitor blood pressure and heart rate.
- Control the patient's body temperature, because skin loss interferes with temperature regulation.
- Use warm fluids, heat lamps, and hyperthermia blankets, as appropriate, to keep the patient's temperature above 97° F (36.1° C), if possible.
- Frequently review laboratory values such as serum electrolyte levels to detect early changes in the patient's condition.
- Infection can increase wound depth, cause rejection of skin grafts, slow healing, worsen pain, prolong hospitalization, and lead to death. For prevention use strict sterile technique during care, dress the burn site as ordered, monitor and rotate I.V. lines regularly, and carefully assess the burn extent, body system function, and the patient's emotional status.
- Other interventions, such as careful positioning and regular exercise for burned extremities, help maintain joint function, prevent contractures, and minimize deformity. (See *Positioning the burn patient to prevent deformity,* pages 342 and 343.)
- Begin discharge planning as soon as the patient enters the facility to help him and his family transition from facility to home.
- To encourage therapeutic compliance, prepare the patient to expect scarring, but advise him that proper therapy can minimize scarring.
- Teach the patient wound management and pain control, and urge him to do the prescribed exercises.
- Provide encouragement and emotional support, and urge the patient to join a burn survivor support group.
- Teach the family or caregivers how to encourage, support, and provide care for the patient.
- Refer the patient and family to home care services for follow-up teaching and therapies as needed.
- Refer the patient and family to burn survivor resources such as Burn Survivors Online, from World Burn Foundation.

Chest physiotherapy

DESCRIPTION

- Used on patients who expectorate large amounts of sputum, such as those with bronchiectasis and cystic fibrosis
- Techniques including postural drainage, chest percussion and vibration, and coughing and deep-breathing exercises
- To mobilize and eliminate secretions, expand lung tissue, and promote efficient use of respiratory muscles
- Important for the bedridden patient; to help prevent or treat atelectasis and possibly prevent pneumonia, which can seriously impede recovery
- Postural drainage done with percussion and vibration, causing peripheral pulmonary secretions to empty into the major bronchi or trachea; accomplished by sequential repositioning of the patient
- Has little value for treating patients with stable, chronic bronchitis
- Contraindicated in active pulmonary bleeding with hemoptysis and at immediate posthemorrhage stage; fractured ribs; unstable chest wall; lung contusions; pulmonary tuberculosis; untreated pneumothorax; acute asthma; bronchospasm; lung abscess; tumor; bony metastasis; head injury; recent myocardial infarction

EQUIPMENT

Stethoscope ◆ pillows ◆ tilt or postural drainage table (if available) or adjustable hospital bed ◆ emesis basin ◆ facial tissues ◆ suction equipment ◆ oral care equipment ◆ trash bag ◆ sterile specimen container ◆ mechanical ventilator ◆ supplemental oxygen (optional)

ESSENTIAL STEPS

- Explain the procedure to the patient, provide privacy, and wash your hands.
- Gather the equipment at the patient's bedside.
- Set up and test the suction equipment.
- Auscultate the patient's lungs to determine baseline respiratory status.
- Position him as ordered.
- In generalized disease, drainage begins with lower lobes, continues with middle lobes, and ends with upper lobes.
- In localized disease, drainage begins with affected lobes and proceeds to other lobes to avoid spreading disease to uninvolved areas.
- Tell the patient to remain in each position for 10 to 15 minutes.

PERFORMING PERCUSSION AND VIBRATION

Instruct the patient to breathe slowly and deeply using the diaphragm to promote relaxation. Percuss each segment with a cupped hand for 1 to 2 minutes. Listen for a hollow sound on percussion to verify correct performance of technique.

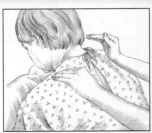

To perform vibration, ask the patient to inhale deeply, then exhale slowly. During exhalation firmly press your hands against the chest wall. Tense the muscles of your arms and shoulders in an isometric contraction to send fine vibrations through the chest wall. Do this during five exhalations over each chest segment.

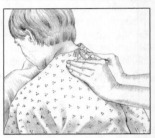

■ Perform percussion and vibration as ordered. (See *Performing percussion and vibration*.)
■ After postural drainage, percussion, or vibration, tell him to cough to remove loosened secretions.
■ Tell the patient to inhale deeply through his nose, then exhale in three short huffs.
■ Have him inhale deeply again and cough through a slightly open mouth. Three consecutive coughs are highly effective. An effective cough sounds deep, low, and hollow; an ineffective cough sounds high-pitched.
■ Have the patient perform exercises for about 1 minute, then rest for 2 minutes. Gradually progress to a 10-minute exercise period four times daily.
■ Provide oral hygiene because secretions may have a foul taste or stale odor.
■ Auscultate the patient's lungs to evaluate effectiveness of therapy.

NURSING CONSIDERATIONS

- For effectiveness and safety, modify chest physiotherapy as needed.
- Chest physiotherapy isn't effective in the patient with status asthmaticus, lobar pneumonia, or acute exacerbations of chronic bronchitis when he has scant secretions and is being mechanically ventilated.
- Suction the patient who has an ineffective cough reflex.
- If he tires quickly during therapy, shorten the sessions because fatigue leads to shallow respirations and increased hypoxia.
- Maintain adequate hydration if he's receiving chest physiotherapy to prevent mucus dehydration and promote mobilization.
- Secretions drain best with the patient positioned so the bronchi are perpendicular to the floor.
- Lower and middle lobe bronchi empty best with the patient in the head-down position; upper lobe bronchi, in the head-up position.
- Percussing the chest with cupped hands mechanically dislodges thick, tenacious secretions from the bronchial walls.
- Vibration can be used with percussion or as an alternative to it in a patient who's frail, in pain, or recovering from thoracic surgery or trauma.
- Avoid postural drainage immediately before or within 1½ hours after meals to avoid nausea, vomiting, and aspiration of food or vomitus.
- To prevent bronchospasm, adjunct treatments — intermittent positive-pressure breathing, aerosol, or nebulizer therapy — should precede chest physiotherapy.
- To avoid injury, don't percuss over the spine, liver, kidneys, or spleen.
- Avoid percussion on bare skin or on a female patient's breasts.
- Percuss over soft clothing or place a thin towel over the chest wall.
- Remove jewelry before percussing.
- Monitor the patient for complications such as impaired respiratory excursion during postural drainage in head-down position; increased intracranial pressure in head-down position; rib fracture caused by vigorous percussion or vibration; pneumothorax caused by coughing.
- Record the date and time of chest physiotherapy.
- Note positions for secretion drainage and length of time for each.
- Document chest segments percussed or vibrated.
- Report color, amount, odor, and viscosity of secretions produced and presence of blood.
- Record complications and nursing actions taken.
- Note the patient's tolerance of treatment.
- Explain coughing and deep-breathing exercises preoperatively so the patient can practice them when he's pain-free and better able to concentrate.
- Postoperatively, splint the patient's incision using your hands, or teach him to splint it himself to minimize pain during coughing.

Closed-wound drain management

DESCRIPTION

- Promotes healing and prevents swelling by suctioning serosanguineous fluid that accumulates at wound site
- Typically inserted during surgery in anticipation of substantial postoperative drainage
- Reduces the risk of infection and skin breakdown and frequency of dressing changes by removing postoperative fluid
- Hemovac and Jackson-Pratt closed drainage systems most commonly used; consisting of perforated tubing connected to a portable vacuum unit
- The distal end of the tubing lying inside the wound and usually exiting the body from a site other than the primary suture line to preserve integrity of the surgical wound
- Drain usually sutured to the skin; tubing exit site treated as an additional surgical wound
- For heavy drainage, a closed-wound drain possibly left in place for longer than 1 week
- Drainage emptied and measured frequently to maintain maximum suction and prevent strain on the suture line

EQUIPMENT

Graduated biohazard cylinder ◆ sterile laboratory container, if needed ◆ alcohol pads ◆ gloves ◆ gown ◆ face shield ◆ trash bag ◆ sterile gauze pads ◆ antiseptic cleaning agent ◆ prepackaged povidone-iodine swabs ◆ label (optional)

ESSENTIAL STEPS

- Check the physician's order and assess the patient's condition.
- Explain the procedure, provide privacy, and wash your hands.
- Unclip the vacuum unit from the patient's bed or gown.
- Using sterile technique, release the vacuum by removing the spout plug on the collection chamber.
- The container expands completely as it draws in air.
- Empty the unit's contents into a graduated biohazard cylinder, and note the amount and appearance of drainage.
- If diagnostic tests will be performed on the specimen, pour the drainage directly into a sterile laboratory container. Note the amount and appearance, label the specimen pad, and send to the laboratory.

USING A CLOSED-WOUND DRAINAGE SYSTEM

This system draws drainage from a wound site, such as the chest wall postmastectomy (shown below top) by means of a Y-tube. To empty the drainage, remove plug and empty into a graduated cylinder. To reestablish suction, compress the drainage unit against a firm surface to expel air and, while holding it down, replace the plug (as shown below left). The same principle is used for the Jackson-Pratt bulb drain (shown below right).

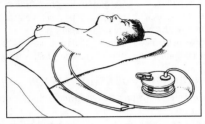

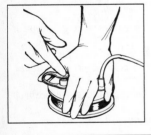
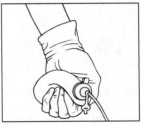

- Clean the unit's spout and plug with an alcohol pad using sterile technique.
- To reestablish the vacuum that creates the drain's suction power, fully compress the vacuum unit.
- Compress the unit with one hand to maintain the vacuum and replace the spout plug. (See *Using a closed-wound drainage system.*)
- Check patency of equipment.
- Make sure tubing is free from twists, kinks, and leaks; the drainage system must be airtight to work properly.
- The vacuum unit should remain compressed when you release manual pressure.

- If rapid reinflation occurs, indicating an air leak, recompress the unit and resecure the spout plug.
- Fasten the vacuum unit to the patient's gown below wound level to promote drainage.
- To prevent dislodgment, don't apply tension on drainage tubing when fastening the unit.
- Remove and discard gloves and wash your hands.
- Check the sutures that secure the drain to the patient's skin.
- Look for signs of pulling or tearing and swelling or infection.
- Gently clean the sutures with sterile gauze pads soaked in an antiseptic cleaning agent or with a povidone-iodine swab.
- Properly dispose of drainage, solutions, and trash bag, and clean or dispose of soiled equipment and supplies according to facility policy.

NURSING CONSIDERATIONS

- Empty drain and measure contents once during each shift, more often if drainage is excessive.
- Removing excess drainage maintains maximum suction and avoids straining the drain's suture line.
- Empty and measure before the patient ambulates to prevent weight of drainage from pulling on the drain.

ALERT *Be careful not to mistake chest tubes for closed-wound drains because the vacuum of a chest tube should never be released.*

- Occlusion of tubing by fibrin, clots, or other particles can reduce or obstruct drainage.
- Record the date and time when you empty the drain.
- Describe appearance of the drain site.
- Note the presence of swelling or signs of infection.
- Document equipment malfunction and nursing action.
- Note the patient's tolerance of treatment.
- Record drainage color, consistency, type, and amount on the input and output sheet.
- If there's more than one closed-wound drain, number the drains and record the information above separately for each drainage site.
- Explain purpose of closed-wound drainage system.
- Explain importance of not pulling on drains and of having the drain emptied before ambulation.
- Explain how to empty the drains and provide site care if the patient is to go home before drains are removed.

Gastric lavage

DESCRIPTION

■ Flushes the stomach and removes ingested substances through a tube (after poisoning or drug overdose or before an endoscopic examination); used in central nervous system depression or inadequate gag reflex or to administer a vasoconstrictive drug to a patient with stomach bleeding before endoscopic examination

■ Can be continuous or intermittent; usually done in the emergency room or intensive care unit by a physician, gastroenterologist, or nurse

■ Contraindicated after ingestion of corrosive substances such as lye, petroleum distillates, ammonia, alkalis, or mineral acids because the lavage tube may perforate the already-compromised esophagus

EQUIPMENT

Lavage setup, consisting of two graduated containers for drainage, three pieces of large-lumen rubber tubing, Y-connector, and clamp or hemostat ◆ 2 to 3 L of normal saline solution, tap water, or appropriate antidote as ordered ◆ Ewald tube or any large-lumen gastric tube, typically #36 to #40 French ◆ I.V. pole ◆ water-soluble lubricant or anesthetic ointment ◆ stethoscope ◆ ½″ hypoallergenic tape ◆ 50-ml bulb or catheter-tip syringe ◆ gloves ◆ face shield ◆ linen-saver pad or towel ◆ Yankauer or tonsil-tip suction device ◆ suction apparatus ◆ labeled specimen container ◆ laboratory request form ◆ norepinephrine ◆ basin of ice, if ordered ◆ patient restraints, charcoal tablets (optional)

Preparation

■ A prepackaged, syringe-type irrigation kit may be used for intermittent lavage. For poisoning or drug overdose, the continuous lavage setup is faster and more effective for diluting and removing the harmful substance.

■ Connect one of the three pieces of large-lumen tubing to the irrigant container. (See *Using wide-bore gastric tubes,* page 352.)

■ Insert the Y-connector stem in the other end of the tubing.

■ Connect the remaining two pieces of tubing to the free ends of the Y connector.

■ Place the unattached end of one of the tubes into one of the drainage containers.

USING WIDE-BORE GASTRIC TUBES

To deliver a large volume of fluid rapidly through a gastric tube (for such conditions as profuse gastric bleeding or poisoning), a wide-bore gastric tube works best. Typically inserted orally, the tube remains in place long enough to complete the lavage and evacuate stomach contents.

Ewald tube
In an emergency, using the Ewald tube—a single-lumen tube with several openings at the distal end—allows you to aspirate large amounts of gastric contents quickly.

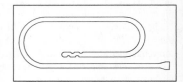

Levacuator tube
The Levacuator tube has two lumens. Use the larger lumen for evacuating gastric contents; the smaller, for instilling an irrigant.

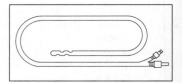

Edlich tube
The Edlich tube is a single-lumen tube that has four openings near the closed distal tip. A funnel or syringe may be connected at the proximal end. Like the Ewald tube, the Edlich tube lets you withdraw large quantities of gastric contents quickly.

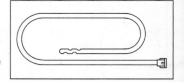

- Clamp the tube leading to the irrigant.
- Suspend the entire setup from the I.V. pole, hanging the irrigant container at the highest level.
- If iced lavage is ordered, chill the ordered irrigant in a basin of ice.
- Lubricate the end of the lavage tube with water-soluble lubricant or anesthetic ointment.

ESSENTIAL STEPS

■ Provide privacy.

■ Wash your hands and put on gloves and a face shield.

■ Place the patient in the left lateral decubitus position.

■ The physician inserts the lavage tube orally and advances it slowly; forceful insertion may injure tissues. Tube placement is checked by aspirating for stomach contents and checking for pH of 5.0 or less on test strip.

■ Correct tube placement is essential; accidental misplacement in the lungs followed by lavage can be fatal.

ALERT *The patient may vomit when the lavage tube reaches the posterior pharynx; be prepared to suction the airway immediately.*

■ After securing the tube with tape and making sure the irrigant inflow tube on the lavage setup is clamped, connect the unattached end of the irrigant inflow tube to the lavage tube.

■ Allow stomach contents to empty into the drainage container before instilling irrigant. This confirms proper tube placement and decreases risk of overfilling the stomach with irrigant and inducing vomiting.

■ If using a syringe irrigation set, aspirate stomach contents with a 50-ml bulb or catheter-tip syringe before instilling irrigant.

■ After you confirm proper tube placement, begin gastric lavage by instilling 100 to 300 ml of irrigant to assess the patient's tolerance and prevent vomiting.

■ If using a syringe, instill about 50 ml of solution at a time until you've instilled between 100 and 300 ml. Clamp the inflow tube and unclamp the outflow tube to allow irrigant to flow out.

■ If using the syringe irrigation kit, aspirate the irrigant with the syringe and empty into a calibrated container. Measure outflow to ensure it at least equals the amount of irrigant instilled. This prevents stomach distention and vomiting.

■ If the drainage amount is significantly less than instilled amount, reposition the tube until sufficient solution flows out. Gently massage the abdomen over the stomach to promote outflow.

■ Repeat the inflow-outflow cycle until returned fluids appear clear, signaling that the stomach no longer contains harmful substances or bleeding has stopped.

■ Assess vital signs, urine output, and level of consciousness (LOC) every 15 minutes. Notify the physician of changes.

■ If ordered, remove the lavage tube.

NURSING CONSIDERATIONS

- Explain the procedure to the patient.
- To control GI bleeding, the physician may order continuous stomach irrigation with a vasoconstrictor. There are two ways to do this:
  - The drug is delivered directly to the liver via the portal septum, thus preventing systemic circulation, which could cause hypertension.
  - The outflow tube is clamped for a prescribed period after instilling the irrigant and vasoconstrictor and before withdrawing them. This allows the mucosa time to absorb the drug.
- Never leave a patient alone during gastric lavage. Watch for changes in LOC and monitor vital signs frequently; the vagal response to intubation can depress the patient's heart rate.
- If you need to restrain the patient, secure restraints on one side of the bed or stretcher so you can free them quickly.
- Keep tracheal suctioning equipment nearby; watch closely for airway obstruction caused by vomiting or excess oral secretions.
- Suction the oral cavity often to ensure an open airway and prevent aspiration.
- If the patient doesn't have an adequate gag reflex, he may need an endotracheal tube before the procedure.
- When aspirating the stomach for ingested poisons or drugs (a rare procedure), save the contents in a labeled container for laboratory analysis.
- If ordered, after lavage to remove poisons or drugs, mix charcoal tablets with the irrigant and administer the mixture through the tube.
- When lavage is performed to stop bleeding, keep precise intake and output records to determine amount of bleeding. When large volumes of fluid are instilled and withdrawn, serum electrolyte and arterial blood gas levels may be measured during or after lavage.
- Monitor for complications, such as vomiting and aspiration, bradyarrhythmias, and cardiac arrhythmias triggered by body temperature dropping after iced lavage.
- Record the date and time of lavage.
- Note the size and type of nasogastric tube used.
- Document volume and type of irrigant.
- Record the amount of drained gastric contents.
- Record information on intake and output record sheet.
- Note the color and consistency of drainage.
- Keep precise records of the patient's vital signs and LOC.
- Document drugs instilled through the tube.
- Note the time the tube was removed.
- Record the patient's tolerance of the procedure.

Gastrostomy feeding button care

DESCRIPTION

- An alternative feeding device for an ambulatory patient receiving long-term enteral feedings
- Approved for 6-month implantation and can replace gastrostomy tubes
- Inserted into an established stoma (takes less than 15 minutes) and lies almost flush with skin; only the top of safety plug visible
- Advantages over ordinary feeding tubes: cosmetic appeal, ease of maintenance, reduced skin irritation and breakdown, and less chance of being dislodged or migrating
- One-way antireflux valve inside a mushroom dome that prevents leakage of gastric contents; usually replaced after 3 to 4 months, typically because the antireflux valve wears out
- Contraindicated in intestinal obstruction that prohibits use of the bowel; diffuse peritonitis; intractable vomiting; paralytic ileus; severe diarrhea that makes metabolic management difficult
- May be used cautiously in severe pancreatitis; enterocutaneous fistulae; gastrointestinal ischemia

EQUIPMENT

Gastrostomy feeding button of correct size (all three sizes, if correct one isn't known) ◆ obturator ◆ water-soluble lubricant ◆ gloves ◆ feeding accessories, including adapter, feeding catheter, food syringe or bag, and formula ◆ catheter clamp ◆ cleaning equipment, including water, a syringe, cotton-tipped applicator, pipe cleaner, and mild soap or povidone-iodine solution ◆ I.V. pole, pump to provide continuous infusion over several hours (optional)

ESSENTIAL STEPS

- Explain the insertion, reinsertion, and feeding procedure to the patient.
- Tell the patient the physician will perform initial insertion. (See *How to reinsert a gastrostomy feeding button*, page 356.)
- Make sure signed consent has been obtained.
- Wash your hands and put on gloves.
- Attach the adapter and feeding catheter to the syringe or feeding bag.
- Clamp the catheter and fill the syringe or bag and catheter with formula.
- Open the safety plug and attach the adapter and feeding catheter to the button.
- Elevate the syringe or feeding bag above stomach level, and gravity-feed the formula for 15 to 30 minutes, varying height as needed to alter flow rate.

HOW TO REINSERT A GASTROSTOMY FEEDING BUTTON

Prepare equipment

- Collect the feeding button (shown below); wash it with soap and water; rinse thoroughly and dry. Obtain an obturator and water-soluble lubricant.

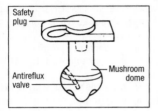

Safety plug

Antireflux valve

Mushroom dome

Insert the button

- Check the depth of the patient's stoma to make sure you have a feeding button of the correct size; clean around the stoma.
- Lubricate the obturator with water-soluble lubricant and distend the button several times to ensure the patency of the antireflux valve within the button.
- Lubricate the mushroom dome and stoma. Push the button through the stoma into the stomach (as shown).

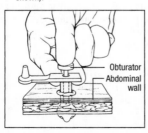

Obturator
Abdominal wall

- Remove the obturator by rotating it as you withdraw it to keep the antireflux valve from adhering to it. If the valve sticks, push the obturator back into the button until the valve closes.
- After removing the obturator, make sure the valve is closed.
- Close the flexible safety plug, which should be relatively flush with the skin surface (as shown).

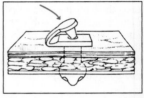

- If you need to give a feeding right away, open the safety plug and attach the feeding adapter and feeding tube (as shown). Deliver feeding as ordered.

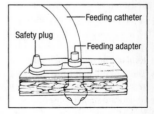

Feeding catheter
Safety plug
Feeding adapter

- Use a pump for continuous infusion or for feedings lasting several hours.
- Refill the syringe before it's empty to prevent air from entering the stomach and distending the abdomen.
- After feeding, flush the button with 10 ml of water.
- Lower the syringe or bag below stomach level to allow burping.
- Remove the adapter and feeding catheter; the antireflux valve should prevent gastric reflux.
- Snap the safety plug in place to keep the lumen clean and prevent leakage if the antireflux valve fails.
- If the patient feels nauseated or vomits after the feeding, vent the button with the adapter and feeding catheter to control emesis.
- Wash the catheter and syringe or feeding bag in warm, soapy water and rinse thoroughly.
- Clean the catheter and adapter with a pipe cleaner.
- Rinse well before using for the next feeding.
- Soak equipment weekly, or according to manufacturer's recommendations.

NURSING CONSIDERATIONS

- If the button pops out while feeding, reinsert it, estimate the formula already delivered, and resume feeding.
- Once daily, clean the peristomal skin with mild soap and water or povidone-iodine, and let the skin air-dry for 20 minutes to avoid skin irritation.
- Clean the peristomal site whenever the feeding bag spills.
- Monitor for complications, such as nausea and vomiting, abdominal distention, exit-site infection, exit-site leakage, and peritonitis.
- Note the date, time, and duration of feeding.
- Record the amount and type of feeding formula used.
- Document the patient's tolerance of the procedure.
- Note intake and output.
- Record the appearance of the stoma and surrounding skin.
- Document skin care.
- Explain to the patient how the gastrostomy feeding button is inserted and cared for.
- Tell the patient how to use the button for feedings.
- Advise the patient how to clean the equipment.
- Explain to the patient peristomal skin care.
- Tell the patient when and whom to call for questions.
- Refer the patient and family to appropriate community support sources.

Halo-vest traction

DESCRIPTION

- Immobilizes the head and neck after traumatic injury to the cervical vertebrae to prevent further spinal cord injury
- Applied by an orthopedic surgeon, with nursing assistance, in the emergency room, a specially equipped room, or operating room after surgical reduction of vertebral injuries
- Consisting of a metal ring that fits over the patient's head and metal bars that connect the ring to a plastic vest that distributes the weight of the entire apparatus around the chest (see *Comparing halo-vest traction devices*)
- Allows greater mobility than traction with skull tongs and has less infection risk because it doesn't require skin incisions and drill holes to position skull pins.

EQUIPMENT

Halo-vest traction unit ◆ halo ring ◆ cervical collar or sandbags (if needed) ◆ plastic vest board or padded headrest ◆ tape measure ◆ halo ring conversion chart ◆ scissors and razor ◆ 4″ × 4″ gauze pads ◆ povidone-iodine solution ◆ sterile gloves ◆ Allen wrench ◆ four positioning pins ◆ multiple-dose vial of 1% lidocaine (with or without epinephrine) ◆ alcohol pads ◆ 3-ml syringe ◆ 25G needles ◆ five sterile skull pins (one more than needed) ◆ torque screwdriver ◆ sheepskin liners ◆ cotton-tipped applicators ◆ ordered cleaning solution ◆ medicated powder or cornstarch ◆ sterile water or normal saline solution ◆ hair dryer, analgesic (optional)

Packaged units that include software, hardware, and tools are commonly used. Obtain a halo-vest traction unit with halo rings and plastic vests in several sizes. Vest sizes are based on the patient's chest and head measurements. Check for sterility and expiration date of the prepackaged tray.

ESSENTIAL STEPS

- Assemble equipment at the patient's bedside.
- Check the support applied to the patient's neck on the way to the hospital. As needed, apply cervical collar or immobilize the head and neck with sandbags.

  ⚠ **ALERT** *Keep cervical collar or sandbags in place until halo is applied; remove to facilitate application of the vest.*
- Because the patient is likely to be frightened, try to reassure him.
- Remove the headboard and furniture near the head of the bed to provide ample working space.

COMPARING HALO-VEST TRACTION DEVICES

Type	Description	Advantages
Low profile (standard) 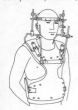	■ Traction and compression are produced by threaded support rods on either side of the halo ring. ■ Flexion and extension are obtained by moving the swivel arm to an anterior or posterior position, depending on location of skull pins.	■ Immobilizes cervical spine fractures while allowing patient mobility ■ Facilitates surgery of cervical spine and permits flexion and extension ■ Allows airway intubation without losing skeletal traction ■ Facilitates necessary alignment by adjustment at the junction of the threaded support rods and horizontal frame
Mark II (type of low profile) 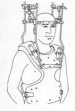	■ Traction and compression are produced by threaded support rods on either side of the halo ring. ■ Flexion and extension are obtained by swivel clamps that allow the bars to intersect and hold at any angle.	■ Enables the physician to assemble metal framework more quickly ■ Allows unobstructed access for anteroposterior and lateral X-rays of cervical spine ■ Allows the patient to wear his usual clothing because uprights are closer to the body
Mark III (update of Mark II) 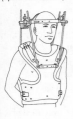	■ Traction and compression are produced by threaded support rods on either side of the halo ring. ■ Flexion and extension are accommodated by a serrated split articulation coupling attached to the halo ring, which can be adjusted in 4-degree increments.	■ Simplifies application while promoting patient comfort ■ Eliminates shoulder pressure and discomfort by using a flexible padded strap instead of the vest's solid plastic shoulder ■ Accommodates the tall patient with modified hardware and shorter uprights ■ Allows unobstructed access for medial and lateral X-rays

(continued)

COMPARING HALO-VEST TRACTION DEVICES *(continued)*

Type	Description	Advantages
Trippi-Wells tongs	■ Traction is produced by four pins that compress the skull. ■ Flexion and extension are obtained by adjusting the midline vertical plate.	■ Makes it possible to change from mobile to stationary traction without interrupting traction ■ Adjusts to three planes for mobile and stationary traction ■ Allows unobstructed access for medial and lateral X-rays

■ Carefully place the patient's head on a board or padded headrest that extends beyond the edge of the bed.

> **ALERT** *To avoid further spinal cord injury, don't put the patient's head on a pillow before applying the halo.*

■ Elevate the bed so the physician has access to the front and back of the halo unit.

■ Stand at the head of the bed and see if the patient's chin lines up with his midsternum, indicating proper alignment.

■ If ordered, support the patient's head in your hands and rotate the neck into alignment without flexing or extending it.

Assisting with halo application

■ Explain the procedure to the patient, wash your hands, and provide privacy.

■ Have an assisting nurse hold the patient's head and neck stable while the physician removes the cervical collar or sandbags. Maintain support until the halo is secure — while you assist with pin insertion.

■ The physician measures the patient's head with a tape measure and refers to the halo ring conversion chart to determine correct ring size.

■ The ring should clear the head by ⅝" (1.6 cm) and fit ½" (1.3 cm) above the bridge of the nose.

■ The physician selects four pin sites: ½" above the lateral one-third of each eyebrow and ½" above the top of each ear in the occipital area.

- He also takes into account the degree and type of correction needed to provide proper cervical alignment.
- Trim and shave hair at the pin sites to facilitate subsequent care and help prevent infection, and put on gloves.
- Use 4″ × 4″ gauze pads soaked in povidone-iodine solution to clean sites.
- Open the halo-vest unit using sterile technique to avoid contamination.
- The physician puts on sterile gloves and removes the halo and Allen wrench.
- He places the halo over the patient's head and inserts the four positioning pins to hold the halo in place temporarily.
- Help the physician prepare anesthetic. Clean the injection port of the multidose vial of lidocaine with an alcohol pad. Invert the vial so the physician can insert a 25G needle attached to the 3-ml syringe and withdraw the anesthetic.
- The physician injects the anesthetic at the four pin sites; he may change needles on the syringe after each injection.
- The physician removes four of the five skull pins from the sterile setup and firmly screws in each pin at a 90-degree angle to the skull.
- When the pins are in place, he removes the positioning pins.
- He tightens the skull pins with the torque screwdriver.

Applying the vest
- After the physician measures the patient's chest and abdomen, he selects an appropriate-sized vest.
- Place sheepskin liners inside the front and back of the vest for comfort and to help prevent pressure ulcers.
- Help the physician to carefully raise the patient while another nurse supports the patient's head and neck; slide the back of the vest under the patient and gently lay him down.
- The physician fastens the front of the vest on the patient's chest using Velcro straps and attaches the metal bars to the halo and vest. He tightens each bolt in turn, avoiding tightening completely, which causes maladjusted tension.

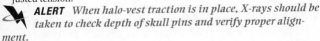 **ALERT** *When halo-vest traction is in place, X-rays should be taken to check depth of skull pins and verify proper alignment.*

Caring for the patient
- Take routine and neurologic vital signs at least every 2 hours for 24 hours, then every 4 hours until stable.

ALERT *Notify the physician immediately of any loss of motor function or decreased sensation from baseline, which could indicate spinal cord trauma.*

- Put on gloves and clean the pin sites every 4 hours with cotton-tipped applicators dipped in cleaning solution.
- Rinse the sites with sterile water or normal saline solution to remove excess cleaning solution.
- Clean pin sites with povidone-iodine or other ordered solution to prevent infection and remove debris that might block drainage and cause abscesses.
- Watch for signs of infection — a loose pin, swelling or redness, purulent drainage, pain at the site — and notify physician if signs develop.
- The physician retightens the skull pins with the torque screwdriver 24 and 48 hours after the halo is applied.
- If the patient complains of headache after the pins are tightened, obtain an order for an analgesic.

ALERT *If pain occurs with jaw movement, notify the physician; this may indicate that pins have slipped onto the thin temporal plate.*

- Examine the halo-vest every shift to ensure everything is secure and the patient's head is centered.
- If the vest fits correctly, you should be able to insert one or two fingers under the jacket at the shoulder and chest when the patient is supine.
- Wash the patient's chest and back daily. Place him on his back, loosening the bottom Velcro straps so you can get to the chest and back.
- Turn the patient on his side — less than 45 degrees — to wash his back. Close the vest.

ALERT *Don't put stress on the apparatus, which could knock it out of alignment and lead to subluxation of the cervical spine.*

- Check for tender areas or pressure spots that may develop into ulcers.
- If necessary, use a hair dryer to dry damp sheepskin; moisture predisposes the skin to pressure ulcer formation.
- Dust the skin with medicated powder or cornstarch to prevent itching. If itching persists, check to see if the patient is allergic to sheepskin or if any drug he's taking might cause skin rash.
- Change the vest lining as necessary, per facility policy.

NURSING CONSIDERATIONS

ALERT *Keep two wrenches available. They may be taped to the halo-vest on the chest area. If cardiac arrest occurs, you'll* *need them to remove the distal anterior bolts. Pull the two upright bars outward, unfasten the straps, and remove the front of the vest. Use the back of the vest as a board for cardiopulmonary resuscitation (CPR); some vests have a hinged front. To prevent subluxating the cervical injury, start CPR with the jaw-thrust maneuver to avoid hyperextending the neck. Pull his mandible forward, while maintaining proper head and neck alignment. This pulls the tongue forward to open the airway.*

ALERT *Always be aware of what type of vest your patient is wearing so that in an emergency, CPR can be performed quickly and effectively.*

ALERT *Never lift the patient up by the vertical bars. This could strain or tear the skin at the pin sites or misalign the traction.*

- To prevent falls, walk with the ambulatory patient. He may have trouble seeing objects at or near his feet, and the weight of the halo-vest unit (about 10 lb [4.5 kg]) may throw him off balance.
- If he's in a wheelchair, lower the leg rests to prevent the chair from tipping backward.
- The vest limits chest expansion; routinely assess pulmonary function, especially in a patient with pulmonary disease.
- Manipulating the patient's neck during application of halo-vest traction may cause subluxation of the spinal cord or push a bone fragment into the spinal cord, possibly causing paralysis below the break.
- Inaccurate skull pin positioning can result in puncturing the skull and dura mater, causing loss of cerebrospinal fluid and central nervous system infection.
- Nonsterile technique during application or inadequate pin-site care can lead to infection at pin sites.
- Record the date and time halo-vest traction was applied.
- Note the length of the procedure and the patient's response.
- After application, record routine and neurologic vital signs.
- Document pin-site care and note signs of infection.
- Teach the patient about pin-site care and shampooing and hair care.
- Teach the patient to turn slowly and incrementally to avoid losing his balance.
- Remind the patient to avoid bending forward; the extra weight of the apparatus may cause him to fall. Teach him to bend at the knees, not the waist.

> **COLLABORATION** *Have a physical therapist teach the patient how to use assistive devices to extend his reach and help him put on socks and shoes.*

■ Suggest to the patient that he wear large shirts that button in front to accommodate the halo-vest.

Knee extension therapy

DESCRIPTION

■ Used to treat patients with joint stiffness and limited range of motion (ROM) from fractures, dislocations, ligament and tendon repairs, joint arthroplasty, burns, total knee replacement, hemophilia, spinal cord injuries, rheumatoid arthritis, tendon release, cerebral palsy, multiple sclerosis, and other traumatic and nontraumatic disorders
■ Involves application of low-load, prolonged-duration stretching force to knee joint
■ Restores functional ROM to limbs stiffened by immobility and possibly contractures or adhesions and helps the patient regain ROM by applying dynamic stress continuously while he's sleeping or resting
■ Provides support to upper and lower limbs by struts fitted with tension rods that apply firm force to coax muscles and connective tissues to stretch
■ Contraindicated in unhealed or unstable fracture; septic joints; acute thrombophlebitis; severe arthritic joint inflammation; recent trauma with possible hidden fractures or internal injuries
■ May be used cautiously in patients with thrombophlebitis, osteoporosis, spasticity, edema, gross ligament instability, and circulatory impairment

EQUIPMENT

Knee extension system ♦ knee extension system and tension adjustment tool ♦ pillow, adhesive tape, marking pen (optional)

ESSENTIAL STEPS

■ Wash your hands.
■ Explain the procedure to the patient.
■ Hold the system so that the adjustment scale is visible on one of the struts.
■ To read the tension, look at the number on the tension scale lined up with the flat top of the tension spacer inside the strut. The tension spacer is visible in the window next to the tension scale.

■ If the top of the tension spacer isn't lined up with the "0" on the tension scale with each strut, adjust the tension screw in the top of each spacer with the tension adjustment tool until they're lined up.

Adjusting strut length

■ To shorten or lengthen the distal strut, first remove the ⅛" screw or screws located near the cam, using the tension adjustment tool.

■ Slide the smaller tube in or out of the larger tube to obtain correct strut length.

■ Line up the screw holes, replace and tighten the screw or screws.

■ Repeat this adjustment on each strut as necessary.

■ Open the front-of-thigh, shin, and over-the-knee straps, pull them out of the D-wire that's attached to the strut, and fold the strap's Velcro closure onto itself.

■ Loosen the back-of-thigh and calf cuffs to widen the splint to accommodate the patient's calf and thigh dimensions.

■ Place the system under his leg.

■ Position the distal struts, which are the larger tubes with the tension adjusters, beneath the calf.

■ Pull the proximal and distal struts up with both hands until the struts are even with the midlines of the sides of the thigh and calf.

■ Align the cams across the knee axis, making sure they're in a straight line.

■ With the cams aligned, close the over-the-knee straps, making sure that you can slide one finger under the upper and lower edges of each strap.

■ Close the front-of-thigh cuffs and shin cuffs.

■ Adjust and close the back-of-thigh cuffs and calf cuffs.

■ If necessary, adjust strut length so that cuffs are positioned on the bulk of the muscle mass at midthigh and midcalf.

> **ALERT** *Elderly patients are at increased risk of skin break-down; assess for pressure ulcer development while using a knee extension system.*

Setting splint tension

■ Insert the tension adjustment tool into the open end of the lower strut.

■ Increase the tension by turning the tool clockwise; reduce the tension by turning it counterclockwise.

■ Make sure the cams are aligned across the knee axis, struts are placed on the medial and lateral axes of the leg, and cuffs are evenly contoured across the leg.

■ Mark the backs of both cuffs to keep the patient from changing the fitting.

- Mark a reference line with a pen on the over-the-knee straps and the front-of-thigh and shin cuffs so the patient knows where to close them.
- Make sure the patient practices applying and removing the splint.

NURSING CONSIDERATIONS

- The system is custom-fitted and tension is adjusted to the patient's tolerance; worn at the optimal tolerable tension for the longest time (8 to 10 hours), preferably at night.
- When applied early in treatment program, duration of rehabilitation is greatly reduced.
- Monitor the patient for complications such as pain and stiffness.
- Note alterations in skin integrity.
- Note the date and time of the procedure.
- Record tension ordered by physician, length of time the patient can tolerate tension, increases or decreases in tension, and reasons for tension changes.
- Document the patient's tolerance of the procedure.
- Record patient teaching.
- Explain the reasons for knee extension therapy.
- Tell the patient how to apply the equipment.
- Advise the patient about the length of time for each session.
- Explain to the patient how to adjust tension settings.
- Inform the patient about signs and symptoms to report.

Nasal packing

DESCRIPTION

- Typically performed with a nurse assisting a physician
- Performed when routine therapeutic measures fail to control epistaxis
- Two main types of epistaxis: anterior bleeding and posterior bleeding
- Contraindicated in nasal trauma that might involve internal structure injury, coagulopathy, potential cerebrospinal fluid leak

EQUIPMENT

For anterior and posterior packing

Gowns ◆ goggles ◆ masks ◆ sterile gloves ◆ emesis basin ◆ facial tissue ◆ patient drape ◆ nasal speculum and tongue depressors ◆ directed illumination source, or fiber-optic nasal endoscope ◆ suction apparatus with sterile suction-connecting tubing and sterile nasal aspirator tip ◆ sterile bowl and sterile normal saline solution for flushing ◆ sterile towels ◆ sterile cotton-

tipped applicators ◆ local anesthetic spray or solution ◆ sedative or analgesic ◆ sterile cotton balls or cotton pledgets ◆ 10-ml syringe with 22G
1½″ needle ◆ silver nitrate sticks ◆ electrocautery device ◆ topical vasoconstrictor ◆ absorbable hemostatic ◆ sterile normal saline solution ◆ hypoallergenic tape ◆ antibiotic ointment ◆ petroleum jelly

For anterior packing
Two packages of 1½″ (4-cm) petroleum strip gauze 36″ to 48″ (0.9 to
1.2 m) ◆ two nasal tampons ◆ anterior nasal packing sponge

For posterior packing
Posterior nasal packing sponge with or without airway or two #14 or #16
French catheters with 30-cc balloon or two single- or double-chamber nasal
balloon catheters ◆ bayonet forceps ◆ marking pen

For assessment and bedside use
Tongue blades ◆ flashlight ◆ long hemostats or sponge forceps ◆ 60-ml syringe for deflating balloons (if applicable)

ESSENTIAL STEPS

■ Wash your hands.
■ Assemble all equipment at the patient's bedside.
■ Plug in and test the suction apparatus, and connect the tubing from the
collection bottle to the suction source.
■ Create a sterile field at the bedside and, using sterile technique, place all
sterile equipment on the sterile field.
■ If the physician will inject a local anesthetic rather than spray, place the
22G 1½″ needle attached to the 10-ml syringe on the sterile field.
■ When the physician readies the syringe, clean the stopper and hold the
vial so he can withdraw the anesthetic.
■ Open the packages containing the sterile suction-connecting tubing and
aspirating tip, and place them on the sterile field.
■ Fill the sterile bowl with normal saline solution to flush the suction tub-
ing.
■ Thoroughly lubricate the anterior or posterior packing with antibiotic
ointment if ordered.
■ Test a balloon for leaks by inflating the catheter with normal saline solu-
tion.
■ Remove the solution before insertion.
■ Wear a gown, gloves, and goggles during insertion of packing to prevent
contamination.
■ Check vital signs, and observe for hypotension with postural changes.

ALERT *Hypotension in a patient with a nosebleed suggests significant blood loss.*

- Monitor airway patency.

ALERT *A patient with an uncontrolled nosebleed is at risk for aspirating or vomiting swallowed blood.*

- Explain the procedure to the patient and offer reassurance.
- If ordered, give a sedative or analgesic to reduce anxiety and pain and decrease sympathetic stimulation, which can exacerbate a nosebleed.
- Help the patient sit with his head tilted forward.
- Turn on the suction apparatus and attach the connecting tubing.
- To inspect the nasal cavity, the physician will use a nasal speculum and an external light source or a fiber-optic nasal endoscope.
- To remove collected blood and help visualize the bleeding vessel, the physician will use suction or cotton-tipped applicators.
- The nose may be treated early with a topical vasoconstrictor such as phenylephrine to slow bleeding and aid visualization.

ALERT *Heavy posterior bleeding that's difficult to treat is most common in elderly patients due to hypertension or coagulopathy.*

For anterior nasal packing

- Help the physician apply a topical vasoconstrictor or use chemical cautery (silver nitrate stick) to control bleeding.
- To enhance the vasoconstrictor's action, apply manual pressure to the nose for about 10 minutes.
- If bleeding persists, you may help insert an absorbable hemostatic nasal tampon directly on the bleeding site.
- If these methods fail, prepare to assist with electrocautery or insertion of petroleum strip gauze or a packing sponge.
- While the anterior pack is in place, apply petroleum jelly to the patient's lips and nostrils to prevent drying and cracking.

For posterior nasal packing

- Wash your hands and put on sterile gloves.
- Lubricate the soft catheters to ease insertion if using a balloon device.
- Instruct the patient to open his mouth and breathe normally.
- Help the physician insert the packing as directed.
- Help the patient assume a position with his head elevated 45 to 90 degrees.
- Assess him for airway obstruction or respiratory changes.
- Monitor vital signs regularly.

NURSING CONSIDERATIONS

ALERT *Nasal packing is very uncomfortable and promotes hypoxia and hypoventilation, which can be fatal if the patient isn't properly monitored.*

■ If mucosal oozing persists, apply a moustache dressing.

■ Change the pad when soiled.

■ Test the patient's call bell to ensure he can summon help.

ALERT *Keep emergency equipment at the patient's bedside to speed packing removal if it becomes displaced and occludes the airway.*

■ Obtain a patient history to determine the underlying cause of nosebleed.

■ Laboratory work may include complete blood count and coagulation profile.

■ A blood transfusion may be necessary.

■ Arterial blood gas analysis may be ordered.

■ Supplemental humidified oxygen with a face mask may be needed.

■ Provide thorough mouth care often.

■ The patient should be on modified bed rest.

■ Give nonaspirin analgesics, decongestants, sedatives, and antibiotics.

■ Nasal packing is usually removed in 2 to 5 days.

■ Monitor the patient for complications such as blood loss; infections such as otitis media and sinusitis; hypoxemia; airway obstruction; mucosal pressure necrosis; hypotension; septal hematoma-perforation; vasovagal episode; and migration of packing.

■ Note the type of pack used to ensure its removal at the appropriate time.

■ Record estimated blood loss and all fluids given.

■ Document vital signs.

■ Note the response to sedation or position changes.

■ Record laboratory results.

■ Document drugs given, including topical agents.

■ Document discharge instructions and clinical follow-up plans.

■ After an anterior pack is removed, tell the patient to avoid picking at, inserting an object into, or blowing his nose forcefully for 48 hours or as ordered.

■ Tell the patient to expect reduced smell and taste ability.

■ Make sure the patient has a working smoke detector at home.

■ Advise the patient to eat soft foods because of eating and swallowing impairment.

■ Instruct the patient to drink fluids or use artificial saliva to cope with dry mouth.

■ Teach the patient how to prevent nosebleeds and have him seek medical help if he can't stop bleeding.

Nasogastric tube insertion and removal

DESCRIPTION

■ Usually inserted to decompress the stomach
■ Can prevent vomiting after major surgery
■ Used to assess and treat upper GI bleeding, collect gastric contents for analysis, perform gastric lavage, aspirate gastric secretions, and give drugs and nutrients
■ Requires close observation of the patient and verification of proper placement
■ Must be inserted with care in pregnant patients and those with increased risk of complications
■ Most common tubes: Levin tube and Salem sump tube
■ Contraindicated in coma, facial or basilar skull fracture with cribriform plate injury, and hypothermia

EQUIPMENT

For inserting a nasogastric tube

Tube (usually #12, #14, #16, or #18 French for a normal adult) ◆ towel or linen-saver pad ◆ facial tissues ◆ emesis basin ◆ penlight ◆ 1″ or 2″ hypoallergenic tape ◆ gloves ◆ water-soluble lubricant ◆ cup or glass of water with straw ◆ pH test strip ◆ tongue blade ◆ catheter-tip or bulb syringe or irrigation set ◆ safety pin ◆ ordered suction equipment

For removing a nasogastric tube

Stethoscope ◆ gloves ◆ catheter-tip syringe ◆ normal saline solution ◆ towel or linen-saver pad ◆ adhesive remover ◆ clamp (optional)

ESSENTIAL STEPS

■ Provide privacy.
■ Wash your hands and put on gloves.
■ Identify the proper tube.
■ Inspect the NG tube for defects.
■ Check the tube's patency by flushing it with water.

Inserting a nasogastric tube

■ Explain the procedure to the patient.
■ Emphasize that swallowing will ease the tube's advancement.

- Agree on a signal the patient can use if he wants you to stop briefly during the procedure.
- Put the patient in high Fowler's position, unless contraindicated.
- Drape the towel or linen-saver pad over his chest.
- Have him blow his nose to clear his nostrils.
- Place the facial tissues and emesis basin within reach.
- Help him face forward with his neck in a neutral position.
- Hold the end of the tube at the tip of his nose, then extend the tube to his earlobe and down to the xiphoid process in order to determine how long the NG tube must be to reach the stomach.
- Mark this distance on the tubing with tape. It may be necessary to add 2″ (5 cm) for tall individuals to ensure entry into the stomach.
- Use a penlight and inspect for a deviated septum or other abnormalities in order to determine which nostril will allow easier access.
- Ask if he ever had nasal surgery or a nasal injury, and assess airflow in both nostrils.
- Lubricate the first 3″ (7.6 cm) of the tube with a water-soluble gel.
- Instruct the patient to hold his head straight and upright.
- Grasp the tube with the end pointing downward, curve it if necessary, and carefully insert it into the more patent nostril.
- Aim the tube downward and toward the ear closer to the chosen nostril.
- Advance it slowly to avoid pressure on the turbinates and resultant pain and bleeding. When the tube reaches the nasopharynx, you'll feel resistance.
- Instruct the patient to lower his head slightly to close the trachea and open the esophagus.
- Rotate the tube 180 degrees toward the opposite nostril.
- Unless contraindicated, offer the patient a cup or glass of water with a straw.
- Direct him to sip and swallow as you slowly advance the tube.
- Watch for respiratory distress as you advance the tube.

   ALERT *If the patient is coughing, choking, or otherwise showing signs of respiratory distress, withdraw the tube until symptoms subside.*

- Stop advancing the tube when the tape mark reaches the patient's nostril.

Ensuring proper tube placement

- Use a tongue blade and penlight to examine the patient's mouth and throat for signs of a coiled section of tubing.
- Attach a catheter-tip or bulb syringe and try to aspirate stomach contents.
- Examine the aspirate and place a small amount on the pH test strip.

- Correct gastric placement is likely if the aspirate has a typical gastric fluid appearance and the pH is 5.0 or less.

  ALERT *When confirming tube placement, never place the tube's end in a container of water. If the tube is in the trachea, the patient may aspirate water. Bubbles don't confirm proper placement as the tube may be coiled in the trachea or the esophagus.*

- Advance the tube 1" to 2" (2.5 to 5 cm) if you still can't aspirate stomach contents. Inject 10 cc of air into the tube.
- Obtain X-ray verification if tests don't confirm proper tube placement.
- Secure the NG tube to the patient's nose with hypoallergenic tape or with a prepackaged product that secures and cushions the tube at the nose.
- Tie a slipknot around the tube with a rubber band; secure the rubber band to the patient's gown with a safety pin.
- Fasten the tape tab to the patient's gown.
- Attach the tube to suction equipment, if ordered, and set the designated suction pressure.
- Provide frequent nose and mouth care while the tube is in place.

Removing a nasogastric tube

- Explain the procedure to the patient.
- Assess bowel function by auscultating for peristalsis or flatus.
- Help the patient into semi-Fowler's position.
- Wash your hands and put on gloves.
- Drape a towel or linen-saver pad across his chest.
- Flush the tube with 10 ml of normal saline solution using a catheter-tip syringe to ensure that the tube doesn't contain stomach contents.
- Untape the tube from the patient's nose and unpin it from his gown.
- Clamp the tube by folding it in your hand.
- Ask the patient to hold his breath to close the epiglottis.
- Withdraw the tube slowly.
- Cover and discard the tube immediately.
- Assist the patient with thorough mouth and skin care.
- Monitor for signs of GI dysfunction for the next 48 hours.
- GI dysfunction may necessitate reinsertion of the tube.

NURSING CONSIDERATIONS

- Pass the tube orally if the patient has a deviated septum or other nasal condition that prevents nasal insertion. Sliding the tube over the tongue, proceed as you would for nasal insertion.
- When using the oral route, coil the end of the tube around your hand.

- If your patient is unconscious, tilt the chin toward his chest to close the trachea.
- Advance the tube between respirations.
- While advancing the tube, watch for signs that it entered the trachea, such as choking or breathing difficulties in a conscious patient and cyanosis in an unconscious patient or a patient without a cough reflex. If these signs occur, remove the tube immediately.
- Allow the patient time to rest; try to reinsert the tube.
- After tube placement, vomiting suggests tubal obstruction or incorrect position. Assess immediately to determine the cause.
- Monitor the patient for complications, such as skin erosion at the nostril, sinusitis, esophagitis, esophagotracheal fistula, gastric ulceration, pulmonary and oral infection, electrolyte imbalances, and dehydration.
- Record the type and size of the NG tube.
- Note the date, time, and route of insertion and removal.
- Note the patient's tolerance of procedure.
- Document type, color, odor, consistency, and amount of gastric drainage.
- Record the patient's tolerance of procedure.
- Note the subsequent irrigation procedures and continuing problems after irrigation.
- Note unusual events following NG removal, such as nausea, vomiting, abdominal distention, and food intolerance.
- Tell the patient what to expect during insertion.
- Explain signs and symptoms to report, as needed.
- Tell the patient to avoid food and drink for several hours after tube removal.

Nephrostomy and cystostomy tube care

DESCRIPTION

- A urinary diversion technique to ensure adequate drainage from kidneys or bladder and help prevent urinary tract infection or kidney failure (see *Urinary diversion techniques*, page 374)
- Nephrostomy tube: drains urine directly from a kidney when a disorder (such as calculi in the ureter or ureteropelvic junction or an obstructing tumor) inhibits normal urine flow
  - Usually placed percutaneously; sometimes surgically inserted
  - Allows kidney tissue damaged by obstructive disease to heal
- Cystostomy tube: drains urine from the bladder, diverting it from the urethra

FOCUS IN
URINARY DIVERSION TECHNIQUES

A cystostomy or a nephrostomy can be used to create a permanent urinary diversion to relieve obstruction from an inoperable tumor or provide an outlet for urine after cystectomy.

A temporary diversion can relieve obstruction from a calculus or ureteral edema.

In a cystostomy, a catheter is inserted percutaneously through the suprapubic area into the bladder. In a nephrostomy, a catheter is inserted percutaneously through the flank into the renal pelvis.

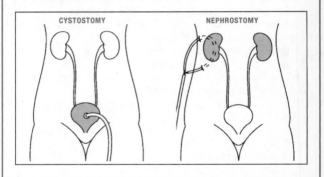

CYSTOSTOMY   NEPHROSTOMY

- Used after certain gynecologic procedures, bladder surgery, prostatectomy, and for severe urethral strictures or traumatic injury
- Inserted about 2" (5 cm) above the symphysis pubis; may be used alone or with an indwelling urethral catheter

EQUIPMENT

For dressing changes

4" × 4" gauze pads ◆ povidone-iodine solution or povidone-iodine pads ◆ sterile cup or emesis basin ◆ paper bag ◆ linen-saver pad ◆ clean gloves (for dressing removal) ◆ sterile gloves (for new dressing) ◆ precut 4" × 4" drain dressings or transparent semipermeable dressings ◆ adhesive tape (preferably hypoallergenic)

For nephrostomy-tube irrigation

3-ml syringe ◆ alcohol pad or povidone-iodine pad ◆ normal saline solution ◆ hemostat (optional)

ESSENTIAL STEPS

- Wash your hands, provide privacy, and explain the procedure to the patient.
- Assemble equipment at the patient's bedside.
- Open several packages of gauze pads, place them in the sterile cup or emesis basin, and pour the povidone-iodine solution over them.
- Open a commercially packaged kit (if available) using sterile technique.
- Fill the cup with antiseptic solution.
- Open the paper bag and place it away from the other equipment to avoid contaminating the sterile field.

Changing a dressing

- Put the patient on his back for a cystostomy tube or the side opposite the tube for a nephrostomy tube.
- Place the linen-saver pad under the patient to absorb drainage.
- Put on clean gloves.
- Carefully remove the tape around the tube.
- Remove wet or soiled dressings.
- Discard the tape and dressing in the paper bag.
- Remove the gloves and discard them in the bag.
- Put on sterile gloves.
- Pick up a saturated pad or dip a dry one into the cup of antiseptic solution.
- To clean the wound, wipe only once with each pad or sponge, moving from the insertion site outward.
- Discard the used pad or sponge in the paper bag.
- To avoid contaminating your gloves, don't touch the bag.
- Pick up a sterile 4″ × 4″ drain dressing and place it around the tube.
- If necessary, overlap two drain dressings to provide maximum absorption. Alternatively, depending on your facility's policy, apply a transparent semipermeable dressing over the site and tubing to allow observation of the site.
- Secure the dressing with hypoallergenic tape.
- Tape the tube to the patient's lateral abdomen to prevent tension.
- Dispose of all equipment appropriately.
- Clean the patient as necessary.

Irrigating a nephrostomy tube

- Fill the 3-ml syringe with the normal saline solution.
- Clean the junction of the nephrostomy tube and drainage tube with the alcohol pad or povidone-iodine pad, and disconnect the tubes.
- Insert the syringe into the nephrostomy tube opening, and instill 2 to 3 ml of normal saline solution into the tube.
- Slowly aspirate the solution back into the syringe.
- Never pull back on the plunger.
- If the solution doesn't return, remove the syringe from the tube and reattach it to the drainage tubing to allow the solution to drain by gravity.
- Dispose of all equipment appropriately.

NURSING CONSIDERATIONS

- Change dressings once per day or more often as needed.

  ALERT *Never irrigate a nephrostomy tube with more than 5 ml of solution because the capacity of the renal pelvis is usually between 4 and 8 ml. (The purpose of irrigation is to keep the tube patent, not to lavage the renal pelvis.)*
- Irrigate a cystostomy tube as you would an indwelling urinary catheter.
- Perform irrigation to avoid damaging suture lines.
- Curve a cystostomy tube to prevent kinks; kinks are likely if the patient lies on the insertion site.
- Check a nephrostomy tube frequently for kinks or obstructions.
- Suspect an obstruction when the amount of urine in the drainage bag decreases or the amount of urine around the insertion site increases.
- If a blood clot or mucus plug obstructs a nephrostomy or cystostomy tube, try milking the tube to restore its patency.
- Check cystostomy hourly for postoperative urologic patients.
- To check tube patency, note the amount of urine in the drainage bag and check the patient's bladder for distention.
- Keep the drainage bag below the level of the kidney at all times.
- Notify the physician immediately if the tube becomes dislodged.
- Cover the site with a sterile dressing.
- While clamping the nephrostomy tube, assess the patient for flank pain and fever, and monitor urine output.
- Monitor the patient for complications such as infection, sepsis, hemorrhage, nephron damage, colonic perforation, and perinephric abscess.
- Record the color and amount of drainage.
- Note the amount and type of irrigant used.
- Document whether you obtained a complete return.
- Document condition of skin around site.

- Document patient teaching.
- Explain how to clean the insertion site with soap and water, check for skin breakdown, and change dressing daily.
- Teach the patient how to change the leg bag or drainage bag.
- Explain how and when to wash the drainage bag.
- Encourage the patient to increase fluid intake to 3 qt (3 L) daily, if no contraindications.
- Explain signs of infection and have the patient report them to his physician.
- Refer the patient and family to appropriate community support sources.

Pacemaker (permanent) insertion and care

DESCRIPTION

- A self-contained heart pacing device implanted in a pocket beneath the patient's skin, designed to operate 3 to 20 years
- Inserted in an operating room or cardiac catheterization laboratory
- Nursing responsibilities: monitoring electrocardiogram (ECG) and maintaining sterile technique
- Used in patients with myocardial infarction, persistent bradyarrhythmia, complete heart block or slow ventricular rates, Stokes-Adams syndrome, Wolff-Parkinson-White syndrome, and sick sinus syndrome
- A biventricular pacemaker possibly benefiting a patient with heart failure
- Functions in the demand mode, which allows the patient's heart to beat on its own but prevents it from falling below a preset level
- Pacing electrodes placed in the atria, ventricles, or in both chambers; most common pacing codes are VVI for single-chamber pacing and DDD for dual-chamber pacing (see *Understanding pacemaker codes*, page 378)

EQUIPMENT

Sphygmomanometer ✦ stethoscope ✦ ECG monitor and strip-chart recorder ✦ sterile dressing tray ✦ povidone-iodine ointment ✦ shaving supplies ✦ sterile gauze dressing ✦ hypoallergenic tape ✦ sedatives ✦ alcohol pads ✦ emergency resuscitation equipment ✦ sterile gown and mask ✦ I.V. line for emergency medications (optional)

ESSENTIAL STEPS

- Explain the procedure to the patient.
- Provide and review literature from the manufacturer or the American Heart Association.

UNDERSTANDING PACEMAKER CODES

A permanent pacemaker uses a three- or five-letter programming code. The first
letter represents the chamber that's paced. The second represents the chamber
that's sensed. The third represents how the pulse generator responds. The fourth
denotes the pacemaker's programmability. The fifth denotes the pacemaker's
response to a tachyarrhythmia.

First letter	Second letter	Third letter
A = atrium	A = atrium	I = inhibited
V = ventricle	V = ventricle	T = triggered
D = dual (both chambers)	D = dual (both chambers)	D = dual (inhibited and
O = not applicable	O = not applicable	triggered)
		O = not applicable

Fourth letter	Fifth letter
P = basic functions programmable	P = pacing ability
M = multiprogrammable parameters	S = shock
C = communicating functions such as telemetry	D = dual ability to shock and pace
R = rate responsiveness	O = none
O = none	

Examples of two common programming codes

DDD	VVI
Pace: Atrium and ventricle	Pace: Ventricle
Sense: Atrium and ventricle	Sense: Ventricle
Response: Inhibited and triggered	Response: Inhibited
This is a fully automatic, or universal, pacemaker	This is a demand pacemaker, inhibited

- Emphasize that the pacemaker augments his natural heart rate.
- Obtain informed consent.
- Ask the patient if he's allergic to anesthetics or iodine.

Preoperative care

For pacemaker insertion

- Shave the patient's chest from the axilla to the midline and from the clavicle to the nipple line on the side selected by the physician.
- Establish an I.V. line at a keep-vein-open rate.

■ Obtain baseline vital signs and a baseline ECG.
■ Provide sedation, as ordered.

In the operating room
■ Put on a gown and a mask.
■ Run a baseline rhythm strip. Check for adequate paper.
■ In transvenous placement, the catheter is guided by a fluoroscope, passes through the cephalic or external jugular vein until it reaches the right ventricle.
■ The catheter is attached to the pulse generator, inserted into the chest wall, and sutured closed. A small drainage tube outlet remains.

Postoperative care
■ Monitor the patient's ECG.
■ Monitor the I.V. flow rate; the I.V. line is usually kept in place for 24 to 48 hours postoperatively to allow for possible emergency treatment of arrhythmias.
■ Check the dressing for signs of bleeding and infection.
■ Prophylactic antibiotics may be ordered for up to 7 days after implantation.
■ Change the dressing and apply povidone-iodine ointment at least once every 24 to 48 hours.
■ If the dressing becomes soiled or the site is exposed to air, change the dressing immediately.
■ Check vital signs and level of consciousness (LOC) every 15 minutes for the first hour, every hour for the next 4 hours, every 4 hours for the next 48 hours, and then once every shift.

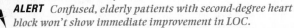 ***ALERT*** *Confused, elderly patients with second-degree heart block won't show immediate improvement in LOC.*

ALERT *Report to the physician signs and symptoms of a perforated ventricle, with resultant cardiac tamponade: persistent hiccups, distant heart sounds, pulsus paradoxus, hypotension with narrow pulse pressure, increased venous pressure, cyanosis, jugular vein distention, decreased urine output, restlessness, or complaints of fullness in the chest.*

NURSING CONSIDERATIONS
■ A biventricular pacemaker has three leads instead of one or two; one lead is placed in the right atrium and the other two are placed in each of the ventricles, improving pumping efficiency.
■ Provide the patient with an identification card that lists the pacemaker

type and manufacturer, serial number, pacemaker rate setting, date implanted, and physician's name.

- Watch for signs of pacemaker malfunction.
- Monitor the patient for complications such as infection; lead displacement; perforated ventricle; cardiac tamponade; and lead fracture and disconnection.
- Record the type, serial number, and manufacturer of pacemaker.
- Document the pacing rate.
- Record the date of implantation.
- Note the physician's name.
- Document whether the pacemaker successfully treated the arrhythmias.
- Tell the patient to inform his physicians, dentist, and other health care personnel that he has a pacemaker.
- Advise the patient to use a cellular phone on the opposite side of his pacemaker.
- Caution the patient to move away from electrical equipment if he experiences light-headedness or dizziness. Moving away should restore normal pacemaker function.
- Teach the patient to clean his pacemaker site gently with soap and water when he takes a shower or a bath. Tell him to leave the incision exposed to the air.
- Instruct the patient to inspect the skin around the incision. Advise him that a slight bulge is normal, but to call the physician if he feels discomfort or notices swelling, redness, discharge, or other problems.
- Teach the patient how to check his pulse for 1 minute on the side of his neck, inside his elbow, or on the thumb side of his wrist. The pulse rate should be the same as his pacemaker rate or faster. Instruct him to contact the physician if he thinks his heart is beating too fast or too slow.
- Advise the patient to take his medications, including those for pain, as prescribed.
- Advise the patient to notify the physician if he experiences signs of pacemaker failure, such as palpitations, a fast heart rate, a slow heart rate (5 to 10 beats less than the pacemaker's setting), dizziness, fainting, shortness of breath, swollen ankles or feet, anxiety, forgetfulness, or confusion.

Postoperative care

DESCRIPTION

- Begins when the patient arrives in the postanesthesia care unit (PACU) and continues as he moves on to the short procedure unit, medical-surgical unit, or critical care area

- To minimize postoperative complications by early detection and prompt treatment
- To treat pain, inadequate oxygenation, or adverse physiologic effects of sudden movement
- Recovery time from general anesthesia varying with the patient's amount of body fat, overall condition, premedication regimen, and type, dosage, and duration of anesthesia; lasts longer than induction because anesthetic is retained in fat and muscle

EQUIPMENT

Thermometer ◆ watch with second hand ◆ stethoscope ◆ sphygmomanometer ◆ postoperative flowchart or documentation tool

ESSENTIAL STEPS

- Assemble the necessary equipment at the patient's bedside.
- Obtain the patient's record from the PACU nurse.
- Transfer the patient from the stretcher to the bed and position him properly.
- Use caution when transferring patients with orthopedic surgery or skeletal traction.
- Provide comfort and ensure safety (raise the bed's side rails).
- Assess level of consciousness, skin color, and mucous membranes.
- Monitor breathing rate, depth, and breath sounds.
- Administer oxygen and initiate oximetry.
- Monitor the patient's pulse rate.
- Make sure that preoperative and postoperative blood pressures are within 20% of each other.
- Make sure the patient's body temperature is at least 95° F (35° C). If it's lower, use blankets or the Bair Hugger patient-warming system.
- Assess infusion sites for redness, pain, swelling, or drainage. If infiltration occurs, discontinue the I.V. and restart.
- Assess wound dressings. If soiled, note the characteristics of drainage and outline the soiled area. Note the date and time of assessment on the dressing.
- If the drainage area enlarges, reinforce the dressing and alert the physician.
- Note the presence and condition of drains and tubes.
- Note the color, type, odor, and amount of drainage and urine output.
- Make sure drains are properly connected and free from obstructions.
- For a vascular or orthopedic surgery, assess all extremities.
- Perform neurovascular checks; assess color, temperature, sensation,

movement, and presence and quality of pulses. Notify the physician of abnormalities.
- Be alert for signs of airway obstruction and hypoventilation.
- Assess for cardiovascular complications (arrhythmias or hypotension).
- Encourage coughing and deep-breathing exercises. (Exceptions: nasal, ophthalmic, or neurologic surgery.)
- Administer postoperative drugs.
- Assess gag reflex before offering fluids.
- Monitor the patient's intake and output.
- Assess for bowel sounds and flatus before offering food.

NURSING CONSIDERATIONS

- Monitor for fear, pain, anxiety, hypothermia, confusion, and immobility, which can affect patient safety and recovery.
- Offer emotional support and refer for ongoing emotional support if indicated.
- Avoid talking about the patient in his presence because hearing returns first.
- Cough and gag reflexes reappear and, if the patient can lift his head, he's usually able to breathe on his own.
- After spinal anesthesia, the patient should remain supine with the bed adjusted between 0 and 20 degrees for at least 6 hours. Reassure him that sensation and mobility will return to his legs.
- Monitor respiratory status for those using epidural analgesia infusion for postoperative pain control.
- Monitor for nausea, vomiting, itching, or sensorimotor loss.
- Monitor the patient for complications such as arrhythmias, hypotension, hypovolemia, septicemia, septic shock, atelectasis, pneumonia, thrombophlebitis, pulmonary embolism, urine retention, wound infection, evisceration, abdominal distention, paralytic ileus, constipation, altered body image, and postoperative psychosis.
- Record vital signs.
- Note the condition of dressings and drains and characteristics of drainage.
- Document interventions taken to alleviate pain and anxiety and the patient's responses to them.
- Record complications and interventions taken.
- Teach the patient how to use the patient-controlled analgesia if one has been ordered.

Preoperative care

DESCRIPTION

■ Begins when surgery is planned and ends with administration of anesthesia

■ Includes an interview and assessment to collect baseline subjective and objective data from the patient and family; diagnostic tests such as urinalysis, electrocardiogram, and chest radiography, preoperative teaching, securing informed consent from the patient, and physical preparation

EQUIPMENT

Thermometer ◆ sphygmomanometer ◆ stethoscope ◆ watch with second hand ◆ weight scale ◆ tape measure

ESSENTIAL STEPS

■ Assemble needed equipment at the patient's bedside or admission area.

■ For same-day surgery, instruct the patient not to eat or drink for 8 hours before surgery.

■ Confirm arrival time and instruct him to leave valuables at home.

■ Verify arrangements for postsurgery transportation.

■ Obtain a health history, including previous medical or surgical procedures.

■ Assess the patient's readiness in knowledge, perceptions, and expectations.

■ Assess psychosocial needs for occupational, financial, support systems, mental status, and cultural areas.

■ Obtain a drug history of prescriptions, over-the-counter drugs, supplements, and herbal preparations.

■ Assess for known allergies to foods, drugs, and latex.

■ Obtain height, weight, and vital signs.

■ Identify risk factors including age, general health, drug use, mobility, nutritional status, fluid and electrolyte disturbances, lifestyle considerations, disorder's duration, location, and nature of the procedure.

■ Explain preoperative procedures to reduce postoperative anxiety and pain, increase compliance, hasten recovery, and decrease length of stay.

■ Explain sequence of events, holding area, surgical dress, equipment, incision, dressings, and staples or sutures.

■ Explain that minimal conversation will help the preoperative medication take effect.

OBTAINING INFORMED CONSENT

Informed consent means that the patient has consented to a procedure after receiving a full explanation of the procedure, its risks and complications, and the risk if the procedure isn't performed at this time. Although obtaining informed consent is the physician's responsibility, the nurse is responsible for verifying that this step has been taken.

You may be asked to witness the patient's signature. However, if you didn't hear the physician's explanation to the patient, you must sign that you're witnessing the patient's signature only.

Consent forms must be signed before the patient receives preoperative medication because forms signed after sedatives are given are legally invalid. Adults and emancipated minors can sign their own consent forms. A consent form for children or adults with impaired mental status must be signed by a parent or guardian.

■ Discuss transfer procedures and techniques; describe sensations the patient will experience.

■ Discuss postoperative exercises such as deep breathing and coughing, extremity exercises, and movement and ambulation to minimize respiratory and circulatory complications.

■ Discuss surgery procedures including morning care, verifying a signed informed consent form, preoperative medications, preoperative checklist, and chart. (See *Obtaining informed consent.*)

■ Discuss preoperative interventions such as restricting food and fluids for about 8 hours before surgery, enemas before abdominal or GI surgery, and antibiotics for 2 or 3 days preoperatively to prevent contamination of the peritoneal cavity by GI bacteria.

■ Remove hairpins, nail polish, and jewelry. Note whether dentures, contact lenses, or prosthetic devices have been removed or left in place. Verify with the patient that the correct surgical site has been marked.

■ Before transport to the surgical area, ensure that the patient's hospital gown and identification band are in place and that his vital signs have been recorded.

NURSING CONSIDERATIONS

■ Administer preoperative medications on time.

■ Make sure the patient has had no food or drink preoperatively.

■ Raise the bed's side rails after giving preoperative medications.

- If present, direct the patient's family to the appropriate waiting area and offer support as needed.
- The chart and the surgical checklist must accompany the patient to surgery.
- Document using preoperative checklist used by your facility.
- Note all nursing care measures.
- Document preoperative drugs.
- Record the results of diagnostic tests.
- Note the time the patient is transferred to the surgical area.
- Teach the patient coughing and deep-breathing exercises before surgery, as appropriate.
- Inform the patient that he may have surgical dressings, surgical drains, an I.V. line, and a urinary catheter after the surgery.
- Advise the patient that he'll feel discomfort but that pain medication will be available and he should ask for it when he feels pain.
- Tell the patient that he'll be in an after-surgery recovery area for at least 1 hour after surgery to monitor his vital signs.

Pressure ulcer care

DESCRIPTION

- Involves relieving pressure, restoring circulation, promoting adequate nutrition, and resolving or managing related disorders
- May require special pressure-reducing devices such as beds, mattresses, mattress overlays, and chair cushions
- Other measures: decreasing risk factors, use of topical treatments, wound cleansing, debridement, and use of dressings to support moist wound healing
- Uses standard precaution guidelines of the Centers for Disease Control and Prevention
- Effectiveness and duration of treatment dependent on the pressure ulcer's characteristics

EQUIPMENT

Hypoallergenic tape or elastic netting ✦ overbed table ✦ piston-type irrigating system ✦ two pairs of gloves ✦ normal saline solution, as ordered ✦ sterile 4″ × 4″ gauze pads ✦ sterile cotton swabs ✦ selected topical dressing ✦ linen-saver pads ✦ impervious plastic trash bag ✦ disposable wound-measuring device

ESSENTIAL STEPS

- Wash your hands.
- Review principles of standard precautions.
- Provide privacy.
- Assemble equipment at the patient's bedside.
- Cut tape into strips.
- Loosen lids on cleaning solutions and drugs.
- Loosen existing dressing edges and tapes.
- Put on gloves.
- Attach an impervious plastic trash bag to the overbed table.

Cleaning the pressure ulcer

- Explain the procedure to allay fear and promote cooperation.
- Position the patient for comfort and easy access to site.
- Cover bed linens with a linen-saver pad to prevent soiling.
- Open the normal saline solution container and the piston syringe.
- Pour solution carefully into a clean or sterile irrigation container.
- Put the piston syringe into the opening of the irrigation container.
- Open the packages of supplies.
- Put on gloves before removing old dressing and exposing the pressure ulcer.
- Discard the soiled dressing in the impervious plastic trash bag.
- Inspect the wound. Note the color, amount, and odor of drainage or necrotic debris.
- Measure the wound perimeter with a disposable wound-measuring device.
- Apply full force of the piston syringe to irrigate the ulcer, remove necrotic debris, and decrease bacteria in the wound.

  ALERT *The benefits of cleaning the wound need to be weighed against the trauma to the tissue bed caused by the cleaning. Don't use povidone-iodine, iodophor, sodium hypochlorite solution, hydrogen peroxide, or acetic acid because they have been shown to be cytotoxic. Use normal saline at a pressure between 4 and 15 pounds per square inch.*

- For nonnecrotic wounds, use minimal pressure to prevent damage.
- Remove and discard your soiled gloves and put on a fresh pair.
- Insert a sterile cotton swab into the wound to assess wound tunneling or undermining.
- Assess and note the condition of clean wound and surrounding skin.

  COLLABORATION *Notify a wound care specialist if adherent necrotic material is present or the ulcer fails to improve.*

- Apply the appropriate topical dressing.

Applying a moist saline gauze dressing
- Irrigate the ulcer with normal saline solution. Blot surrounding skin dry.
- Moisten the gauze dressing with normal saline solution.
- Gently place the dressing over the surface of the ulcer.
- To separate surfaces within the wound, gently place a dressing between opposing wound surfaces. Don't pack the gauze tightly.
- Change the dressing often enough to keep the wound moist.

Applying a hydrocolloid dressing
- Irrigate the ulcer with normal saline solution. Blot surrounding skin dry.
- Choose a clean, dry, presized dressing, or cut one to overlap the pressure ulcer by about 1″ (2.5 cm).
- Remove the dressing from its package, remove the release paper and apply the dressing to the wound. Carefully smooth wrinkles as you apply the dressing.
- If using tape to secure the dressing, apply a skin sealant to the intact skin around the ulcer.
- When dry, tape the dressing to the skin. Avoid tension or pressure.
- Remove and discard your gloves and other refuse.
- Wash your hands.
- Change a hydrocolloid dressing every 2 to 7 days.
- Discontinue if signs of infection are present.

Applying a transparent dressing
- Irrigate the ulcer with normal saline solution. Blot surrounding skin dry.
- Clean and dry the wound as described above.
- Select a dressing to overlap the ulcer by 2″ (5 cm).
- Gently lay the dressing over the ulcer. Don't stretch it.
- Press firmly on the edges of the dressing to promote adherence.
- Tape edges to prevent them from curling.
- If necessary, aspirate accumulated fluid with a 21G needle and syringe.
- Clean the site with an alcohol pad and cover it with a transparent dressing.
- Change the dressing every 3 to 7 days, depending on drainage.

Applying an alginate dressing
- Irrigate the ulcer with normal saline solution. Blot surrounding skin dry.
- Apply alginate dressing to the ulcer surface. Cover with a second dressing. Secure with tape or elastic netting.
- If drainage is heavy, change the dressing once or twice daily for the first 3 to 5 days.

■ As drainage decreases, change the dressing less frequently — every 2 to 4 days or as ordered.

■ When drainage stops or the wound bed looks dry, stop using alginate dressing.

Applying a foam dressing

■ Irrigate the ulcer with normal saline solution. Blot surrounding skin dry.

■ Lay the foam dressing over the ulcer.

■ Use tape, elastic netting, or gauze to hold the dressing in place.

■ Change the dressing when the foam no longer absorbs the exudate.

Applying a hydrogel dressing

■ Irrigate the ulcer with normal saline solution. Blot surrounding skin dry.

■ Apply gel to the wound bed.

■ Cover the area with a second dressing.

■ Change the dressing as needed to keep the wound bed moist.

■ If you choose a sheet form dressing, cut it to match the wound base.

■ Hydrogel dressings also come in a prepackaged, saturated gauze to fill "dead space." Follow the manufacturer's directions.

Preventing pressure ulcers

■ Turn and reposition the patient every 1 to 2 hours unless contraindicated.

■ Use an air, gel, or 4″ foam mattress for those who can't turn themselves or those who are turned on a schedule.

■ Low– or high–air-loss therapy may be indicated.

■ Implement active or passive range-of-motion exercises.

■ To save time, combine exercises with bathing if applicable.

■ Lift rather than slide the patient when turning.

■ Use a turning sheet and get help from coworkers.

■ Use pillows to position the patient and increase his comfort.

> **ALERT** *Don't sit the patient on a rubber or plastic dough-nut, which can increase localized pressure at vulnerable points.*

■ Eliminate sheet wrinkles.

■ Post a turning schedule at his bedside.

■ Avoid the trochanter position. Instead, position at a 30-degree angle.

■ Avoid raising the bed more than 30 degrees for long periods.

■ Adjust or pad appliances, casts, or splints to ensure proper fit.

■ Gently apply lotion after bathing to keep skin moist.

■ Clean and dry soiled skin. Apply a protective moisture barrier.

NURSING CONSIDERATIONS

- Prevention helps avoid extensive therapy; measures include ensuring adequate nourishment and mobility to relieve pressure and promote circulation.
- Direct the patient in a chair or wheelchair to shift his weight every 15 minutes.
- Instruct a paraplegic to shift his weight by doing push-ups.
- Tell the patient to avoid heat lamps and harsh soaps.
- Avoid using elbow and heel protectors with a single narrow strap.
- Avoid using artificial sheepskin. It doesn't reduce pressure.
- Repair of stages 3 and 4 ulcers may require surgical intervention.
- Infection produces foul-smelling drainage, persistent pain, severe erythema, induration, and elevated skin and body temperatures.
- Infection may lead to cellulitis and septicemia.
- Record the date and time of initial and subsequent treatments.
- Detail preventive strategies performed.
- Note the location, size (length, width, depth), color, and appearance of the ulcer.
- Record the amount, odor, color, and consistency of drainage.
- Document condition and temperature of surrounding skin.
- Record body temperature daily.
- Reassess pressure ulcers at least weekly and update the plan.
- Record physician notification.
- Teach the patient and family the importance of prevention, signs and symptoms of infection, position changes, and treatment. Teach proper methods and encourage participation.
- Encourage the patient to follow a diet with adequate calories, protein, and vitamins.
- Refer the patient and his family to home health services for additional follow-up and instruction.

Residual limb and prosthesis care

DESCRIPTION

- Patient care immediately after limb amputation to include monitoring drainage from the residual limb, positioning the affected limb, assisting with exercises prescribed by a physical therapist, and wrapping and conditioning the limb
- Postoperative care slightly variable, depending on the amputation site and whether an elastic bandage or plaster cast is used

- After the residual limb heals, only routine daily care (proper hygiene and continued muscle-strengthening exercises) needed
- Prosthesis to be cleaned and lubricated daily and checked for proper fit

EQUIPMENT

For postoperative residual limb care

Pressure dressing ✦ abdominal pad ✦ suction equipment, if ordered ✦ overhead trapeze ✦ 1" adhesive tape ✦ bandage clips or safety pins ✦ sandbags or trochanter roll (for a leg) ✦ elastic limb shrinker or 4" elastic bandage ✦ tourniquet (optional, as last resort to control bleeding)

For residual limb and prosthesis care

Mild soap or alcohol pads ✦ special limb socks or athletic tube socks ✦ two washcloths ✦ two towels ✦ appropriate lubricating oil

ESSENTIAL STEPS

- Perform routine postoperative care.
- Provide for the patient's comfort, pain management, and safety.

Monitoring residual limb drainage

- Gravity causes fluid to accumulate at the residual limb. Frequently check the amount of blood and drainage on the dressing.
- Notify the physician if accumulations of drainage or blood increase rapidly or excessive bleeding occurs.
- Apply a pressure dressing or compress to the appropriate pressure points.
- Keep a tourniquet available and use it as a last resort.
- Tape the abdominal pad over the moist part of the dressing to provide a dry area to help prevent bacterial infection.
- Monitor the suction drainage equipment and note the amount and type of drainage.

Positioning the extremity

- Elevate the extremity for the first 24 hours.
- To prevent contractures, position the arm with the elbow extended and the shoulder abducted.
- To correctly position the leg, elevate the foot of the bed slightly and place sandbags or a trochanter roll against the hip to prevent external rotation.

  ALERT *Don't place a pillow under the thigh to flex the hip because this can cause hip flexion contracture. For the same reason, tell the patient to avoid prolonged sitting.*

- After a below-the-knee amputation, maintain knee extension to prevent hamstring muscle contractures.

■ After a leg amputation, place the patient on a firm surface in the prone position for at least 2 hours per day, with his legs close together and without pillows under his stomach, hips, knees, or residual limb, unless this position is contraindicated.

Assisting with prescribed exercises

■ After arm amputation, encourage the patient to exercise the residual arm to prevent muscle contractures.

■ Help the patient perform isometric and range-of-motion (ROM) exercises for both shoulders.

■ After leg amputation, stand behind the patient and, if necessary, support him with your hands at his waist during balancing exercises.

■ Instruct the patient to exercise the affected and unaffected limbs to maintain muscle tone and increase muscle strength.

■ The patient with a leg amputation may perform push-ups in the sitting position with his arms at his sides, or pull-ups on the overhead trapeze to strengthen his arms, shoulders, and back, in preparation for using crutches.

Wrapping and conditioning the residual limb

■ If the patient doesn't have a rigid cast, apply an elastic shrinker to prevent edema and shape the limb in preparation for the prosthesis.

■ Wrap the limb so it narrows toward the distal end. (See *Wrapping a residual limb*, page 392.)

■ This helps ensure comfort when the patient wears the prosthesis.

■ If an elastic shrinker isn't available, you can wrap the limb in a 4″ elastic bandage. Stretch the bandage to about two-thirds its maximum length as you wrap it diagonally around the residual limb, with the greatest pressure distally.

■ Make sure the bandage covers all portions of the limb smoothly because wrinkles or exposed areas encourage skin breakdown.

■ If the patient experiences throbbing after the limb is wrapped, the bandage may be too tight. Remove the bandage immediately, reapply it less tightly, and check it regularly.

■ Rewrap it when it begins to bunch up at the end (typically about every 12 hours for a moderately active patient).

■ After removing the bandage to rewrap it, massage the residual limb gently, always pushing toward the suture line rather than away from it.

■ When healing begins, instruct the patient to push the residual limb against a pillow.

■ Have him progress gradually to pushing against harder surfaces.

WRAPPING A RESIDUAL LIMB

Proper residual limb care helps protect the limb, reduces swelling, and
prepares the limb for a prosthesis.
As you perform the procedure,
teach it to the patient.

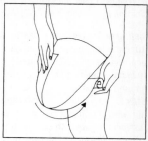

Start by obtaining two 4″ elastic
bandages. Center the end of the
first 4″ bandage at the top of the
patient's thigh. Unroll the bandage
downward over the stump and to
the back of the leg (as shown at
right).

Make three figure-eight turns to adequately cover the ends of the stump. As
you wrap, be sure to include the roll of flesh in the groin area. Use enough pressure to ensure that the stump narrows toward the end so that it fits comfortably
into the prosthesis.

Use the second 4″ bandage to anchor the first bandage around the waist. For
a below-the-knee amputation, use the knee to anchor the bandage in place.
Secure the bandage with clips, safety pins, or adhesive tape. Check the stump
bandage regularly and rewrap it if it bunches at the end.

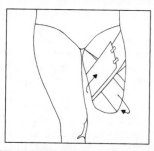
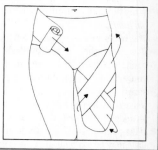

Caring for the healed limb

- Bathe the residual limb at the end of the day because the warm water
  may cause swelling, making reapplication of the prosthesis difficult.
  Don't soak the limb for long periods.
- Don't apply lotion to the limb. This may clog follicles, increasing the risk
  of infection.
- Rub the residual limb with alcohol daily to toughen the skin and reduce
  risk of skin breakdown.

- Instruct the patient to watch for and report severe irritation after rubbing the limb with alcohol.
- Avoid using powders or lotions, which can soften or irritate the skin.
- Inspect the residual limb for redness, swelling, irritation, and calluses. Report these to the physician.
- Change and wash the patient's elastic bandages every day to avoid exposing the skin to excessive perspiration.
- To shape the residual limb, have the patient wear an elastic bandage 24 hours per day except while bathing.
- To prevent infection, never shave the residual limb.
- Tell the patient to avoid putting weight on the residual limb, but continue muscle-strengthening exercises.

Caring for the plastic prosthesis
- Wipe the plastic socket of the prosthesis with a damp cloth and mild soap or alcohol to prevent bacterial accumulation.
- Wipe the insert, if the prosthesis has one, with a dry cloth and dry the prosthesis thoroughly. When possible, allow it to dry overnight.
- Maintain and lubricate the prosthesis and check for malfunctions.
- Frequently check the condition of a shoe on a foot prosthesis and change it as necessary.

Applying the prosthesis
- Apply a residual limb sock, keeping the seams away from bony prominences.
- If the prosthesis has an insert, remove it from the socket, place it over the residual limb, and insert the residual limb into the prosthesis.
- If it has no insert, slide the prosthesis over the residual limb.
- Secure the prosthesis onto the residual limb according to the manufacturer's directions.

NURSING CONSIDERATIONS
- If the patient arrives at the facility with a traumatic amputation, the amputated part may be saved for possible reimplantation. (See *Caring for an amputated body part*, page 394.)
- Exercise of the remaining muscles in an amputated limb must begin the day after surgery.
- Arm exercises progress from isometrics to assisted ROM to active ROM.
- Leg exercises include rising from a chair, balancing on one leg, and ROM exercises of the knees and hips.
- For a below-the-knee amputation, you may substitute an athletic tube sock for a residual limb sock by cutting off the elastic band.

CARING FOR AN AMPUTATED BODY PART

After traumatic amputation, a surgeon may be able to reimplant the severed body part through microsurgery. The chance of successful reimplantation is much greater if the amputated part has received proper care (amputated parts should be placed in a clean plastic bag).

If the patient arrives at the hospital with a severed body part, first make sure that bleeding at the amputation site has been controlled. Follow these guidelines for preserving the body part.

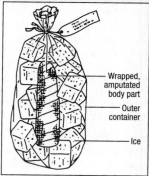

Wrapped, amputated body part

Outer container

Ice

■ Put on sterile gloves. Place several sterile gauze pads and an appropriate amount of sterile roller gauze in a sterile basin and pour sterile normal saline or sterile lactated Ringer's solution over them. Never use any other solution and don't try to scrub or debride the part.

■ Holding the body part in one gloved hand, carefully pat it dry with sterile gauze. Place saline-soaked gauze pads over the stump; wrap the whole body part with saline-soaked roller gauze. Wrap the gauze with a sterile towel, if available. Put this package in a watertight container or bag and seal it.

■ Fill another plastic bag with ice and place the part, still in its watertight container, inside. Seal the outer bag (always protect the part from direct contact with ice—and never use dry ice—to prevent irreversible tissue damage that would make the part unsuitable for reimplantation). Keep this bag ice-cold until reimplantation surgery.

■ Label the bag with the patient's name, identification number, identification of the amputated part, the hospital identification number, and the date and time when cooling began.

■ The body part must be wrapped and cooled quickly. Irreversible tissue damage occurs after only 6 hours at ambient temperature. However, hypothermic management seldom preserves tissues for more than 24 hours.

■ If the patient has a rigid dressing, perform normal cast care.
■ If the cast slips off, apply an elastic bandage immediately and notify the physician because edema will develop rapidly.
■ Monitor the patient for complications, such as hemorrhage, residual limb infection, contractures, swollen or flabby residual limb, skin breakdown or irritation, friction from an irritant in the prosthesis, sebaceous cyst or boil, psychological problems, and phantom limb pain.

- Record the date, time, and specific procedures of postoperative care.
- Note the amount and type of drainage and condition of the dressing.
- Document need for dressing reinforcement.
- Record the appearance and condition of the suture line and surrounding tissue.
- Note pain assessment.
- Record signs of skin irritation or infection, such as redness or tenderness.
- Record complications and nursing actions taken.
- Note the patient's tolerance of exercises, progress in caring for the residual limb or prosthesis, and psychological reaction to the amputation.
- Teach the patient how to care for his residual limb and prosthesis. Encourage proper daily residual limb care.
- Emphasize that proper care of his residual limb can speed healing.
- Tell the patient to inspect his residual limb every day, using a mirror.
- Make sure the patient knows the signs and symptoms that indicate problems in the residual limb.
- Instruct the patient to call the physician if the incision appears to be opening, looks red or swollen, feels warm, is painful to touch, or is seeping drainage.
- Explain to the patient that a 10-lb (4.5-kg) change in body weight will alter his residual limb size and require a new prosthesis socket.
- Tell the patient to massage the residual limb toward the suture line to mobilize the scar and prevent its adherence to bone.
- Advise the patient to avoid exposing the skin around the residual limb to excessive perspiration, which can cause irritation.
- Tell the patient to change his elastic bandages or residual limb socks daily.
- Tell the patient that he may experience twitching, spasms, or phantom limb sensations, such as pain, warmth, cold, or itching, as his residual limb muscles adjust to amputation.
- Discuss measures such as imagery, biofeedback, or distraction to relieve phantom limb pain or other sensations.
- Advise the patient to use heat, massage, or gentle pressure for these symptoms.
- If the patient's residual limb is sensitive to touch, tell him to rub it with a dry washcloth for 4 minutes, three times per day.
- Stress the importance of performing prescribed exercises to help minimize complications, maintain muscle strength and tone, prevent contractures, and promote independence.
- Stress the importance of positioning to prevent contractures and edema.
- Refer the patient and his family to appropriate community support sources, such as home care nursing and physical and occupational therapy as well as prosthetic suppliers.

Skull tong care

DESCRIPTION

- Skeletal traction with skull tongs to immobilize the cervical spine
- Skull tongs applied after a fracture or dislocation, invasion by tumor or infection, or surgery
- Three types of skull tongs: Crutchfield, Gardner-Wells, and Vinke (see *Types of skull tongs*)
- Crutchfield tongs applied by incising the skin with a scalpel, drilling a hole in the exposed skull, and inserting the pins into the hole; Gardner-Wells and Vinke tongs less invasive
- When tongs in place, traction created by extending a rope from the center of the tongs over a pulley and attaching weights to it
- Weights adjusted, using X-ray monitoring to establish reduction and maintain alignment
- Meticulous pin-site care required three times a day
- Frequent observation of the traction apparatus required to make sure that it's working properly

EQUIPMENT

Three sterile specimen containers ◆ one bottle each of ordered cleaning solution ◆ normal saline solution ◆ povidone-iodine solution ◆ sterile, cotton-tipped applicators, sandbags or cervical collar (hard or soft) ◆ fine mesh gauze strips ◆ 4″ × 4″ gauze pads ◆ sterile gloves ◆ sterile basin ◆ sterile scissors ◆ hair clippers ◆ turning frame, antibacterial ointment (optional)

ESSENTIAL STEPS

- Bring the equipment to the patient's room.
- Place the sterile specimen containers on the bedside table.
- Fill one with a small amount of cleaning solution, one with normal saline solution, and one with povidone-iodine solution.
- Set out the cotton-tipped applicators.
- Keep the sandbags or cervical collar handy for emergency immobilization of the head and neck.
- Explain the procedure to the patient.
- Wash your hands.
- Inform the patient that pin sites usually feel tender for several days after the tongs are applied.
- Tell him that he'll also feel some muscular discomfort in the injured area.

TYPES OF SKULL TONGS

Skull (or cervical) tongs consist of a stainless steel body with a pin at the end of each arm. Each pin is about ⅛" (0.5 cm) in diameter with a sharp tip.

On Crutchfield tongs, pins are placed about 5" (12.5 cm) apart in line with the long axis of the cervical spine.

On Gardner-Wells tongs, pins are farther apart. They're inserted slightly above the patient's ears.

On Vinke tongs, pins are placed at the parietal bones, near the widest transverse diameter of the skull, about 1" (2.5 cm) above the helix.

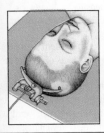 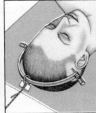 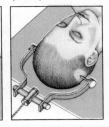

- Before providing care, observe each pin site carefully for signs of infection: loose pins, swelling or redness, or purulent drainage.
- Use hair clippers to trim the patient's hair around the pin sites.
- Put on gloves.
- Wipe pin sites with a cotton-tipped applicator dipped in cleaning solution.
- Repeat with a fresh applicator, as needed, for thorough cleaning.
- Use a separate applicator for each site to avoid cross-contamination.
- Wipe the sites with normal saline solution to remove excess cleaning solution.
- Wipe with povidone-iodine to provide asepsis at the site and prevent infection.
- After providing care, discard all pin-site cleaning materials.
- Apply a povidone-iodine wrap as ordered for infected pin sites.
- Obtain strips of fine mesh gauze or cut a 4" × 4" gauze pad into strips.
- Soak the strips in a sterile basin of povidone-iodine solution or normal saline solution, and squeeze out excess solution.
- Wrap one strip securely around each pin site.
- Leave the strip in place to dry until you provide care again.

- Removing the dried strip aids in debridement and helps clear infection.
- Check the traction apparatus — rope, weights, pulleys — at the start of each shift, every 4 hours, and as necessary.
- Make sure the rope hangs freely.

NURSING CONSIDERATIONS

- Antibacterial ointment for pin-site care may be ordered instead of povidone-iodine solution.
- To remove old ointment, wrap a cotton-tipped applicator with a 4″ × 4″ gauze pad, moisten with cleaning solution, and gently clean each site.
- Keep a box of sterile gauze pads at the patient's bedside.
- Osteoporosis can cause skull pins to slip or pull out, which requires immediate attention to prevent further injury.
- Watch for signs and symptoms of loose pins, such as persistent pain or tenderness at pin sites, redness, drainage, or patient reports of feeling or hearing the pins move.
- If you suspect a pin has loosened or slipped, notify the physician.
- Await the physician's examination before turning the patient.
- If the pins pull out, immobilize the patient's head and neck with sandbags or apply a cervical collar, and carefully remove the traction weights.
- Apply manual traction to the patient's head by placing your hands on each side of the mandible and pulling gently, while maintaining proper alignment.
- After you stabilize the alignment, have someone send for the physician immediately.
- Remain calm and reassure the patient.
- When traction is reestablished, take neurologic vital signs (mental status or Glasgow Coma Scale, and pupillary reflexes).

 ALERT *Never add weights to or subtract weights from the traction apparatus without an order from the physician. Improper procedure can result in neurologic impairment to the patient.*

- Take neurologic vital signs at the beginning of each shift, every 4 hours, and as necessary.
- Carefully assess the function of cranial nerves, which may be impaired by pin placement.
- Note asymmetry, deviation, or atrophy.
- Review the patient's chart to determine baseline neurologic vital signs and those immediately after tongs were applied.
- Monitor respirations closely and keep suction equipment handy.
- Injury to the cervical spine may affect respiration, so be alert for signs of respiratory distress.

- Patients with skull tongs may be placed on a turning frame to facilitate turning without disrupting vertebral alignment. Establish a turning schedule to help prevent complications of immobility.
- Never remove a patient from the bed or turning frame when transporting.
- Monitor for and document signs of infection.
- Monitor for excessive traction force.
- Record the date, time, and type of pin-site care.
- Note the patient's response to the procedure.
- Record whether weights were added or removed.
- Note neurologic vital signs and the patient's respiratory status.
- Explain how skull tong care is performed to lessen the patient's anxiety.
- Tell the patient that pin sites may feel tender for several days after tongs are applied.
- Inform the patient about signs and symptoms of complications, such as pain at pin sites or hearing or feeling the pins move, and to notify the physician or nurse if these occur.
- Teach the patient how to turn and position himself with skull tongs in place.
- Reassure the patient that he'll be closely monitored.

T-tube care

DESCRIPTION

- May be placed in the common bile duct after cholecystectomy or choledochostomy
- The short end inserted into the common bile duct and the long end drawn through the incision; the tube then connected to a closed gravity drainage system
- Facilitates biliary drainage during healing
- Remains in place between 7 and 14 days

EQUIPMENT

Graduated collection container ✦ small plastic bag ✦ sterile gloves and clean gloves ✦ clamp ✦ sterile 4″ × 4″ gauze pads ✦ transparent dressings ✦ rubber band ✦ normal saline solution ✦ sterile cleaning solution ✦ two sterile basins ✦ povidone-iodine pads ✦ sterile precut drain dressings ✦ hypoallergenic paper tape ✦ skin protectant, such as petroleum jelly, aluminum-based gel, or zinc oxide ✦ Montgomery straps (optional)

ESSENTIAL STEPS

- Wash your hands.
- Assemble equipment at the bedside.
- Open all sterile equipment. Place one sterile 4″ × 4″ gauze pad in each sterile basin.
- Using sterile technique, pour 50 ml of cleaning solution into one basin and 50 ml of normal saline solution into the other basin.
- Tape a small plastic bag on the table to use for refuse.
- Provide privacy and explain the procedure to the patient.

Emptying drainage

- Put on clean gloves.
- Place the graduated collection container under the outlet valve of the drainage bag. Without contaminating the clamp, valve, or outlet valve, empty the bag's contents completely into the container and reseal the outlet valve.
- Carefully measure and record the character, color, and amount of drainage.
- Discard gloves.

Redressing the T-tube

- Wash your hands and put on clean gloves.
- Without dislodging the T-tube, remove old dressings, and dispose of them in the small plastic bag. Remove gloves.
- Wash your hands again and put on sterile gloves; follow strict sterile technique to prevent contamination of the incision.
- Inspect the incision and tube site for signs of infection, including redness, edema, warmth, tenderness, induration, or skin excoriation. Assess for wound dehiscence or evisceration.
- Use sterile cleaning solution as prescribed to clean and remove dried matter or drainage from around the tube. Start at the tube site and gently wipe outward in a continuous motion to prevent recontamination of the incision.
- Use normal saline solution to rinse off the prescribed cleaning solution. Dry the area with a sterile 4″ × 4″ gauze pad and discard all used materials.
- Using a povidone-iodine pad, wipe the incision site in a circular motion. Allow the area to dry.
- Apply a skin protectant (petroleum jelly, zinc oxide, or aluminum-based gel) to prevent injury from draining bile.
- Apply a sterile precut drain dressing on each side of the T-tube to absorb drainage.

■ Apply a sterile 4″ × 4″ gauze pad or transparent dressing over the T-tube and the drain dressings.

ALERT *Don't kink the tubing, which can block drainage, and don't put the dressing over the open end of the T-tube because it connects to the closed drainage system.*

■ Secure the dressings with the hypoallergenic paper tape or Montgomery straps if necessary.

Clamping the T-tube

■ As ordered, occlude the tube lightly with a clamp or wrap a rubber band around the end. Clamping the tube 1 hour before and after meals diverts bile back to the duodenum to aid digestion.

■ Monitor the patient's response to clamping.

■ To ensure his comfort and safety, check bile drainage amounts regularly.

ALERT *Report signs of obstructed bile flow: chills, fever, tachycardia, nausea, right-upper-quadrant fullness and pain, jaundice, dark foamy urine, and clay-colored stools.*

NURSING CONSIDERATIONS

■ The T-tube usually drains 300 to 500 ml of blood-tinged bile in the first 24 hours after surgery.

ALERT *Report drainage that exceeds 500 ml in the first 24 hours after surgery; if it's 50 ml or less, notify the physician; the tube may be obstructed. Drainage typically declines to 200 ml or less after 4 days and the color changes to green-brown. Monitor fluid, electrolyte, and acid-base status.*

■ To prevent excessive bile loss (over 500 ml in first 24 hours) or backflow contamination, secure the T-tube drainage system at abdominal level. Bile will flow into bag only when biliary pressure increases.

■ Provide meticulous skin care and frequent dressing changes.

■ Observe for bile leakage, which may indicate obstruction. (See *Managing T-tube obstruction*, page 402.)

■ Assess tube patency and site condition hourly for the first 8 hours, then every 4 hours until the physician removes the tube.

■ Protect the skin edges and avoid excessive taping.

■ Monitor all urine and stools for color changes. Assess for icteric skin and sclera, which may signal jaundice.

■ Monitor the patient for complications, such as obstructed bile flow; skin excoriation or breakdown; tube dislodgment; drainage reflux; and infection.

■ Record the date and time of each dressing change.

■ Note the appearance of the wound and surrounding skin.

MANAGING T-TUBE OBSTRUCTION

If your patient's T-tube blocks after cholecystectomy:
- Notify the physician.
- Unclamp the T-tube (if it was clamped before and after a meal) and connect the tube to a closed gravity-drainage system.
- Inspect the tube to detect any kinks or obstructions.
- Prepare for possible T-tube irrigation or direct X-ray of the common bile duct (cholangiography). Explain the procedure to lessen anxiety and promote cooperation.
- Provide encouragement and support.

- Write down the color, character, and volume of bile collected.
- Record the color of skin and mucous membranes around the T-tube.
- Explain to the patient that loose bowels commonly occur the first few weeks after surgery.
- Teach the patient about signs and symptoms of T-tube and biliary obstruction and to report them to the physician.
- Teach the patient how to care for the tube at home.
- Caution the patient that bile stains clothing.

Tracheostomy care

DESCRIPTION

- Required to ensure airway patency by keeping the tube free of mucus buildup, to maintain mucous membrane and skin integrity, prevent infection, and provide psychological support
- Should be performed using sterile technique until the stoma has healed
- For recent tracheotomies, sterile gloves used for all manipulations at the site; after the stoma has healed, clean gloves may be substituted for sterile ones
- Three types of tracheostomy tube: uncuffed, cuffed, fenestrated (choice dependent on the patient's condition and physician's preference)
  - An uncuffed plastic or metal tube that allows air to flow freely around the tracheostomy tube and through the larynx, reducing risk of tracheal damage
  - A cuffed plastic tube that's disposable; the cuff and tube bonded together to prevent separation inside the trachea, reducing risk of tracheal damage; doesn't require periodic deflating to lower pressure because cuff pressure is low and evenly distributed against the tracheal wall

- A plastic fenestrated tube that permits speech through the upper airway when the external opening is capped and the cuff deflated; also allows easy removal of the inner cannula for cleaning, but may become occluded

EQUIPMENT

For aseptic stoma and outer-cannula care

Waterproof trash bag ◆ two sterile solution containers ◆ sterile normal saline solution ◆ hydrogen peroxide ◆ sterile cotton-tipped applicators ◆ sterile 4" × 4" gauze pads ◆ sterile gloves ◆ prepackaged sterile tracheostomy dressing (or 4" × 4" gauze pad) ◆ supplies for suctioning and mouth care ◆ water-soluble lubricant or topical antibiotic cream ◆ materials for cuff procedures and changing tracheostomy ties (see below)

For aseptic inner-cannula care

All preceding equipment plus a prepackaged commercial tracheostomy care set, or sterile forceps ◆ sterile nylon brush ◆ sterile 6" (15-cm) pipe cleaners ◆ clean gloves ◆ a third sterile solution container ◆ disposable temporary inner cannula (for a patient on a ventilator)

For changing tracheostomy ties

30" (76.2-cm) length of tracheostomy twill tape ◆ bandage scissors ◆ sterile gloves ◆ hemostat

For emergency tracheostomy tube replacement

Sterile tracheal dilator or sterile hemostat ◆ sterile obturator that fits the tracheostomy tube ◆ extra, appropriate-sized, sterile tracheostomy tube and obturator ◆ suction equipment and supplies

For cuff procedures

5- or 10-ml syringe ◆ padded hemostat ◆ stethoscope

ESSENTIAL STEPS

- Assess the patient's condition to determine need for care.
- Explain the procedure, even if the patient is unresponsive. Provide privacy.
- Wash your hands and assemble equipment and supplies in the patient's room.
- Check the expiration date on each sterile package and inspect for tears.
- Place the open waterproof trash bag next to you to avoid reaching across the sterile field or the patient's stoma when discarding soiled items.
- Establish a sterile field near his bed and place equipment and supplies on it.

■ Pour normal saline solution, hydrogen peroxide, or a mixture of equal parts of both solutions into one of the sterile solution containers; pour normal saline solution into the second sterile container for rinsing.

■ For inner-cannula care, use a third sterile solution container to hold the gauze pads and cotton-tipped applicators saturated with cleaning solution.

■ If replacing the disposable inner cannula, open the package containing the new inner cannula while maintaining sterile technique.

■ Obtain or prepare new tracheostomy ties, if indicated.

■ Keep supplies in full view for easy emergency access. Consider taping a wrapped, sterile tracheostomy tube to the head of the bed for emergencies.

■ Place the patient in semi-Fowler's position, unless contraindicated, to decrease abdominal pressure on the diaphragm and promote lung expansion.

■ Remove humidification or ventilation device.

■ Using sterile technique, suction the entire length of the tracheostomy tube to clear the airway of secretions that may hinder oxygenation.

■ Reconnect the patient to the humidifier or ventilator, if necessary.

Cleaning a stoma and outer cannula

■ Put on sterile gloves if you aren't already wearing them.

■ With your dominant hand, saturate a sterile gauze pad or cotton-tipped applicator with the cleaning solution.

■ Squeeze out excess liquid to prevent accidental aspiration.

■ Wipe the patient's neck under the tracheostomy tube flanges and twill tapes.

■ Saturate a second pad or applicator, and wipe until the skin surrounding the tracheostomy is cleaned. Use additional pads or cotton-tipped applicators to clean the stoma site and the tube's flanges.

■ Wipe only once with each pad or applicator to prevent contamination of a clean area.

■ Rinse debris and peroxide you may have used with one or more sterile $4'' \times 4''$ gauze pads dampened in normal saline solution.

■ Dry the area thoroughly with additional sterile gauze pads; apply a new sterile tracheostomy dressing. Remove and discard your gloves.

Cleaning a nondisposable inner cannula

■ Put on sterile gloves. Using your nondominant hand, remove and discard the patient's tracheostomy dressing.

■ With the same hand, disconnect the ventilator or humidification device, and unlock the tracheostomy tube's inner cannula by rotating it counter-clockwise.

■ Place the inner cannula in the container of hydrogen peroxide.

■ Working quickly, use your dominant hand to scrub the cannula with the sterile nylon brush.

■ If the brush doesn't slide easily into the cannula, use a sterile pipe cleaner.

■ Immerse the cannula in the container of normal saline solution, and agitate it for about 10 seconds to rinse it.

■ Inspect the cannula for cleanliness. Repeat the cleaning process if necessary.

■ If it's clean, tap it against the inside edge of the sterile container to remove excess liquid and prevent aspiration.

ALERT *Don't dry the outer surface; a film of moisture acts as a lubricant during insertion.*

■ Reinsert the inner cannula into the patient's tracheostomy tube.

■ Lock it in place and ensure it's positioned securely. Reconnect the mechanical ventilator. Apply a new sterile tracheostomy dressing.

■ If the patient can't tolerate being disconnected from the ventilator for the time it takes to clean the inner cannula, replace the existing inner cannula with a clean one and reattach the mechanical ventilator. Clean the cannula just removed from him, and store it in a sterile container for the next time.

Caring for a disposable inner cannula

■ Put on clean gloves. Using your dominant hand, remove the inner cannula.

■ After evaluating the secretions in the cannula, discard it properly.

■ Pick up the new inner cannula, touching only the outer locking portion. Insert the cannula into the tracheostomy and, following manufacturer's instructions, lock it securely.

Changing tracheostomy ties

■ Get help from another nurse or a respiratory therapist to avoid accidental tube expulsion. Patient movement or coughing can dislodge the tube.

■ Wash your hands and put on sterile gloves if you aren't already wearing them.

■ If you aren't using commercially packaged tracheostomy ties, prepare new ties from a 30" (76.2-cm) length of twill tape by folding one end back 1" (2.5 cm) on itself, and then, with bandage scissors, cutting a 1½" (3.8-cm) slit down the center of the tape from the folded edge.

■ Prepare the other end of the tape the same way.

- Hold both ends together and cut the resulting circle of tape so one piece is about 10" (25.4 cm) long and the other is about 20" (53 cm) long.
- Assist the patient into semi-Fowler's position, if possible.
- After your assistant puts on gloves, instruct her to hold the tracheostomy tube in place to prevent expulsion during replacement of the ties.
- With the assistant's gloved fingers holding the tracheostomy tube in place, cut the soiled tracheostomy ties with bandage scissors or untie them and discard.

 ALERT *Be careful not to cut the tube of the pilot balloon.*

- Thread the slit end of one new tie a short distance through the eye of one tracheostomy tube flange from the underside; use the hemostat, if needed, to pull the tie through. Thread the other end of the tie completely through the slit end and pull it taut so it loops firmly through the flange. This avoids knots that can cause throat discomfort, tissue irritation, pressure, and necrosis.
- Fasten the second tie to the opposite flange in the same manner.
- Instruct the patient to flex his neck while you bring the ties around to the side, and tie them together with a square knot. Flexion produces the same neck circumference as coughing and helps prevent an overly tight tie.
- Have your assistant place one finger under the tapes as you tie them to ensure they're tight enough to avoid slippage but loose enough to prevent choking or jugular vein constriction.
- Placing the closure on the side allows easy access and prevents pressure necrosis at the back of the neck when the patient is recumbent.
- After securing the ties, cut off excess tape with scissors and have your assistant release the tracheostomy tube.
- Make sure the patient is comfortable and can reach the call bell easily.

ALERT *Check tracheostomy tie tension frequently on patients with traumatic injury, radical neck dissection, or cardiac failure because neck diameter can increase from swelling and cause constriction; check neonatal or restless patients frequently because ties can loosen and cause tube dislodgment.*

Concluding tracheostomy care

- Replace humidification device.
- Provide oral care as needed because the oral cavity can become dry and malodorous or develop sores from encrusted secretions.
- Observe soiled dressings and suctioned secretions for amount, color, consistency, and odor. Properly clean or dispose of equipment, supplies, solutions, and trash. Remove and discard your gloves.
- Make sure the patient is comfortable and can reach the call bell easily.

- Make sure necessary supplies are readily available at the bedside.
- Repeat the procedure at least once every 8 hours, or as needed.
- Change the dressing as often as necessary regardless of whether you perform the entire cleaning procedure. A wet dressing with exudate or secretions predisposes the patient to skin excoriation, breakdown, and infection.

Deflating and inflating a tracheostomy cuff

- Read the cuff manufacturer's instructions; cuff types and procedures vary.
- Assess the patient's condition, explain the procedure, and reassure him.
- Wash your hands.
- Help the patient into semi-Fowler's position, if possible, or place him in a supine position so secretions above the cuff site will be pushed up into his mouth if he's receiving positive-pressure ventilation.
- Suction the oropharyngeal cavity to prevent pooled secretions from descending into the trachea after cuff deflation.
- Release the padded hemostat clamping the cuff inflation tubing, if a hemostat is present.
- Insert a 5- or 10-ml syringe into the cuff pilot balloon and slowly withdraw all air from the cuff. Leave syringe attached to tubing for cuff reinflation.
- Slow deflation allows positive lung pressure to push secretions upward from the bronchi. Cuff deflation may also stimulate the cough reflex, producing additional secretions.
- Remove the ventilation device and suction the lower airway through the existing tube to remove all secretions.
- Reconnect the patient to the ventilation device.
- Maintain cuff deflation for the prescribed time.
- Observe for adequate ventilation, and suction as necessary.
- If the patient has difficulty breathing, reinflate the cuff immediately by depressing the syringe plunger very slowly.
- Use a stethoscope to listen over the trachea for the air leak; inject as little air as necessary to achieve an adequate tracheal seal.
- When inflating the cuff, you may use the minimal-leak technique or the minimal occlusive volume technique to help gauge the proper inflation point.
- If inflating the cuff using cuff pressure measurement, don't exceed 25 mm Hg.

ALERT *Recommended cuff pressure is about 18 mm Hg. If pressure exceeds 25 mm Hg, notify the physician. You may need to change to a larger-size tube, use higher inflation pressures, or permit a larger air leak.*

■ After you've inflated the cuff, if the tubing doesn't have a one-way valve at the end, clamp the inflation line with a padded hemostat and remove the syringe.

■ Check for a minimal-leak cuff seal. You shouldn't feel air coming from the patient's mouth, nose, or tracheostomy site, and a conscious patient shouldn't be able to speak.

■ Be alert for air leaks from the cuff itself.

■ Suspect a leak if injection of air fails to inflate the cuff or increase cuff pressure, if you're unable to inject the amount of air you withdrew, if the patient can speak, if ventilation fails to maintain adequate respiratory movement with pressures or volumes previously considered adequate, or if air escapes during the ventilator's inspiratory cycle.

■ Note the exact amount of air used to inflate the cuff to detect tracheal malacia if more air is consistently needed.

■ Make sure the patient is comfortable and can easily reach the call bell and communication aids.

■ Properly clean or dispose of equipment, supplies, and trash according to facility policy.

■ Replenish used supplies and make sure all necessary emergency supplies are at the bedside.

NURSING CONSIDERATIONS

■ Keep appropriate equipment at the patient's bedside for immediate use in an emergency.

■ Consult the physician about first-aid measures you can use for your tracheostomy patient should an emergency occur.

ALERT *Follow facility policy if a tracheostomy tube is expelled or the outer cannula becomes blocked. If breathing is obstructed, call the appropriate code and provide manual resuscitation with a handheld resuscitation bag or reconnect the patient to the ventilator. Don't remove the tracheostomy tube; the airway may close completely. Use caution when reinserting to avoid tracheal trauma, perforation, compression, and asphyxiation.*

■ Don't change tracheostomy ties unnecessarily during the immediate postoperative period before the stoma track is well formed to avoid accidental dislodgment and expulsion of the tube. Unless secretions or drainage is a problem, ties can be changed once per day.

■ Don't change a single-cannula tracheostomy tube or the outer cannula of a double-cannula tube. Because of the risk of tracheal complications, the physician usually changes the cannula; the frequency depends on the patient's condition.

- If the patient's neck or stoma is excoriated or infected, apply a water-soluble lubricant or topical antibiotic cream as ordered. Don't use a powder or oil-based substance on or around a stoma; aspiration can cause infection and abscess.
- Replace all equipment regularly (including solutions) to reduce risk of nosocomial infections.
- Monitor for complications, such as hemorrhage at operative site, bleeding or edema in tracheal tissue, aspiration of secretions, introduction of air into pleural cavity, hypoxia or acidosis, introduction of air into surrounding tissues, secretions under dressings and twill tape, hardened mucus or a slipped cuff, tube displacement, and tracheal erosion and necrosis.
- Record the date, time, and type of procedure.
- Note the amount, consistency, color, and odor of secretions.
- Document stoma and skin condition.
- Record the patient's respiratory status.
- Note change of the tracheostomy tube by the physician.
- Record the duration of cuff deflation.
- Document the amount of cuff inflation.
- Record cuff pressure readings and specific body position.
- Note complications and nursing actions taken.
- Document patient or family teaching and their understanding.
- Record the patient's tolerance of the treatment.
- Explain the procedure, even if the patient is unresponsive.
- If the patient will be discharged with a tracheostomy, start self-care teaching as soon as he's receptive.
- Teach the patient how to change and clean the tube.
- If the patient is being discharged with suction equipment, make sure he and his family are knowledgeable and comfortable about using the equipment.
- Refer the patient and family for home care services for follow-up if tracheotomy is permanent.

Transcutaneous electrical nerve stimulation

DESCRIPTION

- Based on the gate control theory of pain
- Performed with a portable battery-powered device that transmits painless electrical current to peripheral nerves or directly to a painful area over relatively large nerve fibers
- Effectively alters the patient's perception of pain by blocking painful stimuli traveling over smaller fibers

USES OF TENS

Transcutaneous electrical nerve stimulation (TENS) must be prescribed by a
physician and is most successful if administered and taught to the patient by
a skilled therapist. TENS has been used for temporary relief of acute pain,
such as postoperative pain, and for ongoing relief of chronic pain such as sciatica.

Among the types of pain that respond to TENS are:

- arthritis
- bone fracture pain
- bursitis
- cancer-related pain
- lower back pain
- musculoskeletal pain

- myofascial pain
- neuralgias and neuropathies
- phantom limb pain
- postoperative incision pain
- sciatica
- whiplash.

- Used for postoperative patients and those with chronic pain to reduce
  need for analgesics; may allow the patient to resume normal activities
- Treatment typically lasting 3 to 5 days
- Some conditions, such as phantom limb pain, needing continuous stimulation; other conditions, such as a painful arthritic joint, shorter periods
  (see *Uses of TENS*)
- Also known as *TENS*

 ALERT *Cardiac pacemakers can interfere with function.*

EQUIPMENT

Commercial TENS kits are available. They include the stimulator, leadwires,
electrodes, spare battery pack, battery recharger, and adhesive patch.

TENS device ◆ alcohol pads ◆ reusable self-adhesive electrodes ◆ warm
water and soap ◆ leadwires ◆ charged battery pack ◆ battery recharger ◆
skin cleanser and protectant ◆ electrode spray (optional)

 ALERT *Before beginning the procedure, test the battery pack
to ensure it's fully charged.*

ESSENTIAL STEPS

- Wash your hands and follow standard precautions.
- Provide privacy and explain the procedure.
- Thoroughly clean the skin where the electrode will be applied with soap
  and water, dry well. Wipe with skin cleanser and protectant to enhance
  conductivity, if desired.

- If necessary, shave hair at the site where each electrode will be placed.
- Rehydrate electrodes with electrode spray or small amount of water if needed.
- Place the ordered number of electrodes on the proper skin area, leaving at least 2" (5 cm) between them. (See *Positioning TENS electrodes*, page 412.)
- Secure them with the adhesive patch or hypoallergenic tape on all sides evenly, so electrodes are firmly attached to the skin.
- Plug the pin connectors into the electrode sockets.
- To protect the cords, hold the connectors — not the cords themselves — during insertion.
- Turn the channel controls to the OFF position or as recommended in the operator's manual.
- Plug the leadwires into the jacks in the control box.
- Turn the amplitude and rate dials slowly, as the manual directs. The patient should feel a tingling sensation.
- Adjust the control to the prescribed settings or to settings that are most comfortable. Most patients select stimulation frequencies of 60 to 100 Hz.
- Attach the TENS control box to part of the patient's clothing, such as a belt, pocket, or bra.
- To ensure the device is working effectively, monitor for signs of excessive stimulation, such as muscle twitches, and for signs of inadequate stimulation, signaled by the patient not feeling any mild tingling sensation.

After transcutaneous electrical nerve stimulation treatment

- Turn off the controls and unplug the electrode leadwires. If another treatment will be given soon, leave the electrodes in place.
- Replace the electrodes on the plastic pad supplied and enclose in pouch. May refrigerate between uses.
- Don't soak the electrodes in alcohol because it will damage the rubber.
- Remove the battery pack and replace it with a charged battery pack.
- Recharge the used battery pack so it's always ready for use.

NURSING CONSIDERATIONS

- If you must move electrodes during the procedure, turn off the controls first.
- Follow the physician's orders about electrode placement and control settings.

POSITIONING TENS ELECTRODES

In transcutaneous electrical nerve stimulation (TENS), electrodes placed around peripheral nerves (or an incisional site) transmit mild electrical pulses to the brain. The current is thought to block pain impulses. The patient can influence the level and frequency of pain relief by adjusting controls on the device.

Typically, electrode placement varies even though patients may have similar complaints. Electrodes can be placed in several ways:

- They can cover the painful area or surround it, as with muscle tenderness or spasm or painful joints.
- They can "capture" the painful area between electrodes, as with incisional pain.
- In peripheral nerve injury, electrodes should be placed proximal to the injury (between the brain and the injury site) to avoid increasing pain.
- Placing electrodes in a hypersensitive area can also increase pain.
- In an area lacking sensation, electrodes should be placed on adjacent dermatomes.

These illustrations show combinations of electrode placement (colored squares) and areas of nerve stimulation (shaded panels) for low back and leg pain.

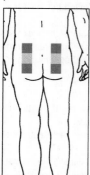 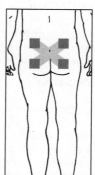 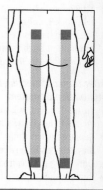

ALERT *Incorrect placement of the electrodes will result in inappropriate pain control. Setting the controls too high can cause pain; setting them too low will fail to relieve pain.*

ALERT *Never place the electrodes near the patient's eyes or over the nerves that innervate the carotid sinus or laryngeal or pharyngeal muscles to avoid interference with critical nerve function.*

- If TENS is used continuously for postoperative pain, remove the electrodes at least daily to check for skin irritation, provide skin care, and to rotate sites of electrode placement.
- Record the electrode sites and control settings.
- Note the patient's tolerance of treatment.
- Record the location of pain and how the patient rates his pain using a pain scale.
- If appropriate, let the patient study the operator's manual.
- Teach the patient how to place the electrodes properly and how to take care of the TENS unit.

Transfusion reaction management

DESCRIPTION

- Condition that stems from a major antigen-antibody reaction and can result from a single or massive transfusion of blood or blood products
- Many reactions occurring during transfusion or within 96 hours afterward
- Requires immediate recognition and prompt nursing action to prevent further complications or death, particularly if the patient is unconscious or heavily sedated and can't report symptoms (see *Guide to transfusion reactions,* pages 414 to 417)

EQUIPMENT

Normal saline solution ◆ I.V. administration set ◆ sterile urine specimen container ◆ needle, syringe, and tubes for blood samples ◆ transfusion reaction report form ◆ oxygen ◆ epinephrine ◆ hypothermia blanket ◆ leukocyte removal filter (optional)

ESSENTIAL STEPS

- If adverse reaction is suspected, stop the transfusion and start the normal saline solution infusion using a new I.V. administration set at a keep-vein-open rate to maintain venous access. Don't discard the blood bag or administration set.
- Notify the physician.
- Monitor vital signs every 15 minutes or as indicated by severity and type of reaction.
- Compare labels on blood containers with corresponding patient identification forms to verify that transfusion was the correct blood or blood product.

(Text continues on page 418.)

GUIDE TO TRANSFUSION REACTIONS

A patient receiving a transfusion of processed blood products risks certain complications; for example, hemosiderosis and hypothermia. The table below describes *endogenous reactions* (those caused by an antigen-antibody reaction in the recipient) and *exogenous reactions* (those caused by external factors in administered blood).

Reaction and causes	Signs and symptoms	Nursing interventions
Endogenous		
Allergic ■ Allergen in donor blood ■ Donor blood hypersensitive to certain drugs	■ Anaphylaxis (chills, facial swelling) ■ Laryngeal edema ■ Pruritus, urticaria, wheezing ■ Fever ■ Nausea and vomiting	■ Administer antihistamines as prescribed. ■ Monitor patient for anaphylactic reaction, and administer epinephrine and corticosteroids if indicated. ■ As prescribed, premedicate him with diphenhydramine before subsequent transfusion.
Bacterial contamination ■ Organisms that can survive cold, such as *Pseudomonas* and *Staphylococcus*	■ Chills ■ Fever ■ Vomiting ■ Abdominal cramping ■ Diarrhea ■ Shock ■ Signs of renal failure	■ Provide broad-spectrum antibiotics, corticosteroids, or epinephrine as prescribed. ■ Maintain strict blood storage control. ■ Change blood administration set and filter every 4 hours or after every 2 units. ■ Infuse each unit of blood over 2 to 4 hours; stop the infusion if the time span exceeds 4 hours. ■ Maintain sterile technique when administering blood products.
Febrile ■ Bacterial lipopolysaccharides ■ Antileukocyte recipient antibodies directed against donor white blood cells	■ Temperature up to 104° F (40° C) ■ Chills ■ Headache ■ Facial flushing ■ Palpitations ■ Cough ■ Chest tightness ■ Increased pulse rate ■ Flank pain	■ Relieve symptoms with an antipyretic, antihistamine, or meperidine, as prescribed. ■ If the patient requires further transfusions, use frozen RBCs, add a special leukocyte removal filter to the blood line, or premedicate him with acetaminophen, as prescribed, before starting another transfusion.

GUIDE TO TRANSFUSION REACTIONS *(continued)*

Reaction and causes	Signs and symptoms	Nursing interventions
Endogenous *(continued)*		
Hemolytic ■ ABO or Rh incompatibility ■ Intradonor incompatibility ■ Improper cross-matching ■ Improperly stored blood	■ Chest pain ■ Dyspnea ■ Facial flushing ■ Fever ■ Chills ■ Shaking ■ Hypotension ■ Flank pain ■ Hemoglobinuria ■ Oliguria ■ Bloody oozing at the infusion site or surgical incision site ■ Burning sensation along vein receiving blood ■ Shock ■ Renal failure	■ Monitor blood pressure. ■ Manage shock with I.V. fluids, oxygen, epinephrine, a diuretic, and a vasopressor, as prescribed. ■ Obtain posttransfusion-reaction blood samples and urine specimens for analysis. ■ Observe for signs of hemorrhage resulting from disseminated intravascular coagulation.
Plasma protein incompatibility ■ Immunoglobulin-A incompatibility	■ Abdominal pain and diarrhea ■ Dyspnea ■ Chills ■ Fever ■ Flushing ■ Hypotension	■ Administer oxygen, fluids, epinephrine, or a corticosteroid, as prescribed.
Exogenous		
Bleeding tendencies ■ Low platelet count in stored blood, causing thrombocytopenia	■ Abnormal bleeding and oozing from a cut ■ A break in the skin surface or the gums; abnormal bruising and petechiae	■ Administer platelets, fresh frozen plasma, or cryoprecipitate, as prescribed. ■ Monitor platelet count.

(continued)

GUIDE TO TRANSFUSION REACTIONS *(continued)*

Reaction and causes	Signs and symptoms	Nursing interventions
Exogenous *(continued)*		
Circulatory overload ■ May result from infusing blood too rapidly or in large volumes	■ Increased plasma volume ■ Back pain ■ Chest tightness ■ Chills ■ Fever ■ Dyspnea ■ Flushed feeling ■ Headache ■ Hypertension ■ Increased central venous pressure and jugular vein pressure	■ Monitor blood pressure. ■ Use packed RBCs instead of whole blood. ■ Administer diuretics, as prescribed.
Elevated blood ammonia level ■ Increased ammonia level in stored donor blood	■ Confusion ■ Forgetfulness ■ Lethargy	■ Monitor ammonia level in blood. ■ Decrease the amount of protein in the patient's diet. ■ If indicated, give neomycin.
Hemosiderosis ■ Increased level of hemosiderin (iron-containing pigment) from red blood cell (RBC) destruction, especially after many transfusions	■ Iron plasma level exceeding 200 mg/dl	■ Perform a phlebotomy to remove excess iron.
Hypocalcemia ■ Citrate toxicity occurs when citrate-treated blood is infused rapidly. Citrate binds with calcium, causing a calcium deficiency, or normal citrate metabolism becomes impeded by hepatic disease.	■ Arrhythmias ■ Hypotension ■ Muscle cramps ■ Nausea ■ Vomiting ■ Seizures ■ Tingling in fingers	■ Slow or stop the transfusion, depending on the patient's reaction. Expect a more severe reaction in hypothermic patients or those with elevated potassium levels. ■ Slowly administer calcium gluconate I.V., if prescribed.

GUIDE TO TRANSFUSION REACTIONS *(continued)*

Reaction and causes	Signs and symptoms	Nursing interventions
Exogenous *(continued)*		
Hypothermia ■ Rapid infusion of large amounts of cold blood, which decreases body temperature	■ Chills; shaking; hypotension; arrhythmias, especially bradycardia ■ Cardiac arrest if core temperature falls below 86° F (30° C)	■ Stop the transfusion. ■ Warm him with blankets. ■ Place the patient in a warm environment if necessary. ■ Obtain an electrocardiogram (ECG). ■ Warm blood if the transfusion is resumed.
Increased oxygen affinity for hemoglobin ■ Decreased level of 2,3-diphosphoglycerate in stored blood, causing an increase in the oxygen's hemoglobin affinity. When this occurs, oxygen stays in the patient's bloodstream and isn't released into body tissues.	■ Depressed respiratory rate, especially in patients with chronic lung disease	■ Monitor arterial blood gas values and provide respiratory support as needed.
Potassium intoxication ■ An abnormally high level of potassium in stored plasma caused by hemolysis of RBCs	■ Diarrhea ■ Intestinal colic ■ Flaccidity ■ Muscle twitching ■ Oliguria ■ Renal failure ■ Bradycardia progressing to cardiac arrest ■ Electrocardiographic changes with tall, peaked T waves	■ Obtain an ECG. ■ Administer sodium polystyrene sulfonate (Kayexalate) orally or by enema. ■ Administer dextrose 50% and insulin, bicarbonate, or calcium, as prescribed, to force potassium into cells.

- Notify the blood bank of a possible transfusion reaction and collect blood samples, as ordered.
- Immediately send the samples, transfusion containers (even if empty), and the administration set to the blood bank; they'll test materials to further evaluate the reaction.
- Collect the first posttransfusion urine specimen, mark the collection slip "Possible transfusion reaction," and send it to the laboratory immediately to test for presence of hemoglobin, which indicates a hemolytic reaction.
- Closely monitor intake and output. Note evidence of oliguria or anuria because hemoglobin deposition in the renal tubules can cause renal damage.
- If prescribed, give oxygen, epinephrine, or other drugs and apply a hypothermia blanket to reduce fever.
- Make the patient as comfortable as possible and provide reassurance as necessary.

NURSING CONSIDERATIONS

- Treat all transfusion reactions as serious until proven otherwise.
- If the physician anticipates a transfusion reaction, he may order prophylactic treatment with antihistamines or antipyretics to precede blood administration.
- To avoid a possible febrile reaction, the physician may order the blood to be washed to remove as many leukocytes as possible, or a leukocyte removal filter may be used during the transfusion.
- Record the time and date of transfusion reaction.
- Note the type and amount of infused blood or blood products.
- Document clinical signs of the transfusion reaction in order of occurrence.
- Record vital signs, specimens sent to the laboratory for analysis, treatment given, and patient response.
- If required by facility policy, complete the transfusion reaction form.
- Tell the patient to report new symptoms promptly.

Part four

Diagnostic tests

Arterial blood gas analysis

PURPOSE

- To measure the partial pressure of arterial oxygen (Pa_{O_2}), the partial pressure of arterial carbon dioxide (Pa_{CO_2}), and the pH of an arterial sample:
  - Pa_{O_2}: amount of oxygen the lungs deliver to the blood
  - Pa_{CO_2}: how efficiently the lungs eliminate carbon dioxide
  - pH: acid-base level of the blood, or the hydrogen ion (H^+) level (acidity indicates H^+ excess; alkalinity, H^+ deficit)
- To measure oxygen content (O_2CT), arterial oxygen saturation (Sa_{O_2}), and bicarbonate (HCO_3^-) values
- To evaluate the efficiency of pulmonary gas exchange
- To assess the integrity of the ventilatory control system
- To monitor respiratory therapy

PATIENT PREPARATION

- Make sure that the patient has signed an appropriate consent form.
- Note and report allergies.
- Explain that arterial blood gas analysis evaluates how well the lungs are delivering oxygen to the blood and eliminating carbon dioxide.
- Tell the patient that the test requires a blood sample. Explain who will perform the arterial puncture, when it will occur, and where the puncture site will be: radial, brachial, or femoral artery.
- Inform the patient that he need not restrict food and fluids.
- Instruct the patient to breathe normally during the test, and warn him that he may experience a brief cramping or throbbing pain at the puncture site.

PROCEDURE

- Wait at least 20 minutes before drawing arterial blood when starting, changing, or discontinuing oxygen therapy; after starting or changing mechanical ventilation settings; or after extubation.
- Use a heparinized blood gas syringe to draw the sample.
- Perform an arterial puncture or draw blood from an arterial line.
- Eliminate air from the sample, place it on ice immediately, and prepare to transport it for analysis.
- Before sending the sample to the laboratory, note on the laboratory request whether the patient was breathing room air or receiving oxygen therapy when the sample was collected.
- Note the flow rate of oxygen therapy and method of delivery. If the pa-

tient is on a ventilator, note the fraction of inspired oxygen, tidal volume mode, respiratory rate, and positive end-expiratory pressure.
■ Note the patient's rectal temperature.

POSTPROCEDURE CARE

■ After applying pressure to the puncture site for 3 to 5 minutes or until bleeding has stopped, tape a gauze pad firmly over it.
■ If the patient is receiving anticoagulants or has a coagulopathy, apply pressure to the puncture site longer than 5 minutes if necessary.
■ If the puncture site is on the arm, don't tape the entire circumference; this may restrict circulation.
■ Monitor the patient's vital signs and observe for signs of circulatory impairment, such as swelling, discoloration, pain, numbness, and tingling in the bandaged arm or leg.
■ Assess bleeding from the puncture site.

NORMAL RESULTS

■ Pao_2: 80 to 100 mm Hg (SI, 10.6 to 13.3 kPa)
■ $Paco_2$: 35 to 45 mm Hg (SI, 4.7 to 5.3 kPa)
■ pH: 7.35 to 7.45 (SI, 7.35 to 7.45)
■ O_2CT: 15% to 23% (SI, 0.15 to 0.23)
■ Sao_2: 94% to 100% (SI, 0.94 to 1)
■ HCO_3^-: 22 to 25 mEq/L (SI, 22 to 25 mmol/L)

ABNORMAL RESULTS

■ Low Pao_2, O_2CT, and Sao_2 levels and a high $Paco_2$ level may result from conditions that impair respiratory function, such as respiratory muscle weakness or paralysis, respiratory center inhibition (from head injury, brain tumor, or drug abuse), and airway obstruction (possibly from mucus plugs or a tumor).
■ Low readings with a high $Paco_2$ level may result from bronchiole obstruction caused by asthma or emphysema, from an abnormal ventilation-perfusion ratio caused by partially blocked alveoli or pulmonary capillaries, or from alveoli that are damaged or filled with fluid because of disease, hemorrhage, or near-drowning.
■ When inspired air contains insufficient oxygen, the Pao_2, O_2CT, and Sao_2 decrease, but the $Paco_2$ may be normal. Such findings are common in pneumothorax, impaired diffusion between alveoli and blood (caused by interstitial fibrosis, for example), or an arteriovenous shunt that permits blood to bypass the lungs.

ABG ANALYSIS INTERFERENCE

- Bicarbonate, ethacrynic acid (Edecrin), hydrocortisone (Cortef), metolazone (Zaroxolyn), prednisone (Deltasone), and thiazides may elevate the partial pressure of arterial carbon dioxide ($Paco_2$).
- Acetazolamide (Diamox), nitrofurantoin (Macrobid), and tetracycline may decrease the $Paco_2$.
- Hypothermia may cause false-low partial pressure of arterial oxygen (Pao_2) and $Paco_2$ levels.
- Fever may cause false-high Pao_2 and $Paco_2$ levels.

- A low O_2CT—with normal Pao_2, Sao_2 and, possibly, $Paco_2$ values—may result from severe anemia, decreased blood volume, and reduced hemoglobin oxygen-carrying capacity. (See *ABG analysis interference*.)

Bone marrow aspiration and biopsy

PURPOSE

- To collect a soft tissue specimen from the medullary canals of long bone and interstices of cancellous bone for histologic and hematologic examination, by aspiration or needle biopsy, under local anesthesia (both methods commonly performed at the same time to obtain the best possible specimen)
- *Aspiration biopsy:* removal of a fluid specimen from the bone marrow
- *Needle biopsy:* removal of a core of marrow cells
- To diagnose thrombocytopenia, leukemias, granulomas, anemias, and primary and metastatic tumors
- To determine causes of infection
- To help stage diseases such as with Hodgkin's disease
- To evaluate chemotherapy
- To monitor myelosuppression

PATIENT PREPARATION

- Make sure that the patient has signed an appropriate consent form.
- Note and report allergies.
- Give a mild sedative 1 hour before the test.
- Explain that collection of a blood sample for laboratory testing is necessary before the biopsy.

- Explain to the patient that he'll feel pressure on insertion of the biopsy needle and a brief pulling pain on removal of the marrow.
- Explain that the test usually takes only 5 to 10 minutes.
- Explain which bone site (sternum, anterior or posterior iliac crest, vertebral spinous process, rib, or tibia) will receive the test. (See *Common bone marrow aspiration and biopsy sites*, page 424.)

PROCEDURE

- The patient is positioned and instructed to remain as still as possible.

Aspiration biopsy

- The biopsy site is prepared and draped, and a local anesthetic is injected. The marrow aspiration needle is inserted through the skin, subcutaneous tissue, and bone cortex, using a twisting motion.
- The stylet is removed from the aspiration needle, and a 10- to 20-ml syringe is attached. From 0.2 to 0.5 ml of marrow is aspirated and the needle is withdrawn.
- If the aspiration specimen is inadequate, the needle may be repositioned within the marrow cavity or removed and reinserted in another anesthetized site. If the second attempt fails, a needle biopsy may be necessary.

Needle biopsy

- The biopsy site is prepared and draped. The skin is marked at the site with an indelible pencil or marking pen. A local anesthetic is injected intradermally, subcutaneously, and at the surface of the bone.
- The biopsy needle is inserted into the periosteum and the needle guard set as indicated. Rotating the inner needle alternately clockwise and counterclockwise directs the needle into the marrow cavity.
- A tissue plug is removed and the needle assembly is withdrawn. The marrow is expelled into a labeled bottle containing a special fixative.

POSTPROCEDURE CARE

- While the marrow slides are being prepared, apply pressure to the biopsy site until bleeding stops.
- Clean the biopsy site and apply a sterile dressing.
- Monitor the patient's vital signs and the biopsy site for signs and symptoms of infection.
- Monitor the patient for hemorrhage and infection.
- Monitor for possible puncture of the mediastinum (sternal site).

COMMON BONE MARROW ASPIRATION AND BIOPSY SITES

These illustrations show commonly used sites for bone marrow aspiration and biopsy.

Usually, the posterior superior iliac spine is preferred for bone marrow aspiration because no vital organs or vessels are located nearby.

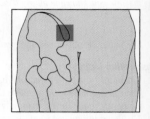

The sternum involves the greatest risk. However, it's commonly used for marrow aspiration because it's near the surface, the cortical bone is thin, and the marrow cavity contains numerous cells and relatively little fat or supporting bone.

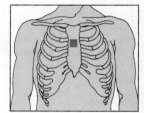

The spinous process is the preferred site if multiple punctures are necessary, if marrow is absent at other sites, or if the patient objects to a sternal puncture.

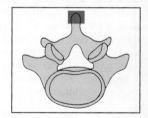

The tibia is the site of choice for infants younger than age 1.

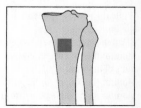

NORMAL RESULTS

- Yellow marrow containing fat cells and connective tissue
- Red marrow containing hematopoietic cells, fat cells, and connective tissue
- The iron stain, which measures hemosiderin (storage iron), at +2
- The Sudan black B stain, which shows granulocytes, negative
- The periodic acid–Schiff (PAS) stain, which detects glycogen reactions, negative

ABNORMAL RESULTS

- Decreased hemosiderin levels in an iron stain, possibly indicating a true iron deficiency
- Increased hemosiderin level, possibly suggesting other types of anemias or blood disorders
- A positive stain, possibly differentiating acute myelogenous leukemia from acute lymphoblastic leukemia (negative stain)
- A positive Sudan black B stain, possibly suggesting granulation in myeloblasts
- A positive PAS stain, possibly suggesting acute or chronic lymphocytic leukemia, amyloidosis, thalassemia, lymphoma, infectious mononucleosis, iron deficiency anemia, or sideroblastic anemia

Bronchoscopy

PURPOSE

- To provide direct visualization of the larynx, trachea, and bronchi using a rigid or fiber-optic bronchoscope
- To allow a better view of the segmental and subsegmental bronchi with less risk of trauma
- To remove foreign objects, excise endobronchial lesions, and control massive hemoptysis; requires general anesthesia (large, rigid bronchoscope)
- To allow a brush, biopsy forceps, or catheter to be passed through the bronchoscope to obtain specimens for cytologic or microbiological examination
- To allow visual examination of tumors, obstructions, secretions, or foreign bodies in the tracheobronchial tree
- To diagnose bronchogenic carcinoma, tuberculosis, interstitial pulmonary disease, and fungal or parasitic pulmonary infections
- To locate bleeding sites in the tracheobronchial tree
- To remove foreign bodies, malignant or benign tumors, mucus plugs, and excessive secretions from the tracheobronchial tree

PATIENT PREPARATION

- Make sure that the patient has signed an appropriate consent form.
- Note and report allergies.
- Obtain results of preprocedure studies; report abnormal results.
- Obtain the patient's baseline vital signs.
- An I.V. sedative may be given.
- Remove the patient's dentures.
- Instruct the patient to fast for 6 to 12 hours before the test.
- Explain to the patient that the test takes 45 to 60 minutes.
- Inform the patient that the airway won't be blocked, but that he may experience hoarseness, loss of voice, hemoptysis, and a sore throat.

PROCEDURE

- Position the patient properly.
- Give the patient supplemental oxygen by nasal cannula, if ordered.
- Monitor the patient's pulse oximetry, vital signs, and cardiac rhythm.
- A local anesthetic is sprayed into the patient's mouth and throat to suppress the gag reflex.
- The bronchoscope is inserted through the mouth or nose; a bite block is placed in the mouth if using the oral approach.
- When the bronchoscope is just above the vocal cords, about 3 to 4 ml of 2% to 4% lidocaine is flushed through the inner channel of the scope to the vocal cords to anesthetize deeper areas.
- A fiber-optic camera is used to take photographs for documentation.
- Tissue specimens are obtained from suspect areas.
- A suction apparatus may remove foreign bodies or mucus plugs.
- Bronchoalveolar lavage may remove thickened secretions or may diagnose infectious causes of infiltrates.
- Specimens are prepared properly and immediately sent to the laboratory.

POSTPROCEDURE CARE

- Position a conscious patient in semi-Fowler's position.
- Position an unconscious patient on one side, with the head of the bed slightly elevated to prevent aspiration.
- Instruct the patient to spit out saliva rather than swallow it.
- Observe the patient for bleeding.
- Resume the patient's usual diet, beginning with sips of clear liquid or ice chips, when the gag reflex returns.
- Provide lozenges or a soothing liquid gargle to ease discomfort when the gag reflex returns.

- Check the follow-up chest X-ray for pneumothorax.
- Monitor the patient's vital signs, characteristics of sputum, and respiratory status.

  ALERT *Monitor the patient for possible subcutaneous crepitus around his face, neck, or chest, which may indicate tracheal or bronchial perforation or pneumothorax.*

  ALERT *Monitor the patient for symptoms of respiratory difficulty as a result of laryngeal edema or laryngospasm, such as laryngeal stridor and dyspnea.*

- Monitor the patient for potential hypoxemia, cardiac arrhythmias, bleeding, and infection.

NORMAL RESULTS

- The bronchi appearing structurally similar to the trachea
- The right bronchus appearing slightly larger and more vertical than the left
- Smaller segmental bronchi branching off from the main bronchi

ABNORMAL RESULTS

- Structural abnormalities of the bronchial wall indicating inflammation, ulceration, tumors, and enlargement of submucosal lymph nodes
- Structural abnormalities of endotracheal origin suggesting stenosis, compression, ectasia, and diverticula
- Structural abnormalities of the trachea or bronchi suggesting calculi, foreign bodies, masses, and paralyzed vocal cords
- Tissue and cell study abnormalities suggesting interstitial pulmonary disease, infection, carcinoma, and tuberculosis

Cardiac blood pool imaging

PURPOSE

- To evaluate regional and global ventricular performance after I.V. injection of human serum albumin or red blood cells (RBCs) tagged with the isotope technetium 99m (^{99m}Tc) pertechnetate
- To calculate the portion of isotope ejected during each heartbeat to determine the ejection fraction and the presence and size of intracardiac shunts
- To provide a higher accuracy rate and less risk to the patient than left ventriculography in assessing cardiac function
- To evaluate left ventricular function

- To detect aneurysms of the left ventricle and other motion abnormalities of the myocardial wall (areas of akinesia or dyskinesia)
- To detect intracardiac shunting

PATIENT PREPARATION

- Make sure that the patient knows that the procedure is contraindicated during pregnancy.
- Make sure that the patient or a responsible family member has signed an informed consent form.
- Explain to the patient that cardiac blood pool imaging permits assessment of the heart's left ventricle.
- Describe the test, including who will perform it, where it will take place, and its expected duration.
- Tell the patient that he need not restrict food and fluids.
- Explain to the patient that he'll receive an I.V. injection of a radioactive tracer and that a detector positioned above his chest will record the circulation of this tracer through his heart.
- Reassure the patient that the tracer poses no radiation hazard and rarely produces adverse effects.
- Inform the patient that he may experience slight discomfort from the needle puncture but that the imaging itself is painless.

PROCEDURE

- The patient is placed in a supine position beneath the detector of a scintillation camera, and 15 to 20 mCi of albumin or RBCs tagged with ^{99m}Tc pertechnetate is injected I.V.
- For the next minute, the scintillation camera records the first pass of the isotope through the heart to locate the aortic and mitral valves.
- Then, using an electrocardiogram, the camera is gated for selected 60 msec intervals, representing end-systole and end-diastole, and 500 to 1,000 cardiac cycles are recorded on X-ray or Polaroid film.
- To observe septal and posterior wall motion, the patient may be assisted to a modified left anterior oblique position or he may be assisted to a right anterior oblique position and given 0.4 mg of nitroglycerin sublingually. The scintillation camera then records additional gated images to evaluate abnormal contraction in the left ventricle.
- The patient may be asked to exercise as the scintillation camera records gated images.

ALERT *If the patient is elderly or physically compromised, help him sit up and make sure that he isn't dizzy. Then help him get off the examination table.*

POSTPROCEDURE CARE

■ Monitor the patient's vital signs and response to the testing.
■ Answer the patient's questions about the test.

NORMAL RESULTS

■ The left ventricle contracting symmetrically and the isotope evenly distributed in the scans
■ Normal ejection fraction: 55% to 65%

ABNORMAL RESULTS

■ In patients with coronary artery disease or pre-existing conditions, such as myocarditis, asymmetrical blood distribution to the myocardium, producing segmental abnormalities of ventricular wall motion
■ In patients with a cardiomyopathy, globally reduced ejection fractions
■ In patients with a left-to-right shunt, the recirculating radioisotope prolonging the down slope of the curve of scintigraphic data; early arrival of activity in the left ventricle or aorta signifying a right-to-left shunt

Cardiac catheterization

PURPOSE

■ To measure pressure in chambers of the heart; to record films of the ventricles and arteries
  – Left-sided heart catheterization: Assesses patency of the coronary arteries and function of the left ventricle
  – Right-sided heart catheterization: Assesses pulmonary artery pressures
■ To evaluate valvular insufficiency or stenosis, septal defects, congenital anomalies, myocardial function, myocardial blood supply, and cardiac wall motion
■ To aid in diagnosing left ventricular enlargement, aortic root enlargement, ventricular aneurysms, and intracardiac shunts

PATIENT PREPARATION

■ Make sure that the patient has signed a consent form.
■ Notify the physician of hypersensitivity to shellfish, iodine, or contrast media.
■ Stop anticoagulants, as ordered, to reduce complications of bleeding.
■ Restrict food and fluids for at least 6 hours before the test.

- Explain that even if a mild sedative is given, the patient remains conscious.
- Warn the patient that a transient hot, flushing sensation or nausea may occur.
- Tell the patient that the test will take 1 to 2 hours.

PROCEDURE

- The patient is placed supine on a padded table and his heart rate and rhythm, respiratory status, and blood pressure are monitored throughout the procedure.
- An I.V. line is started, if not already in place; a local anesthetic is injected at the insertion site.
- A small incision is made into the artery or vein, depending on whether the test is for the left or right side.
- The catheter is passed through the sheath into the vessel and guided using fluoroscopy.
- In right-sided heart catheterization, the catheter is inserted into the antecubital or femoral vein and advanced through the vena cava into the right side of the heart and into the pulmonary artery.
- In left-sided heart catheterization, the catheter is inserted into the brachial or femoral artery and advanced retrograde through the aorta into the coronary artery ostium and left ventricle.
- When the catheter is in place, contrast medium is injected to make visible the cardiac vessels and structures.
- Nitroglycerin is given to eliminate catheter-induced spasm or watch its effect on the coronary arteries.
- After the catheter is removed, direct pressure is applied to the incision site until bleeding stops, and a sterile dressing is applied.

POSTPROCEDURE CARE

- Reinforce the dressing as needed.
- Enforce bed rest for 8 hours.
- If the femoral route was used for catheter insertion, keep the leg straight at the hip for 6 to 8 hours.
- If the antecubital fossa route was used for catheter insertion, keep the arm straight at the elbow for at least 3 hours.
- Resume medications and give analgesics.
- Encourage fluid intake.
- Monitor the patient's vital signs, intake and output, cardiac rhythm, neurologic and respiratory status, and peripheral vascular status distal to the puncture site.

MAXIMUM NORMAL CARDIAC PRESSURES

This chart shows the upper limits of normal pressure in the cardiac chambers and great vessels of recumbent (lying down) adults.

Chamber or vessel	Pressure
Right atrium	6 mm Hg (mean)
Right ventricle	30/6 mm Hg*
Pulmonary artery	30/12 mm Hg* (mean, 18)
Left atrium	12 mm Hg (mean)
Left ventricle	140/12 mm Hg*
Ascending aorta	140/90 mm Hg* (mean, 105)
Pulmonary artery wedge	Almost identical to left atrial mean pressure (±1 to 2 mm Hg)

*Peak systolic and end-diastolic

- Check the catheter insertion site and dressings for signs and symptoms of infection.
- Monitor the patient for the following possible complications:
  - In patients with valvular heart disease: infective endocarditis (administer prophylactic antibiotics)
  - Left- or right-sided heart catheterization: myocardial infarction, arrhythmias, cardiac tamponade, infection, hypovolemia, pulmonary edema, hematoma, blood loss, adverse reaction to contrast media, and vasovagal response
  - Left-sided heart catheterization: arterial thrombus or embolism and stroke
  - Right-sided heart catheterization: thrombophlebitis and pulmonary embolism.

NORMAL RESULTS

- No abnormalities of heart valves, chamber size, pressures, configuration, wall motion or thickness, and blood flow (see *Maximum normal cardiac pressures*)
- Coronary arteries showing smooth and regular outline

ABNORMAL RESULTS

- Coronary artery narrowing greater than 70% suggesting significant coronary artery disease
- Narrowing of the left main coronary artery and occlusion or narrowing high in the left anterior descending artery suggesting the need for revascularization surgery
- Impaired wall motion suggesting myocardial incompetence
- A pressure gradient indicating valvular heart disease
- Retrograde flow of the contrast medium across a valve during systole indicating valvular incompetence

Cerebral angiography

PURPOSE

- Usually performed on patients with suspected abnormalities of the cerebral vasculature, which have been suggested by other imaging studies
- To detect cerebrovascular abnormalities, such as an aneurysm or arteriovenous malformation, thrombosis, narrowing, or occlusion
- To evaluate vascular displacement caused by a tumor, a hematoma, edema, herniation, vasospasm, increased intracranial pressure, or hydrocephalus
- To locate clips applied to blood vessels during surgery and to evaluate the postoperative status of such vessels
- To evaluate the presence and degree of carotid artery disease

PATIENT PREPARATION

- Make sure that the patient has signed an appropriate consent form.
- Note and report drug allergies.
- Have the patient fast for 8 to 10 hours before the test.
- Provide I.V. access and give I.V. fluids.
- Give a sedative.
- Tell the patient that his head will be immobilized and he'll need to lie still.
- Explain to the patient that he'll receive a local anesthetic.
- Warn the patient that nausea, warmth, or burning may occur with the contrast injection.
- Explain to the patient that the test takes 2 to 4 hours.

PROCEDURE

- The patient is placed in a supine position on an X-ray table.
- The access site (usually femoral) is prepared and draped and a local anesthetic is injected.
- The artery is punctured with the appropriate needle and catheterized under fluoroscopic guidance.
- Catheter placement in the carotid or vertebral arteries is verified by fluoroscopy and a contrast medium is injected.
- A series of radiographs is taken and reviewed.
- Arterial catheter patency is maintained by continuous or periodic flushing.
- The patient's vital signs and neurologic status are monitored continuously.
- The catheter is removed, firm pressure is applied to the access site until bleeding stops, and a pressure dressing is applied.

POSTPROCEDURE CARE

- Enforce bed rest and apply an ice bag.
- If active bleeding or expanding hematoma occurs, apply firm pressure to the puncture site and inform the physician immediately.
- Make sure that the patient is adequately hydrated.
- Provide analgesia.
- Monitor the patient's vital signs, along with intake and output.
- Monitor the neurovascular status of the extremity distal to the access site.
- If the femoral approach was used as the access site, keep the involved leg straight at the hip and check pulses distal to the site.
- If the carotid artery was used as the access site, watch for dysphagia or respiratory distress, which can result from hematoma or edema. Also watch for disorientation, weakness, or numbness in the extremities and for arterial spasms, which produce symptoms of transient ischemic attacks (TIAs). Notify the physician immediately if abnormal signs develop.
- If the brachial artery was used as the access site, keep the arm straight at the elbow and assess distal pulses. Avoid venipuncture and blood pressures in the affected arm. Observe the extremity for changes in color, temperature, or sensation. If it becomes pale, cool, or numb, notify the physician immediately.
- Watch for potential adverse reactions to contrast media.
- Watch for potential complications, such as embolism, bleeding, hematoma, infection, vasospasm, thrombosis, TIA, or stroke.

COMPARING CEREBRAL ANGIOGRAMS

The angiograms below show the differences between normal and abnormal cerebral vasculature.

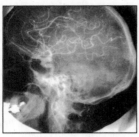

This cerebral angiogram is normal.

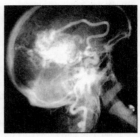

This cerebral angiogram shows occluded blood vessels caused by a large arteriovenous malformation.

NORMAL RESULTS

- Cerebral vasculature normal
- During the arterial phase of perfusion, the contrast medium fills and opacifies superficial and deep arteries and arterioles
- During the venous phase, the contrast medium opacifies superficial and deep veins

ABNORMAL RESULTS

- Changes in the caliber of vessel lumina suggesting vascular disease (see *Comparing cerebral angiograms*)
- Vessel displacement suggesting a possible tumor
- Blockage of vessels suggesting ischemic stroke

Computed tomography

PURPOSE

- To combine radiologic and computer technology to produce cross-sectional images of various layers of tissue, called *computed tomography* (CT)

- To reconstruct cross-sectional, horizontal, sagittal, and coronal plane images
- To accentuate tissue-density differences through the use of an I.V. or oral contrast medium
- To produce tissue images not readily seen on standard radiographs
- Also known as a *CT scan*

PATIENT PREPARATION

- Make sure that the patient has signed an appropriate consent form.
- Note and report allergies.
- A CT scan usually isn't recommended during pregnancy because of the potential risk to the fetus.
- Check the patient's history for hypersensitivity to shellfish, iodine, or iodinated contrast media, and document such reactions on the patient's chart.
- The specific type of CT scan dictates the need for an oral or I.V. contrast medium.
- Warn the patient about transient discomfort from the needle puncture and a warm or flushed feeling from an I.V. contrast medium, if used.

> **ALERT** *Tell the patient to immediately report feelings of nausea, vomiting, dizziness, headache, itching, or hives, indicating a hypersensitivity reaction.*

- Instruct the patient to remain still during the test because movement can limit the accuracy of results.
- Tell the patient he may experience minimal discomfort because of lying still.
- Tell the patient that the study takes from 5 minutes to 1 hour, depending on the type of CT and his ability to remain still.

PROCEDURE

- The patient is positioned on an adjustable table inside a scanning gantry.
- A series of transverse radiographs is taken and recorded.
- The information is reconstructed by a computer and selected images are photographed.
- After the images are reviewed, an I.V. contrast enhancement may be ordered.
- Additional images are obtained after the I.V. contrast injection.
- The patient is observed carefully for adverse reactions to the contrast medium.

POSTPROCEDURE CARE

- Normal diet and activities may resume, unless otherwise ordered.
- Monitor the patient for potential adverse reactions to iodinated contrast media.

NORMAL RESULTS

- Normal findings dictated by specific type of CT scan
- Structures evaluated according to their density, size, shape, and position
- Tissue densities appearing as black, white, or shades of gray on the CT image
- Bone, the densest tissue, appearing white
- Cerebrospinal fluid, the least dense tissue, appearing black

ABNORMAL RESULTS

- Varies with the specific type of CT
- Oral or I.V. contrast media used in previous diagnostic tests (obscures images)

Cultures: Blood, sputum, throat, urine, and wound

PURPOSE

- Bacteriologic examination of blood, sputum, throat tissue or secretions, urine, and wound exudate to identify causative organisms of infection
- Blood culture to confirm bacteremia or determine the cause of fever of unknown origin
- Sputum culture to isolate and identify causes of pulmonary infections; acid-fast sputum smear to disclose evidence of mycobacterial infection such as tuberculosis (TB)
- Throat culture to isolate and identify pathogens, especially group A beta-hemolytic streptococci, and screen asymptomatic carriers of pathogens, especially *Neisseria meningitides;* to make preliminary identification by Gram stain; to detect group A streptococcal antigen in as few as 5 minutes with rapid nonculture antigen-testing methods (all specimens with negative results should be cultured)
- Urine culture to diagnose urinary tract infection (UTI), monitor microorganism colonization after urinary catheter insertion, and identify pathogenic fungi such as *Coccidioides immitis*

- quick urine screen to determine if urine contains high bacteria or white blood cell (WBC) count (only urine with bacteria or WBCs is processed for culture)
- *colony count* to distinguish between true bacteriuria and contamination by estimating numbers of bacteria present in specimen
- quick centrifugation test to determine UTI origin
■ Wound culture to confirm and identify an infectious microbe in a wound; organisms may be aerobic (usually require oxygen to grow and typically appear in a superficial wound) or anaerobic (need little or no oxygen and appear in areas of poor tissue perfusion, such as postoperative wounds, ulcers, or compound fractures)

PATIENT PREPARATION

■ Make sure that the patient has signed an appropriate consent form.
■ Note and report allergies, particularly to antibiotics.
■ Check the patient's history for current use of antimicrobials.
■ Explain that the test requires a specimen of the appropriate material.
■ Tell the patient that he need not restrict food and fluids.
■ Warn the patient of possible discomfort from the needle stick during a blood culture, a gagging feeling during a throat culture, or discomfort if catheterization is required to obtain a urine specimen.

PROCEDURE

See *Obtaining specimens for culture*, pages 438 to 440.

POSTPROCEDURE CARE

■ After blood culture, monitor the venipuncture site for bleeding, hematoma, and signs of infection.
■ After sputum and throat cultures, provide mouth care.
■ After tracheal suctioning to obtain sputum culture, if needed, monitor the patient's vital signs and respiratory status.
■ After urine culture, when specimens are obtained by catheterization, monitor the patient for possible infection.
■ After wound culture, complete the wound care as prescribed and re-dress the wound.

(Text continues on page 440.)

OBTAINING SPECIMENS FOR CULTURE

General procedures for obtaining culture specimens from blood, sputum, throat, urine, and wounds are shown here. Before performing any of these procedures, always check your facility's procedure manual.

Blood
- Put on personal protective equipment (PPE), as appropriate.
- Clean venipuncture site and allow it to dry.
- Perform venipuncture.
- Draw 10 to 20 ml of blood for an adult, 2 to 6 ml for a child.
- Clean diaphragm tops of culture bottles with alcohol or iodine.
- Change needle on syringe.
- For broth, add blood to each bottle until achieving 1:5 or 1:10 dilution.
- For special resin, add blood according to facility protocol; invert gently to mix it.
- For lysis-centrifugation technique, draw blood directly into special collection-processing tube.
- Label specimen with patient's name, prescriber's name, date and time, and origin of specimen.
- Document tentative diagnosis and recent antimicrobial therapy on laboratory request.
- Send to laboratory immediately.
- Repeat culture per facility policy or prescription (commonly 2 consecutive days).

Sputum
- Maintain asepsis; wear PPE.
- Instruct patient to cough deeply and expectorate into container.
- If cough is nonproductive, use chest physiotherapy or nebulization to induce sputum.
- Close containers securely; seal in leak-proof bag.
- *If tracheal suctioning required:* Give oxygen to patient before and after procedure as necessary.
- Attach sputum trap to suction catheter.
- Lubricate catheter with normal saline solution; pass it through patient's nostril without suction.
- Advance catheter into trachea; apply suction only while withdrawing.
- Suction for only 5 to 10 seconds at a time.
- Discard catheter in proper receptacle.
- Detach in-line sputum trap from suction apparatus; cap opening.

OBTAINING SPECIMENS FOR CULTURE *(continued)*

- Label with patient's name, nature and origin of specimen, date and time, initial diagnosis, and current antimicrobial therapy.
- Send to laboratory immediately.

Throat

- Put on gloves; ask patient to tilt his head back and close his eyes.
- Illuminate throat; check for inflamed areas using tongue blade.
- Swab tonsillar areas from side to side; include inflamed or purulent sites.
- Don't touch tongue, cheeks, or teeth with swab.
- Place swab in culture tube immediately.
- If commercial sterile collection and transport system is used, crush ampule and force swab into medium.
- Label specimen with patient's name, prescriber's name, date and time, and origin of specimen.
- Note recent antimicrobial therapy on laboratory request.
- *Corynebacterium diphtheriae* requires two swabs and special growth medium.
- *Neisseria meningitidis* requires enriched selective media.
- Send to laboratory immediately.

Urine

- Collect first-voided mid-stream urine specimen in sterile specimen cup.
- Collect at least 3 ml of urine; don't fill specimen cup more than halfway.
- Seal cup with sterile lid or transfer specimen to culture transport tube per facility policy
- Obtain specimen by sterile straight catheterization if ordered.
- Label specimen with patient's name, prescriber's name, date and time, and origin of specimen.
- Record suspected diagnosis, collection time and method, current antimicrobial therapy, and fluid- or drug-induced diuresis on laboratory request.
- Send to laboratory immediately.
- If transport is delayed for more than 30 minutes, store specimen at 39.2° F (4° C) or place on ice unless urine transport tube contains preservative.

Wound

- Maintain aseptic technique throughout procedure.
- Wear PPE.
- Prepare a sterile field.
- Clean area around wound with antiseptic solution.

(continued)

OBTAINING SPECIMENS FOR CULTURE *(continued)*

- *For aerobic culture:* Express wound and swab as much exudate as possible, or insert swab deep into wound and gently rotate.
- *For anaerobic culture:* Insert swab deep into wound and gently rotate.
- Immediately place swab in aerobic or anaerobic culture tube as appropriate.
- Some anaerobes die in presence of oxygen, so place specimen in culture tube quickly; take care that no air enters tube and check that double stoppers are secure.
- Label specimen container with patient's name, prescriber's name, wound site, and time of collection.
- Record recent antimicrobial therapy, source of specimen, and suspected organism on laboratory request.
- Keep specimen container upright.
- Send to laboratory within 15 minutes.

NORMAL RESULTS

- No pathogenic organisms found in any culture

ABNORMAL RESULTS

Blood culture

- Positive blood cultures not able to confirm pathologic septicemia
- Mild, transient bacteremia that occurs during many infectious diseases or complicates other disorders
- Persistent, continuous, or recurrent bacteremia, reliably confirming the presence of serious infection
- Of cultured blood samples, 2% to 3% contaminated by skin bacteria, such as *Staphylococcus epidermidis*, diphtheroids, and propionibacterium; these organisms clinically significant when isolated from multiple cultures or from immunocompromised patients
- Isolates of *Candida albicans* in debilitated or immunocompromised patients

Sputum culture

- Because sputum invariably contaminated with normal oropharyngeal flora, interpretation of culture isolate dependent on the patient's overall condition
- Isolation of *Mycobacterium tuberculosis*, suggesting TB

■ Isolation of pathogenic organisms, typically suggesting *Streptococcus pneumoniae*, *M. tuberculosis*, *Klebsiella pneumoniae* (and other Enterobacteriaceae), *Haemophilus influenzae*, *Staphylococcus aureus*, and *Pseudomonas aeruginosa*

Throat culture

■ Group A beta-hemolytic streptococci *(Streptococcus pyogenes)*, suggesting possible scarlet fever or pharyngitis
■ *C. albicans*, suggesting possible thrush
■ *Corynebacterium diphtheriae*, suggesting possible diphtheria
■ *Bordetella pertussis*, suggesting possible whooping cough
■ *Legionella* species and *Mycoplasma pneumoniae*, suggesting bacterial pneumonia
■ *Histoplasma capsulatum*, *C. immitis*, and *Blastomyces dermatitidis*, suggesting fungal infections
■ Adenovirus, enterovirus, herpesvirus, rhinovirus, influenza virus, and parainfluenza virus, suggesting viral infections

Urine culture

■ Bacterial count of 100,000 or more organisms of a single microbe species per milliliter, suggesting UTI (less than 100,000/ml may be significant, depending on the patient's age, sex, history, and other individual factors)
■ Bacterial count of less than 10,000/ml, usually suggesting the organisms are contaminants, except in symptomatic patients or those with urologic disorders
■ Isolation of *M. tuberculosis* in a special test for acid-fast bacteria, suggesting TB of the urinary tract
■ Isolation of more than two species of organisms or of vaginal or skin organisms, usually suggesting contamination and requiring a repeat culture

Wound culture

■ The presence of *S. aureus*, group A beta-hemolytic streptococci, *Proteus* species, *Escherichia coli* and other Enterobacteriaceae, and some *Pseudomonas* species, suggesting an aerobic wound infection
■ The presence of *Clostridium*, *Bacteroides*, *Peptococcus*, and *Streptococcus* species, suggesting an anaerobic wound infection

Doppler ultrasound

PURPOSE

- To noninvasively evaluate blood flow in the major veins and arteries of the arms and legs and in the extracranial cerebrovascular system
- To permit direct listening and graphic recording of blood flow by directing high-frequency sound waves to an artery or a vein (see *How the Doppler probe works*)
- To measure systolic pressure to help detect the presence, location, and extent of peripheral arterial occlusive disease
- To detect arteriovenous disease that impairs at least 50% of blood flow (95% accurate)
- To aid in the diagnosis of venous insufficiency, superficial and deep vein thromboses, and peripheral artery disease and arterial occlusion
- To monitor patients who have had arterial reconstruction and bypass grafts
- To detect abnormalities of carotid artery blood
- To evaluate arterial trauma

PATIENT PREPARATION

- Make sure that the patient has signed an appropriate consent form.
- Note and report drug allergies.
- Tell the patient the test takes about 20 minutes.
- Explain that the test doesn't involve risk or discomfort.

PROCEDURE

- Doppler ultrasonography is performed bilaterally.
- The patient is assisted into the supine position on the examination table with his arms at his sides.

Peripheral arterial evaluation

- For peripheral arterial evaluation in the leg, the usual test sites are the common and superficial femoral, popliteal, posterior tibial, and dorsalis pedis arteries.
- For peripheral arterial evaluation in the arm, the usual test sites are the subclavian, brachial, radial, and ulnar arteries.
- Brachial blood pressure is measured, and the transducer is placed at various points along the test arteries.
- The signals are monitored, and the waveforms are recorded for later analysis.
- The blood flow velocity is monitored and recorded over the test artery.

HOW THE DOPPLER PROBE WORKS

The Doppler ultrasonic probe directs high-frequency sound waves through layers of tissue. When these waves strike red blood cells (RBCs) moving through the bloodstream, their frequency changes in proportion to the flow velocity of the RBCs. Recording these waves permits detection of arterial and venous obstruction but not quantitative blood flow measurement.

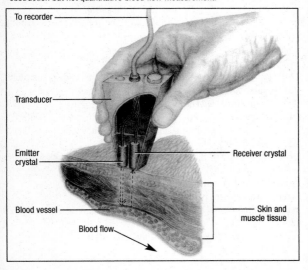

- Segmental limb blood pressures are obtained to localize arterial occlusive disease.

Peripheral venous evaluation

- For peripheral venous evaluation in the leg, the usual test sites are the popliteal, superficial and common femoral veins, and posterior tibial vein.
- For extracranial cerebrovascular evaluation, the usual test sites are the supraorbital artery; the common, external, and internal carotid arteries; the vertebral arteries; and the brachial, axillary, subclavian, and jugular veins.
- The transducer is placed over the appropriate vessel, waveforms are recorded, and respiratory modulations are noted.

- Proximal limb compression maneuvers are performed.
- Augmentation after release of compression is noted to evaluate venous valve competency.
- For tests involving the legs and feet, the patient is asked to perform Valsalva's maneuver, and venous blood flow is recorded.

POSTPROCEDURE CARE

- Remove the conductive jelly from the patient's skin.
- Monitor the patient for bradyarrhythmia, if the probe is placed near the carotid sinus.

NORMAL RESULTS

- Arterial waveforms of the arms and legs multiphasic, with a prominent systolic component and one or more diastolic sounds
- Arm pressure unchanged despite postural changes
- Proximal thigh pressure 20 to 30 mm Hg greater than arm pressure
- Venous blood flow velocity phasic with respiration, with a lower pitch than arterial flow
- Blood flow velocity increasing with distal compression or release of proximal limb compression
- Valsalva's maneuver interrupting venous flow velocity
- In cerebrovascular testing, a strong velocity signal
- In the common carotid artery, blood flow velocity increasing during diastole
- Periorbital arterial flow anterograde out of the orbit
- Ankle-brachial index (ABI): 0.9

ABNORMAL RESULTS

- Diminished blood flow velocity signal suggesting arterial stenosis or occlusion
- Absent velocity signals suggesting complete occlusion and lack of collateral circulation
- ABI 0.5 to 0.9, indicating claudication; ABI 0.5, resting ischemic pain; ABI 0.2, gangrenous foot or leg
- Venous blood flow velocity unchanged by respirations, not increased with compression or Valsalva's maneuver, or absent indicating venous thrombosis
- A reversed flow velocity signal suggesting chronic venous insufficiency and varicose veins
- Absent Doppler signals during cerebrovascular examination implying total arterial occlusion

Echocardiography

PURPOSE

- To noninvasively examine the size, shape, and motion of cardiac structures
- Transducer directs ultra-high–frequency sound waves toward cardiac structures, which reflect these waves; the transducer picks up the echoes, converts them to electrical impulses, and relays them to an echocardiography machine for display
- In M-mode, or motion mode: a single, pencil-like ultrasound beam strikes the heart and produces a vertical view, which is useful for recording the motion and dimensions of intracardiac structures
- In two-dimensional echocardiography: cross-sectional view of cardiac structures used for recording lateral motion and spatial relationship among structures (see *Comparing two types of echocardiography,* page 446)
- To diagnose and evaluate valvular abnormalities
- To measure and evaluate the size of the heart's chambers and valves
- To help diagnose cardiomyopathies and atrial tumors
- To evaluate cardiac function or wall motion after myocardial infarction
- To detect pericardial effusion or mural thrombi

PATIENT PREPARATION

- Tell the patient that he may be asked to breathe in and out slowly, to hold his breath, or to inhale a gas with a slightly sweet odor (amyl nitrite) while changes in heart function are recorded.
- Warn the patient about possible adverse effects of amyl nitrite (dizziness, flushing, and tachycardia), but reassure him that such effects quickly subside.
- Stress the need to remain still during the test because movement may distort results.
- Explain that the test takes 15 to 30 minutes.

PROCEDURE

- The patient is placed in the supine position and conductive gel is applied to the third or fourth intercostal space to the left of the sternum. The transducer is placed directly over it.
- The transducer is systematically angled to direct ultrasonic waves at specific parts of the patient's heart.
- During the test, the oscilloscope screen is observed; significant findings are recorded on a strip chart recorder or videotape recorder.

COMPARING TWO TYPES OF ECHOCARDIOGRAPHY

This illustration shows how M-mode and two-dimensional echocardiography differ. The shaded areas beneath the transducer identify cardiac structures that intercept and reflect the transducer's ultrasonic waves.

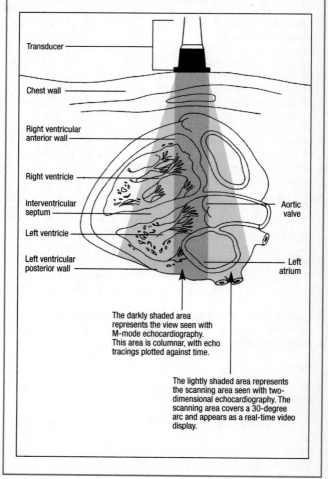

Transducer

Chest wall

Right ventricular anterior wall

Right ventricle

Interventricular septum

Left ventricle

Left ventricular posterior wall

Aortic valve

Left atrium

The darkly shaded area represents the view seen with M-mode echocardiography. This area is columnar, with echo tracings plotted against time.

The lightly shaded area represents the scanning area seen with two-dimensional echocardiography. The scanning area covers a 30-degree arc and appears as a real-time video display.

- For a left lateral view, the patient is placed on his left side.
- Doppler echocardiography may also be used: color flow simulates red blood cell flow through the heart valves. The sound of blood flow may also be used to assess heart sounds and murmurs as they relate to cardiac hemodynamics.

POSTPROCEDURE CARE

- Remove the conductive gel from the patient's skin.

NORMAL RESULTS

- For the mitral valve, anterior and posterior mitral valve leaflets separating in early diastole and attaining maximum excursion rapidly, and then moving toward each other during ventricular diastole; after atrial contraction, the mitral valve leaflets coming together and remaining together during ventricular systole
- For the aortic valve, aortic valve cusps moving anteriorly during systole and posteriorly during diastole
- For the tricuspid valve, valve motion resembling that of the mitral valve
- For the pulmonic valve, moving posterior during atrial diastole and ventricular systole; in right ventricular ejection, the cusp moving anteriorly, attaining its most anterior position during diastole
- For the ventricular cavities, the left ventricular cavity appearing as an echo-free space between the interventricular septum and the posterior left ventricular wall
- The right ventricular cavity appearing as an echo-free space between the anterior chest wall and the interventricular septum

ABNORMAL RESULTS

- In mitral stenosis, the valve narrowing because of the leaflets' thickening and disordered motion; during diastole, both mitral valve leaflets moving anteriorly instead of posteriorly
- In mitral valve prolapse, one or both leaflets ballooning into the left atrium during systole
- In aortic insufficiency, leaflet fluttering of the aortic valve during diastole
- In stenosis, the aortic valve thickening and generating more echoes
- In bacterial endocarditis, valve motion disrupted with fuzzy echoes usually appearing on or near the valve
- A large chamber size suggesting cardiomyopathy, valvular disorders, or heart failure
- A small chamber size suggesting restrictive pericarditis

- Hypertrophic cardiomyopathy causing systolic anterior motion of the mitral valve and asymmetrical septal hypertrophy
- Myocardial ischemia or infarction causing absent or paradoxical motion in ventricular walls
- Fluid accumulation in the pericardial space causing an echo-free space, suggesting pericardial effusion
- In large effusions, pressure exerted by excess fluid restricting pericardial motion
- Movement during test interfering with test results

Echocardiography, exercise

PURPOSE

- To detect changes in cardiac wall motion
- To diagnose and evaluate valvular and wall motion abnormalities
- To identify the causes of chest pain
- To determine chamber size and functional capacity of the heart by collecting images before and after exercise stress testing
- To screen for asymptomatic cardiac disease
- To set limits for an exercise program
- To detect atrial tumors, mural thrombi, vegetative growth on valve leaflets, and pericardial effusions
- To evaluate myocardial perfusion, coronary artery disease (CAD) and obstructions, and the extent of myocardial damage after myocardial infarction (MI)

ALERT *Exercise echocardiography is contraindicated in patients with ventricular or dissecting aortic aneurysms, uncontrolled arrhythmias, pericarditis, myocarditis, severe anemia, uncontrolled hypertension, unstable angina, and heart failure.*

- Stress can be added with medication, such as dobutamine (Dobutrex) or dipyridamole (Persantine), for patients who can't use the treadmill or bicycle for exercise
- Also called *stress echocardiography*

PATIENT PREPARATION

- Make sure that the patient has signed an appropriate consent form.
- Note and report drug allergies.
- The procedure shouldn't be performed without a physician and emergency resuscitation equipment readily available.

- Withhold drugs the patient is currently taking.
- Instruct the patient to refrain from eating, smoking, or drinking alcoholic or caffeinated beverages at least 3 to 4 hours before the test.
- Warn the patient that he might feel tired, diaphoretic, and slightly short of breath. Reassure him that if symptoms become severe or if chest pain develops, the test will stop.
- Explain that the test takes about 60 minutes.

PROCEDURE

- The patient is placed in the supine position and a baseline echocardiogram is obtained.
- An initial baseline electrocardiogram (ECG) and blood pressure reading are obtained.
- The patient is then placed on the treadmill at a slow speed until he becomes acclimated to it.
- The work rate is increased every 3 minutes as tolerated by increasing the speed of the machine slightly and increasing the degree of incline by 3% each time.
- The cardiac monitor is observed continuously for changes, and blood pressure is monitored at predetermined intervals.
- The rhythm strip is checked at preset intervals for arrhythmias, premature ventricular contractions, and ST-segment and T-wave changes.
- The test level and time it took to reach that level are marked on each strip.
- Common responses to maximal exercise include dizziness, lightheadedness, leg fatigue, dyspnea, diaphoresis, and a slightly ataxic gait. If symptoms become severe, the test is stopped.
- The test is stopped for significant ECG changes, arrhythmias, or symptoms, including hypertension, hypotension, or angina.
- After the patient has reached the maximum predicted heart rate, the treadmill is slowed.
- While the patient's heart rate is still elevated, he's helped off the treadmill and placed on a litter for a second echocardiogram.

POSTPROCEDURE CARE

- Remove electrodes and conductive gel.
- Monitor the patient's vital signs, ECG, and heart sounds.
- Monitor the patient for potential complications, such as cardiac arrhythmias, myocardial ischemia or MI, or cardiac arrest.

NORMAL RESULTS

- Increased contractility of the ventricular walls resulting in hyperkinesis linked to sympathetic and catecholamine stimulation
- Heart rate increasing in direct proportion to the workload and metabolic oxygen demand; systolic blood pressure also increasing as the workload increases
- The endurance level appropriate for the patient's age and exercise limits attained

ABNORMAL RESULTS

- Exercise-induced myocardial ischemia suggesting disease in the coronary artery supplying the involved area of myocardium
- Hypokinesis or akinesis of the myocardium indicating significant CAD
- Exercise-induced hypotension, ST-segment depression of 2 mm or more, or down-sloping ST segments appearing within the first 3 minutes of exercise and lasting 8 minutes after the test ends suggesting multivessel or left CAD
- ST-segment elevation suggesting critical myocardial ischemia or injury
- Wolff-Parkinson-White syndrome, electrolyte imbalance, or the use of digoxin preparations (may give false-positive results)
- Conditions that cause left ventricular hypertrophy interfering with results

Electroencephalography

PURPOSE

- To record a portion of the brain's electrical activity through electrodes attached to the scalp
- To record EEG changes for localization of seizure focus through surgically implanted intracranial electrodes
- To determine the presence and type of epilepsy
- To aid in the diagnosis of intracranial lesions
- To evaluate brain activity in metabolic disease, head injury, meningitis, encephalitis, and psychological disorders by electrical impulses transmitted, magnified, and recorded as brain waves
- To help confirm brain death

PATIENT PREPARATION

- Make sure that the patient or a family member has signed an appropriate consent form.

- Note and report drug allergies.
- Wash and dry the patient's hair to remove hairsprays, creams, or oils.
- Withhold tranquilizers, barbiturates, and other sedatives for 24 to 48 hours before the test.
- Minimize sleep (4 to 5 hours) the night before the study.
- If a sleep EEG is ordered, give a sedative to promote sleep during the test.
- The patient need not restrict food and fluids before the test, but stimulants such as caffeinated beverages, chocolate, and nicotine aren't permitted for 8 hours before the study.
- Reassure the patient that the electrodes won't shock him.
- If the test will involve needle electrodes, warn the patient that he might feel pricking sensations during insertion.
- Explain that the test takes about 1 hour.

ALERT *Infants and very young children may require sedation to prevent crying and restlessness; however, sedatives may alter test results.*

PROCEDURE

- The patient is positioned and electrodes are attached to the scalp.
- During recording, the patient is carefully observed and movement, such as blinking, swallowing, or talking, are noted; these movements can cause artifacts.
- The patient may undergo testing in various stress situations, including hyperventilation and photic stimulation, to elicit abnormal patterns not obvious in the resting stage.

POSTPROCEDURE CARE

- Tell the patient that he may resume drug therapy.
- Provide a safe environment.
- Monitor the patient for seizures and maintain seizure precautions.
- Help the patient remove electrode paste from his hair.
- Monitor the patient for adverse effects of sedation, if used.
- If brain death is confirmed, provide emotional support to the family and refer them to social services and a transplant team if appropriate.

NORMAL RESULTS

- Alpha waves (8 to 13 cycles/second in a regular rhythm) when the patient is awake and alert but with eyes closed, usually disappearing with visual activity or mental concentration
- Alpha waves decreased by apprehension or anxiety and most prominent in the occipital leads

COMPARING EEG TRACINGS

The EEG tracings below compare a normal tracing with tracings associated with various seizure types.

This is a normal tracing. The top tracing reflects the right temporal area; the bottom tracing, the parietal-occipital area.

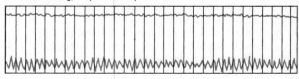

This tracing demonstrates spikes and waves, which occur during absence seizures.

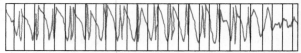

Generalized tonic-clonic seizures create multiple high-voltage spiked waves like those in this tracing.

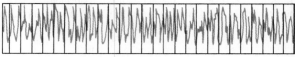

These focal spiked waves indicate right temporal lobe epilepsy.

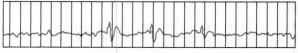

- Beta waves (13 to 30 cycles/second) when the patient is alert with eyes open, most commonly seen in the frontal and central regions of the brain
- Theta waves (4 to 7 cycles/second) most common in children and young adults, primarily in the parietal and temporal regions
- Theta waves indicating drowsiness or emotional stress in adults
- Delta waves (fewer than 4 cycles/second) visible in deep sleep stages and in serious brain dysfunction

ABNORMAL RESULTS

- Spikes and waves at a frequency of 3 cycles/second suggesting absence seizures (see *Comparing EEG tracings*)
- Multiple, high-voltage, spiked waves in both hemispheres suggesting generalized tonic-clonic seizures
- Spiked waves in the affected temporal region suggesting temporal lobe epilepsy
- Localized, spiked discharges suggesting focal seizures
- Slow waves (usually delta waves but possibly unilateral beta waves) suggesting intracranial lesions
- Focal abnormalities in the injured area suggesting vascular lesions
- Generalized, diffuse, and slow brain waves suggesting metabolic or inflammatory disorders or increased intracranial pressure
- An absent EEG pattern or a flat tracing (except for artifacts) suggesting brain death
- Hypoglycemia and altered brain wave patterns caused by skipping the meal before the test
- Interference by anticonvulsants, tranquilizers, barbiturates, and other sedatives

Electromyography

PURPOSE

- To record the electrical activity of selected skeletal muscle groups at rest and during voluntary contraction
- To measure nerve conduction time
- To differentiate between primary muscle disorders, such as muscular dystrophy, and certain metabolic disorders
- To identify diseases characterized by central neuronal degeneration such as amyotrophic lateral sclerosis (ALS)
- To aid in diagnosing neuromuscular disorders such as myasthenia gravis
- To aid in diagnosing radiculomyopathies

PATIENT PREPARATION

- Tell the patient that the test is contraindicated if he has a bleeding disorder.
- Make sure that the patient has signed an appropriate consent form.
- Note and report drug allergies.
- Check for and note drugs that may interfere with test results, such as

cholinergics, anticholinergics, anticoagulants, and skeletal muscle relaxants.

- Tell the patient that he need not restrict food and fluids before the test, but that it may be necessary to restrict nicotine and caffeine for 2 to 3 hours beforehand.
- Warn the patient that he might experience discomfort as a needle is inserted into selected muscles.
- Explain that the test takes at least 1 hour.

PROCEDURE

- The patient is positioned in a way that relaxes the muscle to be tested.
- Needle electrodes are quickly inserted into the selected muscle.
- A metal plate lies under the patient to serve as a reference electrode.
- The resulting electrical signal is recorded during rest and contraction, amplified 1 million times, and displayed on an oscilloscope or computer screen.
- Leadwires are usually attached to an audio-amplifier so that voltage fluctuations within the muscle are audible.

POSTPROCEDURE CARE

- Apply warm compresses and give analgesics for discomfort.
- Resume drugs that were withheld before the test.
- Monitor the patient for signs and symptoms of infection at the insertion site.
- Monitor the patient's pain level and response to analgesics.

NORMAL RESULTS

- At rest, minimal electrical activity in muscle
- During voluntary contraction, electrical activity increasing markedly
- In a sustained contraction, or one of increasing strength, a rapid "train" of motor unit potentials

ABNORMAL RESULTS

- Short motor unit potentials, with frequent, irregular discharges suggesting primary muscle disease such as muscular dystrophy
- Isolated and irregular motor unit potentials with increased amplitude and duration suggesting ALS and peripheral nerve disorders
- Initially normal motor unit potentials that progressively diminish in amplitude with continuing contractions suggesting myasthenia gravis

Endoscopic retrograde cholangiopancreatography

PURPOSE

- To visualize via X-ray the pancreatic ducts and hepatobiliary tree after injection of a contrast medium into the duodenal papilla
- To evaluate obstructive jaundice
- To diagnose cancer of the duodenal papilla, pancreas, and biliary ducts
- To locate calculi and stenosis in the pancreatic ducts and hepatobiliary tree
- Also known as *ERCP*

PATIENT PREPARATION

- Make sure that the patient has signed an appropriate consent form.
- Note and report allergies.
- Inform the physician about the patient's hypersensitivity to iodine, seafood, or iodinated contrast media.
- Give the patient a sedative.
- Tell the patient to fast after midnight before the test.
- Explain the use of a local anesthetic spray to suppress the gag reflex and the use of a mouth guard to protect the teeth.
- Provide reassurance that oral insertion of the endoscope doesn't obstruct breathing and that the patient will remain conscious during the procedure.
- Explain that the test takes 1 to 1½ hours or longer if a procedure such as stent placement is performed.
- Explain that the patient may have a sore throat for 3 to 4 days after the examination.
- Explain that avoidance of alcohol and driving is necessary for 24 hours after the test.

PROCEDURE

- An I.V. infusion is started.
- The patient is given a local anesthetic and I.V. sedation.
- The patient's vital signs, cardiac rhythm, and pulse oximetry are continuously monitored.
- The patient is placed in a left lateral position.
- The endoscope is inserted into the mouth and advanced, using fluoroscopic guidance, into the stomach and duodenum.
- The patient is helped into the prone position.

- An I.V. anticholinergic or glucagon may be given to decrease GI motility.
- A cannula is passed through the biopsy channel of the endoscope, into the duodenal papilla, and into the ampulla of Vater; contrast medium is injected.
- The pancreatic duct and hepatobiliary tree become visible.
- Rapid-sequence X-rays are taken after each contrast injection.
- A tissue specimen or fluid may be aspirated for histologic and cytologic examination.
- Therapeutic measures (sphincterectomy, stent placement, stone removal, or balloon dilatation) may be performed before endoscope withdrawal, as indicated.
- After the films are reviewed, the cannula is removed.

POSTPROCEDURE CARE

- Withhold food and fluids until the gag reflex returns; then have the patient resume his usual diet.
- Provide soothing lozenges and warm saline gargles for sore throat.
- Monitor the patient's vital signs, cardiac rhythm, and pulse oximetry.
- Observe the patient's level of consciousness.
- Monitor the patient for abdominal distention and bowel sounds.
- Watch for adverse drug reactions.
- Emergency resuscitation equipment and a benzodiazepine and opioid antagonist should be immediately available during and after the test.
- Monitor the patient for possible complications, including ascending cholangitis, pancreatitis, adverse drug reactions, cardiac arrhythmias, bowel perforation, respiratory depression, and urine retention.

NORMAL RESULTS

- Duodenal papilla appearing as a small red or pale erosion protruding into the lumen
- Pancreatic and hepatobiliary ducts usually joining and emptying through the duodenal papilla; separate orifices sometimes present
- Contrast medium uniformly filling the pancreatic duct, hepatobiliary tree, and gallbladder

ABNORMAL RESULTS

- Hepatobiliary tree filling defects, strictures, or irregular deviations suggesting biliary cirrhosis, primary sclerosing cholangitis, calculi, or cancer of the bile ducts

- Filling defects, strictures, and irregular deviations of the pancreatic duct suggesting pancreatic cysts and pseudocysts, pancreatic tumors, chronic pancreatitis, pancreatic fibrosis, calculi, or papillary stenosis

Endoscopy

PURPOSE

- To transmit light into the viscus through a cablelike cluster of glass fibers in the endoscope; the image then returns to the scope's optical head or video monitor, which shows the lining of a hollow viscus
- To diagnose inflammatory, ulcerative, and infectious diseases
- To diagnose benign and malignant tumors and other lesions of the mucosa

PATIENT PREPARATION

- Make sure that the patient has signed an appropriate consent form.
- Note and report drug allergies.
- Explain that the study takes about 1 hour.
- Give the patient an I.V. sedative to help him relax before the endoscope insertion.
- For a patient taking an anticoagulant, it may be necessary to adjust his dosage.
- For high-risk procedures, the patient should stop taking warfarin 3 to 5 days before the procedure; an appropriate drug, such as low-molecular-weight heparin, should be ordered.
- Stop aspirin or nonsteroidal anti-inflammatory drugs 3 to 7 days before the study.

PROCEDURE

- Provide I.V. access, if indicated.
- The patient's vital signs, pulse oximetry, and cardiac rhythm are monitored throughout the procedure.
- The procedure is followed for the specific endoscopy to be performed: arthroscopy, bronchoscopy, colonoscopy, colposcopy, cystourethroscopy, endoscopic retrograde cholangiopancreatography, esophagogastroduodenoscopy, hysteroscopy, laparoscopy, laryngoscopy, mediastinoscopy, proctosigmoidoscopy, sigmoidoscopy, or thoracoscopy.

POSTPROCEDURE CARE

- Provide a safe environment.
- Withhold food and fluids until the gag reflex returns, if indicated.
- Have the patient resume his usual diet.
- Monitor the patient's vital signs.
- Monitor the patient's respiratory and neurologic status.
- Monitor the patient's cardiac rhythm.
- Monitor the patient for possible complications, such as an adverse reaction to sedation, cardiac arrhythmias, respiratory depression, and bleeding.

NORMAL RESULTS

Varies with the specific endoscopy procedure

ABNORMAL RESULTS

Varies with the specific endoscopy procedure

Holter monitoring

PURPOSE

- To record heart activity continuously, as the patient follows his normal routine, usually for 24 hours
- Patient-activated monitor: worn for 5 to 7 days, to allow patient to manually initiate recording of heart activity when he experiences symptoms
- To detect cardiac arrhythmias
- To evaluate chest pain
- To evaluate the effectiveness of antiarrhythmic drug therapy
- To monitor pacemaker function
- To correlate symptoms and palpitations with actual cardiac events and patient activities
- To detect sporadic arrhythmias missed by an exercise or resting electrocardiogram (ECG)
- Also known as *ambulatory ECG* or *dynamic monitoring*

PATIENT PREPARATION

- Make sure that the patient has signed an appropriate consent form.
- Note and report allergies.
- Provide bathing instructions because some equipment must not get wet.
- Instruct the patient to avoid magnets, metal detectors, high-voltage areas, and electric blankets.

- Explain the importance of keeping a log of daily activities as well as emotional upsets, physical symptoms, and ingestion of medication.
- Explain how to mark the tape at the onset of symptoms, if applicable.
- Explain how to check the recorder to make sure that it's working properly.

PROCEDURE

- Electrodes are applied to the chest wall and securely attached to the leadwires and monitor.
- Placing electrodes over large muscles masses, such as the pectorals, is avoided to limit artifact.
- A new or fully charged battery is inserted in the recorder.
- A tape is inserted and the recorder is turned on.
- The electrode attachment circuit is tested by connecting the recorder to a standard ECG machine, noting artifact during normal patient movement.

POSTPROCEDURE CARE

- Remove all chest electrodes.
- Clean the electrode sites.
- Check for skin sensitivity to the electrodes.

NORMAL RESULTS

- No significant arrhythmias or ST-segment changes on ECG
- Changes in heart rate during various activities

ABNORMAL RESULTS

- Abnormalities in cardiac rate or rhythm suggesting serious symptomatic or asymptomatic arrhythmias
- ST-T wave changes coinciding with patient symptoms or increased patient activity and suggesting myocardial ischemia

Lumbar puncture

PURPOSE

- To sample cerebrospinal fluid (CSF) for qualitative analysis
- To measure CSF pressure
- To aid in the diagnosis of viral or bacterial meningitis, subarachnoid or intracranial hemorrhage, tumors and brain abscesses, or neurosyphilis and chronic central nervous system infections
- Also known as a *spinal tap*

PATIENT PREPARATION

- Make sure that the patient has signed an appropriate consent form.
- Note and report allergies.
- Inform the patient that he need not restrict food and fluids.
- Explain that the test takes at least 15 minutes.
- Explain that headache is the most common adverse effect.

PROCEDURE

- Position the patient on his side at the edge of the bed with his knees drawn up to his abdomen and his chin tucked against his chest (the fetal position); or position the patient sitting while leaning over a bedside table.
- If the patient is in a supine position, provide pillows to support the spine on a horizontal plane.
- The skin site is prepared and draped.
- A local anesthetic is injected.
- The spinal needle is inserted midline between the spinous processes of the vertebrae, usually between L3 and L4 or L4 and L5.
- The stylet is removed from the needle; CSF will drip out of the needle if properly positioned.
- A stopcock and manometer are attached to the needle to measure initial CSF pressure.
- Specimens are collected and placed in the appropriate containers.
- The needle is removed and a small sterile dressing is applied.
- An epidural blood patch may be placed after needle removal to decrease the risk of postprocedural headache.

   ALERT *During the procedure, observe the patient closely for signs of an adverse reaction, such as an elevated pulse rate, pallor, or clammy skin.*

POSTPROCEDURE CARE

- Keep the patient lying flat if indicated (some prescribers prefer early ambulation).
- Inform the patient that he can turn from side to side if his movement should be restricted.
- Encourage the patient to drink fluids and assist him as needed.
- Give an analgesic, such as caffeine sodium benzoate, if needed, for persistent headache.
- Monitor the patient's vital signs, neurologic status, and intake and output.
- Monitor the puncture site for redness, swelling, and drainage.

■ Monitor the patient for possible complications, such as an adverse reaction to the anesthetic, infection, meningitis, bleeding into the spinal canal, CSF leakage, cerebellar herniation, and medullary compression.

ALERT *In a patient with increased pressure, CSF should be removed with extreme caution because cerebellar herniation and medullary compression can result.*

NORMAL RESULTS

■ Pressure: 50 to 180 mm H_2O
■ Appearance of CSF: clear, colorless
■ Protein: 15 to 45 mg/dl
■ Gamma globulin: 3% to 12% of total protein
■ Glucose: 50 to 80 mg/dl (or about 60% of serum glucose level)
■ Cell count: 0 to 5 white blood cells; no red blood cells (RBCs)
■ Venereal Disease Research Laboratory (VDRL) test: nonreactive
■ Chloride: 118 to 130 mEq/L
■ Gram stain: showing no organisms

ABNORMAL RESULTS

■ Increased intracranial pressure (ICP), indicating tumor, hemorrhage, or edema caused by trauma
■ Decreased ICP, indicating spinal subarachnoid obstruction
■ Cloudy appearance, suggesting infection
■ Yellow or bloody appearance, suggesting intracranial hemorrhage or spinal cord obstruction
■ Brown or orange appearance, indicating increased protein levels or RBC breakdown
■ Increased protein level, suggesting tumor, trauma, diabetes mellitus, or blood in CSF
■ Decreased protein level, indicating rapid CSF production
■ Increased gamma globulin level, associated with demyelinating disease or Guillain-Barré syndrome
■ Increased glucose level, suggesting hyperglycemia
■ Decreased glucose level, which could result from hypoglycemia, infection, or meningitis
■ Increased cell count, indicating meningitis, tumor, abscess, or demyelinating disease
■ The presence of RBCs from hemorrhage or traumatic entry
■ A positive VDRL test result, indicating neurosyphilis
■ Decreased chloride level, pointing to infected meninges
■ Gram-positive or gram-negative organisms, indicating bacterial meningitis

Lung perfusion scan

PURPOSE

- To produce a visual image of pulmonary blood flow after I.V. injection of a radiopharmaceutical
- To assess arterial perfusion of the lungs
- To detect pulmonary emboli
- To evaluate pulmonary function

PATIENT PREPARATION

- Make sure that the patient has signed an appropriate consent form.
- Note and report allergies.
- Tell the patient that he need not restrict food and fluids before the test.
- Stress the importance of lying still during imaging.
- Explain that the test takes about 30 minutes.
- Explain that the amount of radioactivity is minimal.

PROCEDURE

- The patient is assisted into the supine position on a nuclear medicine table.
- The radiopharmaceutical is injected I.V.
- A gamma camera takes a series of images in various views.
- Images projected on an oscilloscope screen show the distribution of radioactive particles.

POSTPROCEDURE CARE

- Monitor the injection site for a hematoma and apply warm soaks if one develops.
- Monitor the patient for sensitivity to the radiopharmaceutical.

NORMAL RESULTS

- Hot spots (areas of high uptake) indicating normal blood perfusion
- Uniform uptake pattern

ABNORMAL RESULTS

- Cold spots (areas of low uptake) indicating poor perfusion and possibly an embolism
- Decreased regional blood flow, without vessel obstruction, suggesting pneumonitis

Lung ventilation scan

PURPOSE

- To differentiate areas of ventilated lung from areas of underventilated lung
- To diagnose pulmonary emboli when used in combination with a lung perfusion scan
- To identify areas of the lung that are capable of ventilation
- To evaluate regional respiratory function
- To locate regional hypoventilation

PATIENT PREPARATION

- Make sure that the patient has signed an appropriate consent form.
- Note and report allergies.
- Tell the patient that he need not restrict food and fluids.
- Stress the importance of lying still during imaging.
- Tell the patient that he will wear a tight-fitting mask during the study.
- Explain that the test takes 15 to 30 minutes.

PROCEDURE

- The patient is assisted into the supine position on a nuclear medicine table.
- A tight-fitting mask is applied, covering the patient's nose and mouth.
- The patient inhales air mixed with a small amount of radioactive gas through the tightly fitted mask.
- Distribution of the gas in the lungs is monitored on a nuclear scanner.
- The patient's chest is scanned as the gas is exhaled.

POSTPROCEDURE CARE

- Reinstate oxygen therapy as appropriate.
- Monitor the patient's vital signs and respiratory status.
- Monitor the patient for panic attacks from wearing the tight-fitting mask.

NORMAL RESULTS

- Gas equally distributed in both lungs (see *Comparing normal and abnormal ventilation scans,* page 464)

ABNORMAL RESULTS

- Gas distributed unequally in both lungs, suggesting poor ventilation or airway obstruction in areas with low radioactivity

COMPARING NORMAL AND ABNORMAL VENTILATION SCANS

The normal ventilation scan on the left, taken 30 minutes to 1 hour after the wash-out phase, shows equal gas distribution. The abnormal scan on the right, taken 1½ to 2 hours after the start of the wash-out phase, shows unequal gas distribution, represented by the area of poor wash-out on the left and right sides.

NORMAL SCAN

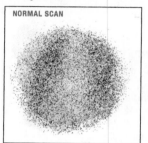

ABNORMAL SCAN

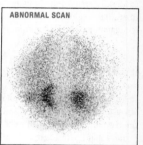

- When performed with a lung perfusion scan, vascular obstruction with normal ventilation, suggesting decreased perfusion such as in pulmonary embolism
- Ventilation and perfusion abnormalities, suggesting parenchymal disease

Magnetic resonance imaging

PURPOSE

- To produce computerized images of internal organs and tissues by using a powerful magnetic field and radiofrequency waves
- To obtain images of internal organs and tissues not readily visible on standard X-rays
- To obtain images of internal organs and tissues without harming cells and eliminating the other risks associated with exposure to X-ray beams
- Also known as *MRI*

PATIENT PREPARATION

- Patients that need life-support equipment, including ventilators, require special preparation; contact MRI staff ahead of time.

■ Make sure that the patient has signed an appropriate consent form.
■ Note and report allergies.
■ A claustrophobic patient may require sedation or an open MRI to reduce anxiety. (See *Open MRI: A better choice for claustrophobes.*)
■ Instruct the patient to remove metal objects he's wearing or carrying.
■ Advise the patient that he'll be asked to remain still during the procedure.
■ Warn the patient that the machine makes loud clacking sounds.
■ Explain that the test takes about 30 to 90 minutes.
■ Tell the patient that he need not restrict food and fluids.

PROCEDURE

■ If the patient is to receive a contrast medium, an I.V. line is started and the medium is administered before the procedure.
■ The patient is checked for metal objects at the scanner room door.
■ The patient is placed in the supine position on a padded scanning table.
■ The table is positioned in the opening of the scanning gantry.
■ A call bell or intercom is used to maintain verbal contact.
■ The patient may wear earplugs if needed.
■ Varying radiofrequency waves are directed at the area being scanned.
■ A computer reconstructs information as images on a television screen.

POSTPROCEDURE CARE

■ Tell the patient to resume his normal diet and activities unless otherwise indicated.
■ Monitor the patient's vital signs.
■ Watch for orthostatic hypotension.

OPEN MRI: A BETTER CHOICE FOR CLAUSTROPHOBES

With an open magnetic resonance imaging (MRI) unit, the patient isn't completely enclosed in a tunnel. This is ideal for a patient with claustrophobia. Open MRI units are low-field units (0.2 to 0.5 Tesla), whereas closed MRI units are typically high-field units (1.0 to 1.5 Tesla or greater).

But not ideal

Image quality is almost always better in a high-field unit because of field strength, gradient speed and strength, surface coils, and software. Also, accurate diagnosis may be difficult unless the interpreting radiologist has experience reading low-field units.

NORMAL RESULTS

- Varies with the specific type of MRI

ABNORMAL RESULTS

- Varies with the specific type of MRI
- Metal objects, such as I.V. pumps, ventilators, other metallic equipment, or computer-based equipment, in the MRI area interfering with test results

Mammography

PURPOSE

- To screen for malignant breast tumors
- To detect breast cysts or tumors, especially those not palpable on physical examination
- To investigate breast masses, breast pain, or nipple discharge
- To differentiate between benign breast disease and malignant tumors
- To be never substituted for biopsy; mammography may not reveal all cancers and may produce many false-positive results
- To monitor patients with breast cancer who are treated with breast-conserving surgery and radiation

PATIENT PREPARATION

- When scheduling the test, inform the staff if the patient has breast implants.
- Make sure that the patient has signed an appropriate consent form.
- Note and report allergies.
- Instruct the patient to avoid using underarm deodorant or powder the day of the examination.
- Explain that the test takes about 15 minutes.
- Explain to the patient that she may be asked to wait while the films are checked.

PROCEDURE

- The patient rests one breast on a table above the X-ray cassette.
- The compressor is placed on the breast.
- The patient holds her breath until the X-ray is taken and she's told to breathe again.
- An X-ray of the craniocaudal view is taken.

- The machine is rotated, and the breast is compressed again.
- An X-ray of the lateral view is taken.
- The procedure is repeated for the other breast.
- The film is developed and checked for quality.

POSTPROCEDURE CARE

- Answer the patient's questions about the test.

NORMAL RESULTS

- Normal ducts, glandular tissue, and fat architecture revealed
- No abnormal masses or calcifications present

ABNORMAL RESULTS

- Irregular, poorly outlined, opaque areas suggesting a malignant tumor, especially if solitary and unilateral
- Well-outlined, regular, clear spots possibly benign, especially if bilateral

Nuclear medicine scans

PURPOSE

- To provide imaging of specific body organs or systems by a scintillating scanning camera after I.V. injection, inhalation, or oral ingestion of a radioactive tracer compound
- To produce tissue analysis and images not readily seen on standard X-rays
- To detect or rule out malignant lesions when X-ray findings are normal or questionable

PATIENT PREPARATION

- Make sure that the patient has signed an appropriate consent form.
- Note and report allergies.
- Note if the patient has had previous nuclear medicine procedures.
- Make sure that the patient isn't scheduled for more than one radionuclide scan on the same day.
- Advise the patient that he'll be asked to take various positions on a scanner table.
- Stress the importance that the patient remain still during the procedure.
- Explain that the study takes about 1½ hours, but the time varies depending on the specific nuclear medicine scan.

PROCEDURE

- If the patient will receive an I.V. tracer isotope, an I.V. line is started.
- The detector of a scintillation camera is directed at the area being scanned and displays the image on a monitor.
- Scintigraphs are obtained and reviewed for clarity.
- If necessary, additional views are obtained.

POSTPROCEDURE CARE

- Tell the patient to resume his normal diet and activities.
- Monitor the patient's vital signs.
- Observe the injection site.
- Watch the patient for infection and orthostatic hypotension.

NORMAL RESULTS

- Varies with the specific nuclear medicine scan

ABNORMAL RESULTS

- Varies with the specific nuclear medicine scan

Paracentesis

PURPOSE

- To obtain samples of ascitic fluid for diagnostic and therapeutic purposes by insertion of a trocar and cannula through the abdominal wall
- In four-quadrant tap, to aspirate fluid from each quadrant of the abdomen to verify abdominal trauma and the need for surgery
- In peritoneal fluid analysis, to assess gross appearance, red blood cell (RBC) and white blood cell (WBC) counts, cytologic studies, microbiological studies for bacteria and fungi, and determinations of protein, glucose, amylase, ammonia, and alkaline phosphatase levels
- To determine the cause of ascites
- To detect abdominal trauma
- To remove accumulated ascitic fluid

PATIENT PREPARATION

- Make sure that the patient has signed an appropriate consent form.
- Note and report allergies, use of nonsteroidal anti-inflammatory drugs or anticoagulants, and possibility of pregnancy.
- Tell the patient that he need not restrict food and fluids.
- Inform the patient that he'll receive a local anesthetic.

- If the patient has severe ascites, inform him that the procedure will relieve his discomfort and allow him to breathe easier.
- Explain that a blood sample may be taken for analysis.
- Explain that the test takes 45 to 60 minutes.
- Have the patient empty his bladder just before the procedure.

PROCEDURE

- Obtain the patient's baseline vital signs, weight, and abdominal girth measurement.
- Assist the patient onto a bed or chair.
- If the patient can't tolerate being out of bed, assist him into high Fowler's position.
- Prepare and drape the puncture site.
- Local anesthetic is injected.
- The needle or trocar and cannula are inserted, usually 1″ to 2″ (2.5 to 5 cm) below the umbilicus, or in each quadrant of the abdomen.
- Fluid samples are aspirated; additional fluid may be drained.
- Specimens are placed in appropriately labeled containers.
- The trocar or needle is removed and a dressing is applied.

POSTPROCEDURE CARE

- Instruct the patient to resume his previous activity.
- Give I.V. infusions and albumin.
- Monitor the patient's vital signs and intake and output.
- Observe the puncture site and drainage for bleeding and infection.
- Measure the patient's weight and abdominal girth daily.
- Observe the patient for hematuria, which may indicate bladder trauma.
- Monitor serum electrolyte (especially sodium) and protein levels.
- If a large amount of fluid was removed, watch for signs of vascular collapse (tachycardia, tachypnea, hypotension, dizziness, and mental status changes).
- Watch the patient for signs and symptoms of hemorrhage and shock and for increasing pain and abdominal tenderness. These may indicate a perforated intestine or, depending on the site of the tap, puncture of the inferior epigastric artery, hematoma of the anterior cecal wall, or rupture of the iliac vein or bladder.
- Observe the patient with severe liver disease for signs of hepatic coma, which may result from a loss of sodium and potassium accompanying hypovolemia. Watch for mental status changes, drowsiness, and stupor. Such a patient is also prone to uremia, infection, hemorrhage, and protein depletion.

■ Monitor the patient for possible complications, such as hemorrhage, infection, bladder trauma, shock, a perforated intestine, inferior epigastric artery puncture, anterior cecal wall hematoma, and iliac vein rupture.

NORMAL RESULTS

■ Fluid that's odorless, clear to pale yellow

ABNORMAL RESULTS

■ Milk-colored fluid indicating chylous ascites
■ Bloody fluid indicating a benign or malignant tumor, hemorrhagic pancreatitis, a perforated intestine, or a duodenal ulcer
■ Cloudy or turbid fluid suggesting peritonitis or an infectious process
■ RBC count greater than 100/µl suggesting neoplasm or tuberculosis
■ RBC count greater than 100,000/µl suggesting intra-abdominal trauma
■ WBC count greater than 300/µl, with more than 25% neutrophils, suggesting spontaneous bacterial peritonitis or cirrhosis
■ A high percentage of lymphocytes suggesting tuberculous peritonitis or chylous ascites
■ A protein ascitic fluid–serum ratio of 0.5 or greater and a lactate dehydrogenase (LD) ascitic fluid–serum ratio greater than 0.6, suggesting malignant, tuberculous, or pancreatic ascites
■ Albumin gradient between ascitic fluid and serum greater than 1 g/dl indicating chronic liver disease
■ Gram-positive cocci commonly indicating primary peritonitis; gram-negative organisms indicating secondary peritonitis
■ Fungi indicating histoplasmosis, candidiasis, or coccidioidomycosis

Pulmonary function tests

PURPOSE

■ To evaluate pulmonary function through a series of spirometric measurements
■ To assess the effectiveness of a specific therapeutic regimen
■ To evaluate the patient's pulmonary status
■ Also known as *PFTs*

ALERT PFTs may be contraindicated in patients with acute coronary insufficiency, angina, or recent myocardial infarction (MI). Watch for respiratory distress, changes in pulse rate and blood pressure, coughing, and bronchospasm in these patients.

PATIENT PREPARATION

- Make sure that the patient has signed an appropriate consent form.
- Note and report allergies.
- Withhold bronchodilators for 8 hours.
- Stress the need for the patient to avoid smoking for 12 hours before the tests.
- Stress the need to avoid a heavy meal before the tests.

PROCEDURE

- For tidal volume (V_T), the patient breathes normally into the mouthpiece 10 times.
- For expiratory reserve volume (ERV), the patient breathes normally for several breaths and then exhales as completely as possible.
- For vital capacity (VC), the patient inhales as deeply as possible and exhales into the mouthpiece as completely as possible. This is repeated three times, and the largest volume is recorded.
- For inspiratory capacity (IC), the patient breathes normally for several breaths and inhales as deeply as possible.
- For functional residual capacity (FRC), the patient breathes normally into a spirometer. After a few breaths, the levels of gas in the spirometer and in the lungs reach equilibrium. The FRC is calculated by subtracting the spirometer volume from the original volume.
- For forced vital capacity (FVC) and forced expiratory volume (FEV), the patient inhales as slowly and deeply as possible and then exhales into the mouthpiece as quickly and completely as possible. This is repeated three times, and the largest volume is recorded. The volume of air expired at 1 second (FEV_1), at 2 seconds (FEV_2), and at 3 seconds (FEV_3) during all three repetitions is recorded.
- For maximal voluntary ventilation, the patient breathes into the mouthpiece as quickly and deeply as possible for 15 seconds.
- For diffusing capacity for carbon monoxide, the patient inhales a gas mixture with a low level of carbon monoxide and holds his breath for 10 to 15 seconds before exhaling.

POSTPROCEDURE CARE

- Resume regular medications.

NORMAL RESULTS

- Results based on age, height, weight, and sex; values expressed as a percentage

- V_T: 5 to 7 mg/kg of body weight
- ERV: 25% of VC
- IC: 75% of VC
- FEV_1: 83% of VC after 1 second
- FEV_2: 94% of VC after 2 seconds
- FEV_3: 97% of VC after 3 seconds

ABNORMAL RESULTS

- FEV_1 less than 80%, suggesting obstructive pulmonary disease
- FEV_1 to FVC ratio greater than 80% suggesting restrictive pulmonary disease
- Decreased V_T suggesting restrictive disease
- Decreased minute volume (MV) suggesting disorders such as pulmonary edema
- Increased MV suggesting acidosis, exercise, or low compliance states
- Reduced carbon dioxide response suggesting emphysema, myxedema, obesity, hypoventilation syndrome, or sleep apnea
- Residual volume greater than 35% of total lung capacity after maximal expiratory effort suggesting obstructive disease
- Decreased IC suggesting restrictive disease
- Increased FRC suggesting obstructive pulmonary disease
- Low total lung capacity (TLC) suggesting restrictive disease
- High TLC suggesting obstructive disease
- Decreased FVC suggesting flow resistance from obstructive or restrictive disease
- Low forced expiratory flow suggesting obstructive disease of the small and medium-sized airways
- Decreased peak expiratory flow rate suggesting upper airway obstruction
- Decreased diffusing capacity for carbon monoxide suggesting possible interstitial pulmonary disease

Thallium imaging

PURPOSE

- To evaluate myocardial blood flow after I.V. injection of the radioisotope thallium-201 or Cardiolyte
- Also known as *cardiac nuclear imaging*, *cold spot myocardial imaging*, or *myocardial perfusion scan*

Cardiolyte

■ To allow for imaging myocardial blood flow before and after reperfusion
■ To assess myocardial perfusion
■ To demonstrate the location and extent of a myocardial infarction (MI)
■ To diagnose coronary artery disease (CAD) (stress imaging)
■ To evaluate coronary artery patency following surgical revascularization
■ To evaluate the effectiveness of antianginal therapy or percutaneous revascularization interventions (stress imaging)

Thallium

■ Concentrates in healthy myocardial tissue but not in necrotic or ischemic tissue: Taken up rapidly in areas of the heart with a normal blood supply and intact cells; fails to be taken up by areas with poor blood flow and ischemic cells, which appear as cold spots on a scan

Rest imaging

■ Can disclose an acute MI within the first few hours of symptoms but doesn't distinguish an old from a new infarct

Stress imaging

■ Performed after exercise stress testing or after pharmacologic stress testing; used to assess known or suspected CAD

PATIENT PREPARATION

■ Make sure that the patient has signed an appropriate consent form.
■ Note and report allergies.
■ For stress imaging: Instruct the patient to wear comfortable walking shoes during the treadmill exercise.
■ Inform the patient that he must restrict his use of alcohol, tobacco, and nonprescription medications for 24 hours before the test.
■ Tell the patient to fast after midnight the night before the test.
■ Tell the patient to report fatigue, pain, shortness of breath, or other anginal symptoms immediately.

PROCEDURE

■ Stress imaging: The patient walks on a treadmill at a regulated pace that's gradually increased while his electrocardiogram (ECG), blood pressure, and heart rate are monitored.
■ When the patient reaches peak stress, give him 1.5 to 3 mCi of thallium.
■ The patient exercises an additional 45 to 60 seconds to permit circulation and uptake of the isotope.

ALERT *Stop the stress imaging immediately if the patient develops chest pain, dyspnea, fatigue, syncope, hypotension, ischemic ECG changes, significant arrhythmias, or other critical signs and symptoms (confusion, staggering, or pale, clammy skin).*

■ Disconnect the patient from monitoring equipment as long as he's clinically stable, and position him on his back under the nuclear medicine camera.
■ Additional scans may be taken after the patient rests and occasionally after 24 hours.
■ Scanning after rest is helpful in differentiating between an ischemic area and an infarcted or scarred area of the myocardium.
■ Resting imaging: The patient is given an injection of thallium I.V. or Cardiolyte.
■ Scanning is performed as in stress imaging.

POSTPROCEDURE CARE

■ If further scanning is required, have the patient rest and restrict foods and beverages other than water.
■ Monitor the patient's vital signs and ECG.
■ Monitor the patient for possible complications, such as cardiac arrhythmias, myocardial ischemia, respiratory distress, cardiac arrest, and hypotension or hypertension.

NORMAL RESULTS

■ Normal distribution of the isotope throughout the myocardium without defects (cold spots)
■ After coronary artery bypass surgery, improved regional perfusion, suggesting graft patency
■ Improved perfusion after nonsurgical revascularization interventions, suggesting increased coronary flow

ABNORMAL RESULTS

■ Persistent defects suggesting MI
■ Transient defects (those that disappear after a 3- to 6-hour rest) suggesting myocardial ischemia caused by CAD

Part five

Clinical tools

Abdominal quadrants

Right upper quadrant
- Right lobe of the liver
- Gallbladder
- Pylorus
- Duodenum
- Head of the pancreas
- Hepatic flexure of the colon
- Portions of the transverse and ascending colon

Left upper quadrant
- Left lobe of the liver
- Stomach
- Body of the pancreas
- Spleen
- Splenic flexure of the colon
- Portions of the transverse and descending colon

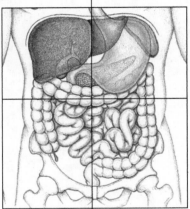

Right lower quadrant
- Cecum and appendix
- Portion of the ascending colon
- Portion of the small intestine

Left lower quadrant
- Sigmoid colon
- Portion of the descending colon
- Portion of the small intestine

Antidotes to drug or toxin overdoses

Drug or toxin	Antidote
Acetaminophen	Acetylcysteine (Mucomyst)
Anticholinergics	Physostigmine (Antilirium)
Benzodiazepines	Flumazenil (Romazicon)
Calcium channel blockers	Calcium chloride
Cyanide	Amyl nitrate, sodium nitrite, and sodium thiosulfate (Cyanide Antidote Kit); methylene blue
Digoxin, cardiac glycosides	Digoxin immune Fab (Digibind)
Ethylene glycol	Ethanol
Heparin	Protamine sulfate
Insulin-induced hypoglycemia	Glucagon
Iron	Deferoxamine mesylate (Desferal)
Lead	Edetate calcium disodium (Calcium Disodium Versenate)
Opioids	Naloxone (Narcan), nalmefene (Revex), naltrexone (ReVia)
Organophosphates, anticholinesterases	Atropine, pralidoxime (Protopam)
Warfarin	Vitamin K

Arterial blood gas results

Disorder	ABG findings	Possible causes
Respiratory acidosis (excess CO_2 retention)	■ pH < 7.35 ■ HCO_3^- > 26 mEq/L (if compensating) ■ $Paco_2$ > 45 mm Hg	■ Central nervous system depression from drugs, injury, or disease ■ Hypoventilation from respiratory, cardiac, musculoskeletal, or neuromuscular disease
Respiratory alkalosis (excess CO_2 loss)	■ pH > 7.45 ■ HCO_3^- < 22 mEq/L (if compensating) ■ $Paco_2$ < 35 mm Hg	■ Hyperventilation due to anxiety, pain, or improper ventilator settings ■ Respiratory stimulation from drugs, disease, hypoxia, fever, or high room temperature ■ Gram-negative bacteremia
Metabolic acidosis (HCO_3^- loss or acid retention)	■ pH < 7.35 ■ HCO_3^- < 22 mEq/L ■ $Paco_2$ < 35 mm Hg (if compensating)	■ Depletion of HCO_3^- from renal disease, diarrhea, or small-bowel fistulas ■ Excessive production of organic acids from hepatic disease, endocrine disorders such as diabetes mellitus, hypoxia, shock, or drug toxicity ■ Inadequate excretion of acids due to renal disease
Metabolic alkalosis (HCO_3^- retention or acid loss)	■ pH > 7.45 ■ HCO_3^- > 26 mEq/L ■ $Paco_2$ > 45 mm Hg (if compensating)	■ Loss of hydrochloric acid from prolonged vomiting or gastric suctioning ■ Loss of potassium from increased renal excretion (as in diuretic therapy) or corticosteroid overdose ■ Excessive alkali ingestion

Arterial blood gas results in respiratory acidosis

This table shows typical arterial blood gas findings in uncompensated and compensated respiratory acidosis.

	Uncompensated	Compensated
pH	< 7.35	Normal
$Paco_2$ (mm H)	> 45	> 45
HCO_3^- (mEq/L)	Normal	> 26

Arterial blood gas results in respiratory alkalosis

This table shows typical arterial blood gas findings in uncompensated and compensated respiratory alkalosis.

	Uncompensated	Compensated
pH	> 7.45	Normal
$Paco_2$ (mm H)	< 35	< 35
HCO_3^- (mEq/L)	Normal	< 22

Bioterrorism agents

Listed below are potentially threatening biological (bacterial and viral) agents as well as treatments and vaccines currently available.

Implement standard precautions for all cases of suspected exposure. For cases of smallpox, institute airborne precautions for the duration of the illness and until all scabs fall off. For pneumonic plague cases, institute droplet precautions for 72 hours after initiation of effective therapy.

Biological agent (condition)	Signs and symptoms	Treatment
Bacillus anthracis (anthrax)	Abdominal pain, low blood pressure, chest pain, chills, cough, bloody diarrhea, dyspnea, fever, headache, hematemesis, lymphadenopathy, malaise, nausea, papular rash, stridor, vomiting, weakness	■ Ciprofloxacin, doxycycline, or amoxicillin ■ Vaccine: Limited supply available; not recommended in absence of exposure to anthrax
Clostridium botulinum (botulism)	Diplopia, dysarthria, dysphagia, dyspnea, ptosis, unsteady gait, symmetrical descending weakness, possible progression to flaccid paralysis and respiratory paralysis	■ Supportive: ET intubation and mechanical ventilation ■ Passive immunization with equine antitoxin to lessen nerve damage ■ Vaccine: Postexposure prophylaxis with equine botulinum antitoxin; botulinum toxoid available from CDC; recombinant vaccine under development
Francisella tularensis (tularemia)	Chest pain, chills, cough, dyspnea, fever, headache, myalgias, diarrhea, progressive weakness	■ Gentamicin or streptomycin; alternatively, doxycycline, chloramphenicol, or ciprofloxacin ■ Vaccine: Live, attenuated vaccine currently under investigation and review by the Food and Drug Administration (FDA)
Variola major (smallpox)	Abdominal pain, back pain, high fever, headache, malaise, rash that starts out papular and becomes vesicular and pustular	■ No FDA-approved antiviral available; cidofovir may be therapeutic if given 1 to 2 days after exposure ■ Vaccine: Prophylaxis within 3 to 4 days of exposure
Yersinia pestis (pneumonic plague)	Chest pain, chills, cough, dyspnea, fever, headache, hemoptysis, myalgias, tachypnea, nausea, vomiting; purpuric skin lesions and respiratory failure if advanced	■ Streptomycin or gentamicin; alternatively, doxycycline, or chloramphenicol ■ Vaccine: Under investigation

Blood and selected component transfusion

Blood component	Nursing considerations
Whole blood Complete (pure) blood Volume: 500 ml	■ Administer only with 0.9% saline solution. ■ Use a straight-line or Y-type I.V. set to infuse blood over 2 to 4 hours. ■ Monitor the patient for tolerance of the circulatory volume. ■ Add a microfilter to the administration set to remove platelets. ■ Warm blood if a large quantity is being given.
Packed red blood cells (RBCs) Same RBC mass as whole blood, but with 80% of the plasma removed Volume: 250 ml	■ Administer only with 0.9% saline solution. ■ Use a straight-line or Y-type I.V. set to infuse blood over 2 to 4 hours.
White blood cells (WBCs or leukocytes) Whole blood with all of the RBCs and about 80% of the supernatant plasma removed Volume: usually 150 ml	■ Use a straight-line I.V. set with a standard in-line blood filter to provide 1 unit daily for 5 days or until the infection resolves. ■ As prescribed, premedicate with diphenhydramine. ■ Administer an antipyretic if fever occurs. Don't discontinue the transfusion; instead, reduce the flow rate as ordered for patient comfort. ■ Agitate the container to prevent the WBCs from settling, thus preventing the delivery of a bolus infusion of WBCs.
Leukocyte-poor RBCs Same as packed RBCs, with about 95% of the leukocytes removed Volume: 200 ml	■ Use a straight-line or Y-type I.V. set to infuse blood over 1½ to 4 hours. ■ Use a 40-micron filter that's suitable for hard-spun, leukocyte-poor RBCs.
Platelets Platelet sediment whole blood Volume: 35 to 50 ml/unit; 1 unit of platelets = 7×10^7 platelets	■ Use a filtered component drip administration set to infuse 100 ml over 15 minutes. ■ As prescribed, premedicate with antipyretics and antihistamines if the patient's history includes a platelet transfusion reaction. ■ Avoid administering platelets when the patient has a fever. ■ Prepare to draw blood for a platelet count as ordered, 1 hour after the platelet transfusion.

(continued)

Blood component	Nursing considerations
Fresh frozen plasma (FFP) Uncoagulated plasma separated from RBCs and rich in coagulation factors V, VIII, and IX Volume: 200 to 250 ml	■ Use a straight-line I.V. set, and administer the infusion rapidly. ■ Keep in mind that large-volume transfusions of FFP may require correction for hypocalcemia because citric acid in FFP binds calcium. ■ Must be infused within 24 hours of being thawed.
Albumin 5% (buffered saline); albumin 25% (salt poor) A small plasma protein prepared by fractionating pooled plasma Volume: 5% = 12.5 g/250 ml; 25% = 12.5 g/50 ml	■ Use a straight-line I.V. set, with the rate and volume dictated by the patient's condition and response. ■ Reactions to albumin (fever, chills, nausea) are rare. ■ Avoid mixing albumin with protein hydrolysates and alcohol solutions. ■ Monitor for signs and symptoms of circulatory overload.
Factor VIII (concentrate) Recominant genetically engineered product, derivative obtained from plasma Volume: about 30 ml	■ Use the administration set supplied by the manufacturer and administer with a filter, or administer by I.V. injection.
Factors II, VII, IX, X complex (prothrombin complex) Lyophilized, commercially prepared solution drawn from pooled plasma	■ Administer with a straight-line I.V. set, basing the dose on the desired factor level and the patient's body weight. ■ Recognize that a high risk of hepatitis accompanies this type of transfusion. ■ Draw blood for a coagulation assay before administration and at ordered intervals during treatment.

Blood transfusion compatibility

		Compatible donors							
	(universal donor)	O-	O+	B-	B+	A-	A+	AB-	AB+
(universal recipient)	AB+	✔	✔	✔	✔	✔	✔	✔	✔
	AB-	✔		✔		✔		✔	
	A+	✔	✔			✔	✔		
	A-	✔				✔			
	B+	✔	✔	✔	✔				
	B-	✔		✔					
	O+	✔	✔						
	O-	✔							

Patient's ABO group

Body surface area estimation in adults

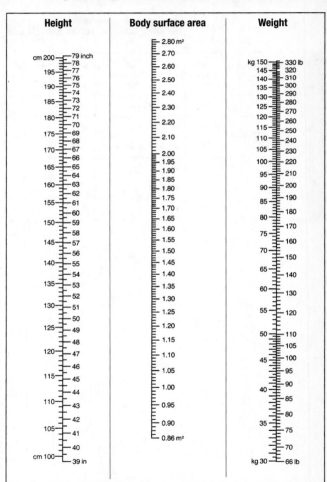

Burns classification and estimation

Burns are classified according to the depth of the injury, as follows:

- First-degree burns are limited to the epidermis. Sunburn is a typical first-degree burn. These burns are painful but self-limiting. They don't lead to scarring and require only local wound care.
- Second-degree burns extend into the dermis but leave some residual dermis viable. These burns are very painful and the skin will appear swollen and red with blister formation.
- Third-degree, or full-thickness, burns involve destruction of the entire dermis, leaving only subcutaneous tissue exposed. These burns look dry and leathery and are painless because the nerve endings are destroyed.
- Fourth-degree burns are a rare type of burn usually associated with lethal injury. They extend beyond the subcutaneous tissue, involving the muscle, fasciae, and bone. Occasionally termed transmural burns, these injuries are commonly associated with complete transection of an extremity.

RULE OF NINES

Use to estimate the extent of an adult patient's burns.

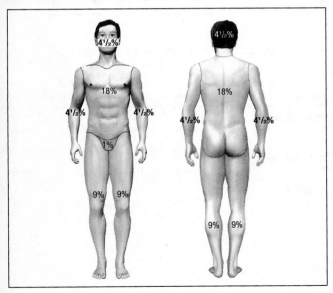

LUND AND BROWDER CHART

Use to estimate the extent of an infant's or a child's burns, or more accurately estimate an adult's burns.

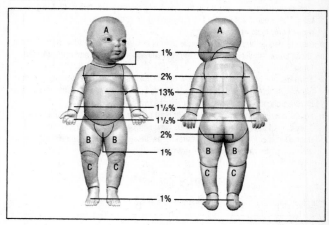

RELATIVE PERCENTAGES OF AREAS AFFECTED BY AGE

	At birth	0 to 1 yr	1 to 4 yr	5 to 9 yr	10 to 15 yr	Adult
A: Half of head	9½%	8½%	6½%	5½%	4½%	3½%
B: Half of thigh	2¾%	3¼%	4%	4¼%	4½%	4¾%
C: Half of leg	2½%	2½%	2¾%	3%	3¼%	3½%

Calcium disorders

CLINICAL EFFECTS OF HYPERCALCEMIA

Body system	Effects
Cardiovascular	■ Signs of heart block, cardiac arrest, hypertension
Gastrointestinal	■ Anorexia, nausea, vomiting, constipation, dehydration, polydipsia
Musculoskeletal	■ Weakness, muscle flaccidity, bone pain, pathologic fractures
Neurologic	■ Drowsiness, lethargy, headaches, depression or apathy, irritability, confusion
Other	■ Renal polyuria, flank pain and, eventually, azotemia

CLINICAL EFFECTS OF HYPOCALCEMIA

Body system	Effects
Cardiovascular	■ Arrhythmias, hypotension
Gastrointestinal	■ Increased GI motility, diarrhea
Musculoskeletal	■ Paresthesia, tetany or painful tonic muscle spasms, facial spasms, abdominal cramps, muscle cramps, spasmodic contractions
Neurologic	■ Anxiety, irritability, twitching around mouth, laryngospasm, seizures, Chvostek's sign, Trousseau's sign
Other	■ Blood-clotting abnormalities

Cardiac monitoring lead placement

Five-leadwire system

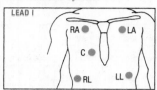
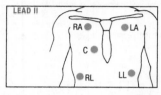
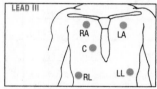
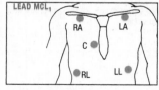
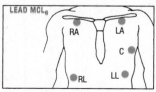

Three-leadwire system

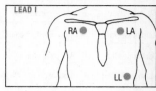
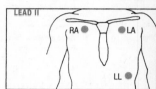
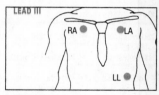
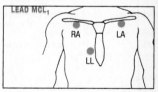
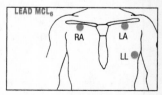

PRECORDIAL LEAD PLACEMENT FOR 12-LEAD ECG

To record the precordial chest leads, place the electrodes as follows:

V_1 . . .Fourth intercostal space (ICS), right sternal border
V_2 . . .Fourth ICS, left sternal border
V_3 . . .Midway between V_2 and V_4
V_4 . . .Fifth ICS, left midclavicular line
V_5 . . .Fifth ICS, left anterior axillary line
V_6 . . .Fifth ICS, left midaxillary line

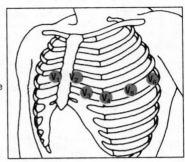

RIGHT PRECORDIAL LEAD PLACEMENT FOR 12-LEAD ECG

To record the right precordial chest leads, place the electrodes as follows:

V_1R . . .Fourth ICS, left sternal border
V_2R . . .Fourth ICS, right sternal border
V_3R . . .Halfway between V_2R and V_4R
V_4R . . .Fifth ICS, right midclavicular line
V_5R . . .Fifth ICS, right anterior axillary line
V_6R . . .Fifth ICS, right midaxillary line

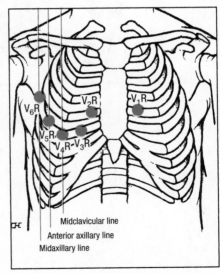

Midclavicular line
Anterior axillary line
Midaxillary line

POSTERIOR LEAD PLACEMENT

To ensure an accurate ECG reading, make sure the posterior electrodes V_7, V_8, and V_9 are placed at the same level horizontally as the V_6 lead at the fifth intercostal space. Place lead V_7 at the posterior axillary line, lead V_9 at the paraspinal line, and lead V_8 halfway between leads V_7 and V_9.

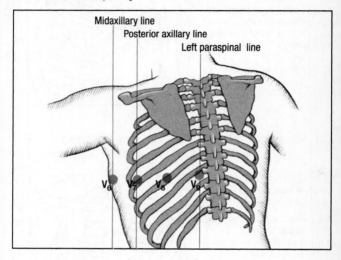

Cardiovascular system assessment

HEART SOUND SITES

When auscultating for heart sounds, place the stethoscope over the four sites circled below.

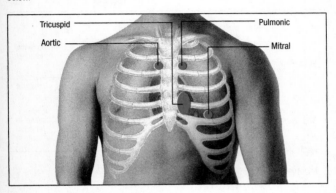

GRADING MURMURS

Use the system outlined below to describe the intensity of a murmur:

- Grade I is a barely audible murmur.
- Grade II is audible but quiet and soft.
- Grade III is moderately loud without a thrust or thrill.
- Grade IV is loud with a thrill.
- Grade V is very loud with a thrust or a thrill.
- Grade VI is loud enough to be heard before the stethoscope comes into contact with the chest.

When recording your findings, use Roman numerals as part of a fraction, always with VI as the denominator. For instance, a grade III murmur would be recorded as "grade III/VI."

Continuous bladder irrigation setup

In continuous bladder irrigation, a triple-lumen catheter allows irrigating solution to flow into the bladder through one lumen and flow out through another, as shown in the inset. The third lumen is used to inflate the balloon that holds the catheter in place.

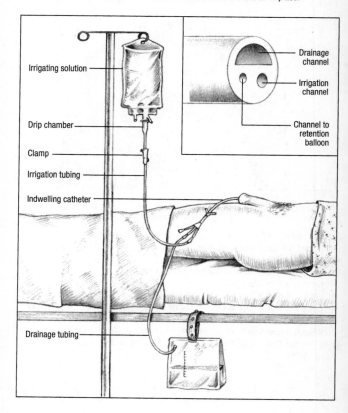

Defibrillator paddle placement

Here's a guide to correct paddle placement for defibrillation.

ANTEROLATERAL PLACEMENT

Place one paddle to the right of the upper sternum, just below the right clavicle, and the other over the fifth or sixth intercostal space at the left anterior axillary line.

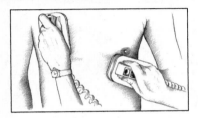

ANTEROPOSTERIOR PLACEMENT

Place the anterior paddle directly over the heart at the precordium, to the left of the lower sternal border. Place the flat posterior paddle under the patient's body beneath the heart and immediately below the scapula (but not under the vertebral column).

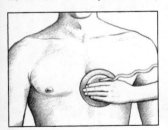 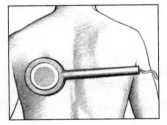

Diabetes: HHNS versus DKA

Hyperosmolar hyperglycemic nonketotic syndrome (HHNS) and diabetic ketoacidosis (DKA), both acute complications of diabetes, share some similarities, but they're two distinct conditions. Use this flowchart to help determine which condition your patient is experiencing.

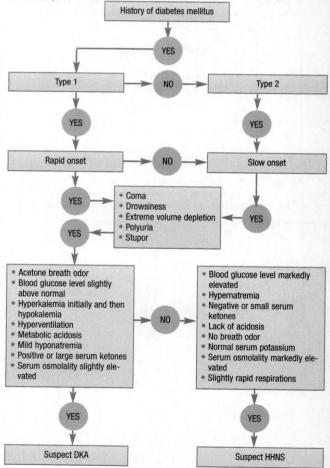

Dosage calculations

$$\text{Body surface area in } m^2 = \sqrt{\frac{\text{height in cm} \times \text{weight in kg}}{3,600}}$$

$$\text{mcg/ml} = \text{mg/ml} \times 1,000$$

$$\text{ml/minute} = \frac{\text{ml/hour}}{60}$$

$$\text{mg/minute} = \frac{\text{mg in bag}}{\text{ml in bag}} \times \text{flow rate} \div 60$$

$$\text{mcg/minute} = \frac{\text{mg in bag}}{\text{ml in bag}} \div 0.06 \times \text{flow rate}$$

$$\text{mcg/kg/minute} = \frac{\text{mcg/ml} \times \text{ml/minute}}{\text{weight in kg}}$$

Drip rate calculations

When calculating the flow rate of I.V. solutions, remember that the number of drops required to deliver 1 ml varies with the type of administration set you're using. To calculate the drip rate, you must know the drops per milliliter for each specific manufacturer's product. As a quick guide, refer to the chart below. Use this formula to calculate specific drip rates:

$$\frac{\text{infusion volume (in ml)}}{\text{time (in minutes)}} \times \text{drip factor (in drops/ml)} = \textbf{drops/minute}$$

Ordered volume

500 ml/24 hr or 21 ml/hr	1,000 ml/24 hr or 42 ml/hr	1,000 ml/20 hr or 50 ml/hr	1,000 ml/10 hr or 100 ml/hr	1,000 ml/6 hr or 166 ml/hr

Drops/ml	Drops/min to infuse				
Macrodrip					
10	3	7	8	17	28
15	5	11	13	25	42
20	7	14	17	34	56
Microdrip					
60	21	42	50	100	166

Drug administration safety guidelines

When administering a drug, be sure to adhere to set practices to avoid potential problems. You can help prevent drug mistakes by following these guidelines as well as your facility's policies.

DRUG ORDERS

- Don't rely on the pharmacy computer system to detect all unsafe orders. Before you give a drug understand the correct dosage, indications, and adverse effects. If necessary, check a current drug reference guide.
- Be aware of the drugs your patient takes regularly, and question any deviation from his regular routine. As with any drug, take your time and read the label carefully.
- Ask all prescribers to spell out drug names and any error-prone abbreviations.
- Before you give drugs that are ordered in units, such as insulin and heparin, always check the prescriber's written order against the provided dose. Never abbreviate the word "units."
- If you must accept a verbal order, have another nurse listen in; then transcribe that order directly into an order form and repeat it to the prescriber to ensure that you've transcribed it correctly.
- To prevent an acetaminophen overdose from combined analgesics, note the amount of acetaminophen in each drug. Beware of substitutions by the pharmacy because the amount of acetaminophen might vary.
- Keep in mind that lipid-based products have different dosages than their conventional counterparts. Check the prescriber's orders and labels carefully to avoid confusion.

DRUG PREPARATION

- If a familiar drug has an unfamiliar appearance, find out why. If the pharmacist cites a manufacturing change, ask him to double-check whether he has received verification from the manufacturer. Document the appearance discrepancy, your actions, and the pharmacist's response in the patient record.
- Obtain a new allergy history with each admission. If the patient's history must be faxed, name the drugs, note how many are included, and follow your facility's faxing safeguards. If the pharmacy also adheres to strict guidelines, the computer-generated medication administration record should be accurate.

GIVING DRUGS

- Use two patient identifiers, such as the patient's name and assigned medical record number, to identify the patient before administering drug or treatment. Teach the patient to offer his identification bracelet for inspection when anyone arrives with drugs and to insist on having it replaced if it's removed.
- Ask the patient about his use of over-the-counter and alternative therapies, including herbs, and record your findings in his medical record. Monitor the patient carefully and report unusual events. Ask the patient to keep a diary of all therapies he uses and to take the diary for review each time he visits a health care professional.

CALCULATION ERRORS

- Writing the mg/kg or mg/m² dose and the calculated dose provides a safeguard against calculation errors. Whenever a prescriber provides the calculation, double-check it and document that the dose was verified.
- Don't assume that liquid drugs are less likely to cause harm than other forms, including parenteral ones. Pediatric and geriatric patients commonly receive liquid drugs and may be especially sensitive to the effects of an inaccurate dose. If a unit-dose form isn't available, calculate carefully and double-check your math and the drug label.
- Leaving potentially dangerous chemicals near a patient is extremely risky, especially when the container labels don't indicate toxicity. To prevent problems, never leave drug containers near a patient.
- Read the label on every drug you prepare and never administer any drug that isn't labeled.

DOSAGE EQUATIONS

- After you calculate a drug dosage, always have another nurse calculate it independently to double-check your results. If doubts or questions remain or if the calculations don't match, ask a pharmacist to calculate the dose before you give the drug.

AIR BUBBLES IN PUMP TUBING

- To clear bubbles from I.V. tubing, never increase the pump's flow rate to flush the line. Instead, remove the tubing from the pump, disconnect it from the patient, and use the flow-control clamp to establish gravity flow.
- When the bubbles have been removed, return the tubing to the pump, restart the infusion, and recheck the flow rate.

INCORRECT ADMINISTRATION ROUTE

- When a patient has multiple I.V. lines, label the distal end of each line.
- Use of a parenteral syringe to prepare oral liquid drugs increases the chance for error because the syringe tip fits easily into I.V. ports. To safely give an oral drug through a feeding tube, use a dose prepared by the pharmacy and a syringe with the appropriate tip.

Drug pregnancy risk categories

Pregnancy risk categories were designed to alert prescribers to the risks associated with drugs administered during pregnancy. The categories include:

- **A:** Adequate studies in pregnant women have failed to show a risk to the fetus.
- **B:** Animal studies haven't shown a risk to the fetus, but controlled studies haven't been conducted in pregnant women; or animal studies have shown an adverse effect on the fetus, but adequate studies in pregnant women have not shown a risk to the fetus.
- **C:** Animal studies have shown an adverse effect on the fetus, but adequate studies haven't been conducted in humans. The benefits from use in pregnant women may be acceptable despite potential risks.
- **D:** The drug may cause risk to the fetus, but the potential benefits of use in pregnant women may be acceptable despite the risks (such as in life-threatening situations or serious disease for which safer drugs can't be used or are ineffective).
- **X:** Studies in animals and humans show fetal abnormalities, or adverse reaction reports indicate evidence of fetal risk. The risks involved clearly outweigh potential benefits.
- **NR:** Not rated.

ECG rhythm strips

NORMAL SINUS RHYTHM

Normal sinus rhythm, shown below, represents normal impulse conduction through the heart.

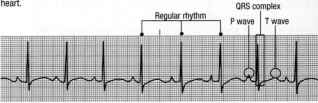

Lead II
- Atrial and ventricular rhythms regular
- Atrial and ventricular rates 60 to 100 beats/minute (80 beats/minute shown)
- Normal P wave preceding each QRS complex
- Normal PR interval (0.12 to 0.20 second)
- QRS complex within normal limits (0.06 to 0.10 second)
- T wave normally shaped (upright and rounded); follows each QRS complex
- QT interval within normal limits and constant (0.36 to 0.44 second)

SINUS BRADYCARDIA

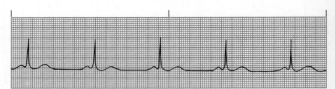

Rhythm . . . . regular
Rate . . . . < 60 beats/minute
P wave . . . . Normal
PR interval . . . . . . 0.12 to 0.20 second
QRS complex . . . . . 0.06 to 0.10 second

SINUS TACHYCARDIA

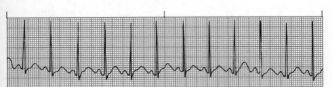

Rhythm . . . . regular
Rate . . . . 100 to 160 beats/minute
P wave . . . . normal
PR interval . . . . 0.12 to 0.20 second
QRS complex . . . . . 0.06 to 0.10 second

PREMATURE ATRIAL CONTRACTIONS (PACs)

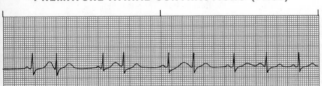

Rhythm . . . . irregular
Rate . . . . varies with underlying rhythm
P wave . . . . premature and abnormally shaped with premature atrial contractions
PR interval . . . . usually within normal limits, but varies depending on ectopic focus
QRS complex . . . . . 0.06 to 0.10 second

ATRIAL TACHYCARDIA

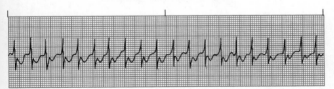

Rhythm . . . . regular
Rate . . . . 150 to 250 beats/minute; ventricular rate depends on atrioventricular
                         conduction rates
P wave . . . . hidden in the preceding T wave
PR interval . . . . not visible
QRS complex . . . . . 0.06 to 0.10 second

ATRIAL FLUTTER

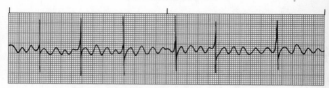

Rhythm . . . . atrial—regular; ventricular—typically irregular
Rate . . . . atrial—250 to 400 beats/minute; ventricular—usually 60 to
                        100 beats/minute; ventricular rate depends on degree of atrio-
                        ventricular block
P wave . . . . classic saw tooth appearance
PR interval . . . . . . unmeasurable
QRS complex . . . . . 0.06 to 0.10 second

ATRIAL FIBRILLATION

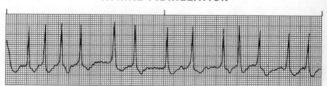

Rhythm . . . . irregularly irregular
Rate . . . . atrial—usually > 400 beats/minute; ventricular—varies
P wave . . . . absent; replaced by fine fibrillatory waves, or f waves
PR interval . . . . . . indiscernible
QRS complex . . . . . 0.06 to 0.10 second

PREMATURE JUNCTIONAL CONTRACTIONS (PJCs)

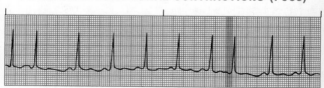

Rhythm . . . . irregular atrial and ventricular rhythms during PJCs
Rate . . . . reflects the underlying rhythm
P wave . . . . usually inverted and may occur before or after or be hidden within the
                        QRS complex (see shaded area)
PR interval . . . . . . < 0.12 second if P wave precedes QRS complex; otherwise unmeasurable
QRS complex . . . . . 0.06 to 0.10 second

JUNCTIONAL ESCAPE RHYTHM

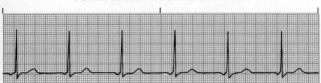

Rhythm . . . . regular
Rate . . . . 40 to 60 beats/minute
P wave . . . . usually inverted and may occur before or after or be hidden within QRS
complex
PR interval . . . . < 0.12 second if P wave precedes QRS complex; otherwise unmeasurable
QRS complex . . . . . 0.06 to 0.10 second

ACCELERATED JUNCTIONAL RHYTHM

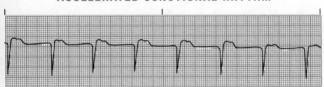

Rhythm . . . . regular
Rate . . . . 60 to 100 beats/minute
P wave . . . . usually inverted and may occur before or after or be hidden within QRS
complex
PR interval . . . . < 0.12 second if P wave precedes QRS complex; otherwise unmeasurable
QRS complex . . . . . 0.06 to 0.10 second

PREMATURE VENTRICULAR CONTRACTIONS (PVCs)

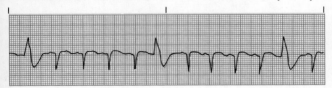

Rhythm . . . . irregular
Rate . . . . reflects the underlying rhythm
P wave . . . . none with PVC, but P wave present with other QRS complexes
PR interval . . . . unmeasurable except in underlying rhythm
QRS complex . . . . . early, with bizarre configuration and duration of > 0.12 second; QRS
complexes are normal in underlying rhythm

VENTRICULAR TACHYCARDIA

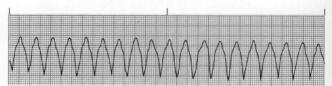

Rhythm . . . . regular
Rate . . . . atrial—can't be determined; ventricular—100 to 250 beats/minute
P wave . . . . absent
PR interval . . . . . . unmeasurable
QRS complex . . . . . > 0.12 second; wide and bizarre

VENTRICULAR FIBRILLATION

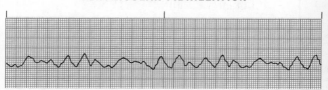

Rhythm . . . . chaotic
Rate . . . . can't be determined
P wave . . . . absent
PR interval . . . . . . unmeasurable
QRS complex . . . . . indiscernible

ASYSTOLE

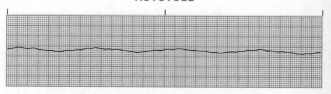

Rhythm . . . . atrial—usually indiscernible; ventricular—absent
Rate . . . . atrial—usually indiscernible; ventricular—absent
P wave . . . . may be present
PR interval . . . . . . unmeasurable
QRS complex . . . . . absent or occasional escape beats

FIRST-DEGREE ATRIOVENTRICULAR BLOCK

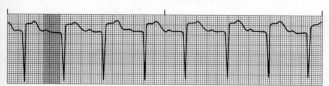

Rhythm . . . . regular
Rate . . . . within normal limits
P wave . . . . normal
PR interval . . . . > 0.20 second (see shaded area) but constant
QRS complex . . . . . 0.06 to 0.10 second

TYPE I SECOND-DEGREE ATRIOVENTRICULAR BLOCK

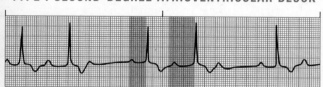

Rhythm . . . . atrial—regular; ventricular—irregular
Rate . . . . atrial—exceeds ventricular rate; both remain within normal limits
P wave . . . . normal
PR interval . . . . progressively prolonged (see shaded areas) until a P wave appears
without a QRS complex
QRS complex . . . . . 0.06 to 0.10 second

TYPE II SECOND-DEGREE ATRIOVENTRICULAR BLOCK

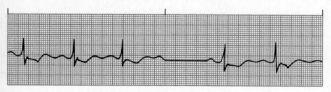

Rhythm . . . . atrial—regular; ventricular—irregular
Rate . . . . atrial—within normal limits; ventricular—slower than atrial but may be
within normal limits
P wave . . . . normal
PR interval . . . . constant for conducted beats
QRS complex . . . . . within normal limits; absent for dropped beats

THIRD-DEGREE ATRIOVENTRICULAR BLOCK

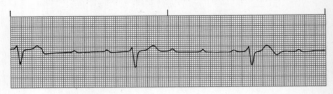

Rhythm .... regular
Rate .... atria and ventricles beat independently; atrial—60 to 100 beats/
minute; ventricular—40 to 60 beats/minute intranodal block (junctional
escape rhythm) < 40 beats/minute intranodal block (ventricular escape
rhythm)
P wave .... normal
PR interval .... varied; not applicable or measurable
QRS complex ..... normal or widened

Gastrostomy feeding button reinsertion

If a gastrostomy feeding button pops out, follow these procedures to reinsert the device.

PREPARE EQUIPMENT

- Collect the feeding button (shown below); wash it with soap and water; rinse thoroughly and dry. Obtain an obturator and water-soluble lubricant.

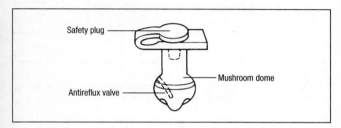

INSERT THE BUTTON

- Check the depth of the patient's stoma to make sure you have a feeding button of the correct size; clean around the stoma.
- Lubricate the obturator with water-soluble lubricant and distend the button several times to ensure the patency of the antireflux valve within the button.
- Lubricate the mushroom dome and stoma. Push the button through the stoma into the stomach (as shown).
- Remove the obturator by rotating it as you withdraw it, to keep the antireflux valve from adhering to it. If the valve sticks, push the obturator back into the button until the valve closes.

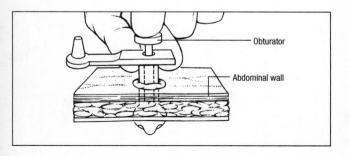

- After removing the obturator, make sure the valve is closed.
- Close the flexible safety plug, which should be relatively flush with the skin surface (as shown).

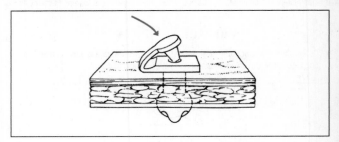

- If you need to give a feeding right away, open the safety plug and attach the feeding adapter and feeding tube (as shown). Deliver feeding as ordered.

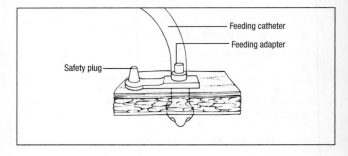

Glasgow Coma Scale

In this test of baseline mental status, a score of 15 indicates that the patient is alert, can follow simple commands, and is oriented to person, place, and time. A decreased score in one or more categories may signal an impending neurologic crisis. A score of 7 or less indicates severe neurologic damage.

Test	Score	Patient response
Eye-opening response		
Spontaneously	4	Opens eyes spontaneously
To speech	3	Opens eyes when instructed
To pain	2	Opens eyes only to painful stimulus
None	1	Doesn't open eyes to stimuli
Motor response		
Obeys	6	Shows two fingers when asked
Localizes	5	Reaches toward painful stimulus and tries to remove it
Withdraws	4	Moves away from painful stimulus
Abnormal flexion	3	Assumes a decorticate posture
Abnormal extension	2	Assumes a decerebrate posture
None	1	No response; just lies flaccid
Verbal response (to question "What year is this?")		
Oriented	5	States correct date
Confused	4	States incorrect year
Inappropriate words	3	Replies randomly with incorrect words
Incomprehensible	2	Moans or screams
No response	1	No response
Total score		

Height and weight conversions

HEIGHT CONVERSION

To convert a patient's height from inches to centimeters, multiply the number of inches by 2.54. To convert a patient's height from centimeters to inches, multiply the number of centimeters by 0.394.

Imperial	Inches	Metric (cm)
4'8"	56	142
4'9"	57	144.5
4'10"	58	147
4'11"	59	150
5'	60	152.5
5'1"	61	155
5'2"	62	157.5
5'3"	63	160
5'4"	64	162.5
5'5"	65	165
5'6"	66	167.5
5'7"	67	170
5'8"	68	172.5
5'9"	69	175
5'10"	70	177.5
5'11"	71	180
6'	72	183
6'1"	73	185.5
6'2"	74	188
6'3"	75	190.5

WEIGHT CONVERSION

To convert a patient's weight from pounds to kilograms, divide the number of pounds by 2.2 kg; to convert a patient's weight from kilograms to pounds, multiply the number of kilograms by 2.2 lb.

Pounds	Kilograms
10	4.5
20	9
30	13.6
40	18.1
50	22.7
60	27.2
70	31.8
80	36.3
90	40.9
100	45.4
110	49.9
120	54.4
130	59
140	63.5
150	68
160	72.6
170	77.1
180	81.6
190	86.2
200	90.8
210	95.5
220	100
230	104.5
240	109.1
250	113.6
260	118.2

Herb-drug interactions

Herb	Drug	Possible effects
echinacea	hepatotoxic drugs	May increase risk of liver damage
	immunosuppressants	Herb may counteract drugs
	warfarin	Increases bleeding time without increased International Normalized Ratio
ginkgo	anticoagulants, antiplatelets	May lead to increased anticoagulation
	anticonvulsants	May decrease effectiveness of drugs
	drugs known to lower seizure threshold	May further reduce seizure threshold
	insulin	Ginkgo leaf extract can affect glucose level
	thiazide diuretics	Ginkgo leaf may increase blood pressure
ginseng	anabolic steroids, hormones	May potentiate effects of drugs
	antibiotics	May enhance effects of some antibiotics
	anticoagulants, antiplatelets	May decrease platelet adhesiveness
	antidiabetics	May enhance glucose-lowering effects
	digoxin	May falsely elevate drug level
	furosemide	May decrease diuretic effect
	warfarin	May reverse drug effects
kava	benzodiazepines	Concurrent use may result in comalike state
	hepatotoxic drugs	May increase the risk of liver damage
	levodopa	Decreases effectiveness of drug

Herb	Drug	Possible effects
St. John's wort	cyclosporine	Reduces drug levels below therapeutic levels
	digoxin	Decreases therapeutic effects of drug
	human immunodeficiency virus protease inhibitors, indinavir, nonnucleoside reverse transcriptase inhibitors	Decreases therapeutic effects of drug
	hormonal contraceptives	Decreases effects of drug
	theophylline	Decreases effects of drug
	warfarin	Decreases effects of drug

Herb usage: Signs and symptoms

Listed below are commonly used herbs and the signs and symptoms that may develop as a result of an adverse reaction to the herb.

Herbs	Major associated signs and symptoms						
	Bleeding	Blood pressure, decreased	Blood pressure, increased	Confusion	Diarrhea	Dizziness	
Aloe					●		
Capsicum	●				●		
Chamomile							
Echinacea							
Ephedra		●	●	●		●	
Evening primrose oil					●		
Fennel							
Feverfew	●					●	
Garlic	●				●		
Ginger	●						
Ginkgo	●				●	●	
Ginseng (Asian, Siberian)		●	●		●	●	
Goldenseal		●	●		●		
Kava	●						
Milk thistle					●		
Passion flower		●		●			
St. John's wort					●		
SAM-e					●		
Saw palmetto			●		●		
Valerian					●		

Dyspnea	Edema, generalized	Erythema	Fatigue	Flatulence	Headache	Insomnia	Level of consciousness, decreased	Nausea	Palpitations	Pulse rhythm abnormalities	Seizure	Tachycardia	Vomiting
	•									•			
•		•											
		•						•					•
								•					•
		•			•	•		•	•	•	•	•	
				•	•			•					•
•		•						•			•		•
		•						•				•	
•		•	•	•	•	•		•				•	•
							•			•			
					•	•		•	•				•
	•				•	•						•	•
		•					•	•		•			•
			•				•						
								•					•
•					•			•		•		•	•
			•		•			•					
					•			•					
					•			•					
		•	•		•	•		•		•			•

I.V. and syringe drug compatibility

KEY	atropine sulfate	butorphanol tartrate	chlorpromazine HCl	cimetidine HCl	codeine phosphate	dexamethasone sodium phosphate	dimenhydrinate	diphenhydramine HCl	droperidol	fentanyl citrate	glycopyrrolate	heparin Na	hydromorphone HCl	hydroxyzine HCl	meperidine HCl	metoclopramide HCl
atropine sulfate		Y	P	Y			P	P	P	P	Y	$P_{(5)}$	Y	P*	P	P
butorphanol tartrate	Y		Y	Y			N	Y	Y	Y				Y	Y	Y
chlorpromazine HCl	P	Y		N			N	P	P	P	Y	N	Y	P	P	P
cimetidine HCl	Y	Y	N					Y	Y	Y	Y	$P_{(5)}$	Y	Y	Y	
codeine phosphate										Y				Y		
dexamethasone sodium phosphate							N*			N			N*			Y
dimenhydrinate	P	N	N					P	P	P	N	$P_{(5)}$	Y	N	P	P
diphenhydramine HCl	P	Y	P	Y		N*	P		P	P	Y		Y	P	P	Y
droperidol	P	Y	P	Y			P	P		P	Y	N	P	P	P	P
fentanyl citrate	P	Y	P	Y			P	P	P			$P_{(5)}$	Y	P	P	P
glycopyrrolate	Y		Y	Y	Y	N	N	Y	Y				Y	Y	Y	
heparin Na	$P_{(5)}$		N	$P_{(5)}$*			$P_{(5)}$		N	$P_{(5)}$					N	$P_{(5)}$*
hydromorphone HCl	Y		Y	Y		N*	Y	Y		Y	Y			Y		
hydroxyzine HCl	P*	Y	P	Y	Y		N	P	P	P	Y		Y		P	P
meperidine HCl	P	Y	P	Y			P	P	P	P		N		P	P	P
metoclopramide HCl	P	Y	P			Y	P	P	P	P		$P_{(5)}$*		P	P	
midazolam HCl	Y	Y	Y	Y			N	Y	Y	Y	Y		Y	Y	Y	Y
morphine sulfate	P	Y	P	Y			P	P	P	P	Y	N*		P	N	P
nalbuphine HCl	Y			Y				Y	Y		Y			Y		
pentazocine lactate	P	Y	P	Y			P	P	P	P	N	N	Y	P	P	P
pentobarbital Na	P	N	N	N			N	N	N	N	N		Y	N	N	
perphenazine	Y	Y	Y	Y			Y	Y	Y	Y				Y	Y	P*
phenobarbital Na												$P_{(5)}$	N			
prochlorperazine edisylate	P	Y	P	Y			N	P	P	P	Y		N*	P	P	P
promazine HCl	P		P	Y			N	P	P	P	Y			P	P	P
promethazine HCl	P	Y	P	Y			N	P	P	P	Y	N	P	P	P	P*
ranitidine HCl	Y		N*		Y		Y	Y	Y		Y		Y	N	Y	Y
scopolamine HBr	P	Y	P	Y			P	P	P	P	Y		Y	P	P	P
secobarbital Na			N									N				
sodium bicarbonate											N					N
thiethylperazine maleate		Y												Y		
thiopental Na			N				N	N			N				N	

KEY
Y = compatible for at least 30 minutes
P = provisionally compatible; administer within 15 minutes
$P_{(5)}$ = provisionally compatible; administer within 5 minutes
N = not compatible
* = conflicting data (A blank space indicates no available data.)

midazolam HCl	morphine sulfate	nalbuphine HCl	pentazocine lactate	pentobarbital Na	perphenazine	phenobarbital Na	prochlorperazine edisylate	promazine HCl	promethazine HCl	ranitidine HCl	scopolamine HBr	secobarbital Na	sodium bicarbonate	thiethylperazine maleate	thiopental Na	
Y	P	Y	P	P	Y		P	P	P	Y	P					atropine sulfate
Y	Y		Y	N	Y		Y		Y		Y			Y		butorphanol tartrate
Y	P		P	N	Y		P	P	P	N*	P				N	chlorpromazine HCl
Y	Y	Y	Y	N	Y		Y	Y	Y		Y	N				cimetidine HCl
																codeine phosphate
										Y						dexamethasone sodium phosphate
N	P		P	N	Y		N	N	N	Y	P				N	dimenhydrinate
Y	P	Y	P	N	Y		P	P	P	Y	P				N	diphenhydramine HCl
Y	P	Y	P	N	Y		P	P	P		P					droperidol
Y	P		P	N	Y		P	P	P	Y	P					fentanyl citrate
Y	Y	Y	N	N			Y	Y	Y	Y	Y	N	N		N	glycopyrrolate
	N*		N			P(5)	N									heparin Na
Y			Y	Y		N	N*		Y	Y	Y			Y		hydromorphone HCl
Y	P	Y	P	N	Y		P	P	P	N	P					hydroxyzine HCl
Y	N		P	N	Y		P	P	P	P	P				N	meperidine HCl
Y	P		P		P*		P	P	P*	Y	P		N			metoclopramide HCl
	Y	Y		N	N		N	Y	Y	N	Y			Y		midazolam HCl
Y			P	N*	Y		P*	P	P*	Y	P				N	morphine sulfate
Y				N			Y		N*	Y	Y			Y		nalbuphine HCl
	P			N	Y		P	P*	P*		Y					pentazocine lactate
N	N*	N	N		N		N	N	N	N	P		Y		Y	pentobarbital Na
N	Y		Y	N			Y		Y	Y	Y		N			perphenazine
											N					phenobarbital Na
N	P*	Y	P	N	Y			P	P	Y	P				N	prochlorperazine edisylate
Y	P		P*	N			P			P	P					promazine HCl
Y	P*	N*	P*	N	Y		P	P		Y	P				N	promethazine HCl
N	Y	Y	Y	Y	N	Y	Y		Y		Y			Y		ranitidine HCl
Y	P	P	P	P	Y		P	P	P	Y					Y	scopolamine HBr
															N	secobarbital Na
				Y												sodium bicarbonate
Y		Y		N						Y						thiethylperazine maleate
	N			Y			N		N			N				thiopental Na

I.V. drug compatibility

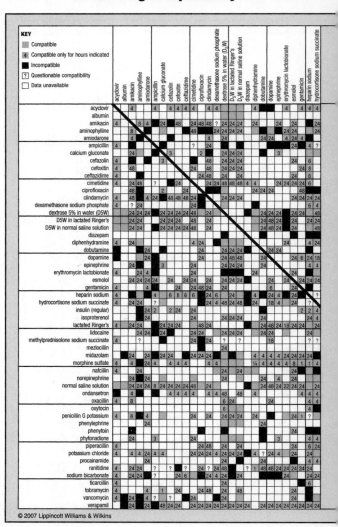

KEY
- Compatible
- 4 Compatible only for hours indicated
- Incompatible
- ? Questionable compatibility
- Data unavailable

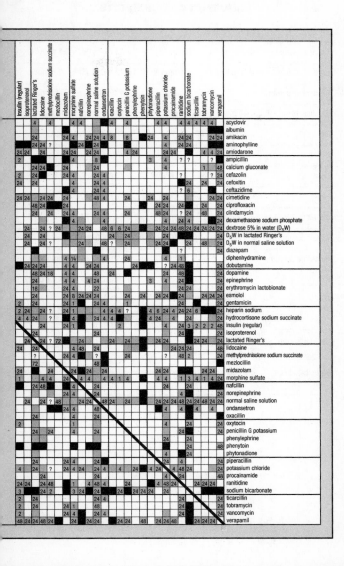

Laboratory values, crisis

Test	Low value	High value
Calcium, serum	< 6 mg/dl (SI, < 1.5 mmol/L)	> 13 mg/dl (SI, > 3.2 mmol/L)
Carbon dioxide	< 10 mEq/L (SI, < 10 mmol/L)	> 40 mEq/L (SI, > 40 mmol/L)
Creatinine, serum	—	> 4 mg/dl (SI, > 353.6 µmol/L)
Glucose, blood	< 40 mg/dl (SI, 2.2 mmol/L)	> 300 mg/dl (SI, > 16.6 mmol/L)
Hb	< 8 g/dl (SI, < 80 g/L)	> 18 g/dl (SI, > 180 g/L)
INR	—	> 3.0
$Paco_2$	< 20 mm Hg (SI, < 2.7 kPa)	> 70 mm Hg (SI, > 9.3 kPa)
Pao_2	< 50 mm Hg (SI, < 6.7 kPa)	—
pH, blood	< 7.2 (SI, < 7.2)	> 7.6 (SI, > 7.6)
Platelet count	< 50,000/µl	> 500,000/mm³
Potassium, serum	< 3 mEq/L (SI, < 3 mmol/L)	> 6 mEq/L (SI, > 6 mmol/L)
PT	—	> 14 sec (SI, > 14 s); for patient on warfarin, > 20 sec (SI, > 20 s)
PTT	—	> 40 sec (SI, > 40 s); for patient on heparin, > 70 sec (SI, > 70 s)
Sodium, serum	< 120 mEq/L (SI, < 120 mmol/L)	> 160 mEq/L (SI, > 160 mmol/L)
White blood cell count	< 2,000/mm³ (SI, < 2 × 10⁹/L)	> 20,000/mm³ (SI, > 20 × 10⁹/L)

Laboratory values, normal

ANTIBIOTIC PEAKS AND TROUGHS

Test	Conventional units	SI units
Amikacin		
Peak	20 to 30 mcg/ml	34 to 52 µmol/L
Trough	1 to 4 mcg/ml	2 to 7 µmol/L
Chloramphenicol		
Peak	15 to 25 mcg/ml	46.4 to 77 µmol/L
Trough	5 to 15 mcg/ml	15.5 to 46.4 µmol/L
Gentamycin		
Peak	4 to 8 mcg/ml	8.4 to 16.7 µmol/L
Trough	1 to 2 mcg/ml	2.1 to 4.2 µmol/L
Tobramycin		
Peak	4 to 8 mcg/ml	8.6 to 17.1 µmol/L
Trough	1 to 2 mcg/ml	2.1 to 4.3 µmol/L
Vancomycin		
Peak	25 to 40 mcg/ml	14 to 27 µmol/L
Trough	5 to 10 mcg/ml	3.4 to 6.8 µmol/L

CARDIAC BIOMARKERS

	Conventional units	SI units
Protein		
Troponin-I	< 0.35 mcg/L	< 0.35 mcg/L
Troponin-T	< 0.1 mcg/L	< 0.1 mcg/L
Myoglobin	< 55 ng/ml	< 55 mcg/L
Hs-CRP	0.020 to 0.800 mg/dl	0.2 to 8 mg/L
Enzyme		
CK	Male: 55 to 170 units/L Female: 30 to 135 units/L	0.94 to 2.89 μkat/L 0.51 to 2.3 μkat/L
CK-MB	< 5%	< 0.05
LD	140 to 280 units/L	2.34 to 4.68 μkat/L
Hormone		
BNP	100 pg/ml	< 100 ng/L

Initial evaluation	Peak	Time to return to normal
4 to 6 hr	12 hr	3 to 10 days
4 to 8 hr	12 to 48 hr	7 to 10 days
2 to 4 hr	8 to 10 hr	24 hr
—	—	Depends on degree of inflammation
—	—	—
—	—	—
4 to 8 hr	12 to 24 hr	72 to 96 hr
2 to 5 days	—	10 days
—	—	Depends on severity of heart failure

CHEMISTRY TESTS, OTHER

Test	Conventional units	SI units
A/G ratio	3.4 to 4.8 g/dl	34 to 38 g/dl
Ammonia	< 50 ng/dl	< 36 µmol/L
Amylase	26 to 102 units/L	0.4 to 1.74 µkat/L
Anion gap	8 to 14 mEq/L	8 to 14 mmol/L
Bilirubin, direct	< 0.5 mg/dl	< 6.8 µmol/L
Calcitonin	Male: < 16 pg/ml Female: < 8 pg/ml	< 16 ng/L < 8 ng/L
Calcium, ionized	4.65 to 5.28 mg/dl	1.1 to 1.25 mmol/L
Cortisol	a.m.: 7 to 25 mcg/dl p.m.: 2 to 14 mcg/dl	0.2 to 0.7 µmol/L 0.06 to 0.39 µmol/L
C-reactive protein	< 0.8 mg/dl	< 8 mg/L
Ferritin	Male: 20 to 300 ng/ml Female: 20 to 120 ng/ml	20 to 300 mcg/L 20 to 120 mcg/L
Folate	2 to 20 ng/ml	4.5 to 45.3 nmol/L
GGT	Male: 7 to 47 units/L Female: 5 to 25 units/L	0.12 to 1.80 µkat/L 0.08 to 0.42 µkat/L
HbA$_{1c}$	4% to 7%	0.04 to 0.07
Homocysteine	< 12 µmol/L	< 12 µmol/L
Iron	Male: 65 to 175 mcg/dl Female: 50 to 170 mcg/dl	11.6 to 31.3 µmol/L 9 to 30.4 µmol/L
Iron-binding capacity	250 to 400 mcg/dl	45 to 72 µmol/L
Lactic acid	0.5 to 2.2 mEq/L	0.5 to 2.2 mmol/L
Lipase	10 to 73 units/L	0.17 to 1.24 µkat/L
Magnesium	1.3 to 2.2 mg/dl	0.65 to 1.05 mmol/L
Osmolality	275 to 295 mOsm/kg	275 to 295 mOsm/kg
Phosphate	2.7 to 4.5 mg/dl	0.87 to 1.45 mmol/L
Prealbumin	19 to 38 mg/dl	190 to 380 mg/L
Uric acid	Male: 3.4 to 7 mg/dl Female: 2.3 to 6 mg/dl	202 to 416 µmol/L 143 to 357 µmol/L

COAGULATION STUDIES

Test	Conventional units	SI units
ACT	107 sec ± 13 sec	107 sec ± 13 sec
Bleeding time	3 to 6 min	3 to 6 min
D-dimer	< 250 mcg/L	< 1.37 nmol/L
Fibrinogen	200 to 400 mg/dl	2 to 4 g/L
INR (target therapeutic)	2.0 to 3.0	2.0 to 3.0
Plasminogen	80% to 130%	—
PT	10 to 14 sec	10 to 14 sec
PTT	21 to 35 sec	21 to 35 sec
Thrombin time	10 to 15 sec	10 to 15 sec

COMPLETE BLOOD COUNT WITH DIFFERENTIAL

Test	Conventional units	SI units
Hemoglobin	Male: 14 to 17.4 g/dl Female: 12 to 16 g/dl	140 to 174 g/L 120 to 160 g/L
Hematocrit	Male: 42% to 52% Female: 36% to 48%	0.42 to 0.52 0.36 to 0.48
RBC	Male: 4.2 to 5.4 $\times$ 10^6/mm^3 Female: 3.6 to 5 $\times$ 10^6/mm^3	4.2 to 5.4 $\times$ 10^{12}/L 3.6 to 5 $\times$ 10^{12}/L
MCH	26 to 34 pg/cell	0.40 to 0.53 fmol/cell
MCHC	32 to 36 g/dl	320 to 360 g/L
MCV	82 to 98 mm^3	82 to 98 fL
WBC	Black: 3.2 to 10 $\times$ 10^3/cells/mm^3 Nonblack: 4.5 to 10.5 $\times$ 10^3/cells/mm^3	3.2 to 10 $\times$ 10^9/L 4.5 to 10.5 $\times$ 10^9/L
Bands	0% to 3%	0 to 0.03
Basophils	0% to 1%	0 to 0.01
Eosinophils	0% to 3%	0 to 0.03
Lymphocytes	25% to 40%	0.25 to 0.40
Monocytes	3% to 7%	0.03 to 0.07
Neutrophils	54% to 75%	0.54 to 0.75
Platelets	140,000 to 400,000/mm^3	140 to 400 $\times$ 10^9/L

COMPREHENSIVE METABOLIC PANEL

Test	Conventional units	SI units
Albumin	3.5 to 5 g/dl	35 to 50 g/L
Alkaline phosphatase	45 to 115 units/L	45 to 115 units/L
ALT	Male: 10 to 40 units/L Female: 7 to 35 units/L	0.17 to 0.68 µkat/L 0.12 to 0.60 µkat/L
AST	12 to 31 units/L	0.21 to 0.53 µkat/L
Bilirubin, total	0.2 to 1 mg/dl	3.5 to 17 µmol/L
BUN	6 to 20 mg/dl	2.1 to 7.1 mmol/L
Calcium	8.2 to 10.2 mg/dl	2.05 to 2.54 mmol/L
Carbon dioxide	22 to 26 mEq/L	22 to 26 mmol/L
Chloride	100 to 108 mEq/L	100 to 108 mmol/L
Creatinine	Male: 0.8 to 1.2 mg/dl Female: 0.6 to 0.9 mg/dl	62 to 115 µmol/L 53 to 97 µmol/L
Glucose	70 to 100 mg/dl	3.9 to 6.1 mmol/L
Potassium	3.5 to 5 mEq/L	3.5 to 5 mmol/L
Protein, total	6.3 to 8.3 g/dl	64 to 83 g/L
Sodium	135 to 145 mEq/L	135 to 145 mmol/L

CSF ANALYSIS

Test	Normal	Abnormal	Implications
Pressure	50 to 180 mm H_2O	Increase	Increased ICP
		Decrease	Spinal subarachnoid obstruction above puncture site
Appearance	Clear, colorless	Cloudy Xanthochromic or bloody	Infection Subarachnoid, intracerebral, or intraventricular hemorrhage; spinal cord obstruction; traumatic lumbar puncture (only in initial specimen)
		Brown, orange, or yellow	Elevated protein levels, RBC breakdown (blood present for at least 3 days)
Protein	15 to 50 mg/dl (SI, 0.15 to 0.5 g/L)	Marked increase	Tumors, trauma, hemorrhage, diabetes mellitus, polyneuritis, blood in CSF
		Marked decrease	Rapid CSF production
Gamma globulin	3% to 12% of total protein	Increase	Demyelinating disease, neurosyphilis, Guillain-Barré syndrome
Glucose	50 to 80 mg/dl (SI, 2.8 to 4.4 mmol/L)	Increase	Systemic hyperglycemia
		Decrease	Systemic hypoglycemia, bacterial or fungal infection, meningitis, mumps, postsubarachnoid hemorrhage
Cell count	0 to 5 WBCs	Increase	Active disease: meningitis, acute infection, onset of chronic illness, tumor, abscess, infarction, demyelinating disease
	No RBCs	RBCs	Hemorrhage or traumatic lumbar puncture
VDRL	Nonreactive	Positive	Neurosyphilis
Chloride	118 to 130 mEq/L (SI, 118 to 130 mmol/L)	Decrease	Infected meninges
Gram stain	No organisms	Gram-positive or gram-negative organisms	Bacterial meningitis

HEMATOLOGY TESTS, OTHER

Test	Conventional units	SI units
Erythrocyte sedimentation rate	Male: 0 to 10 mm/hr Female: 0 to 20 mm/hr	0 to 10 mm/hr 0 to 20 mm/hr
Pyruvate kinase	2.8 to 8.8 units/g Hb	46.7 to 146.7 μkat/g Hb

LIPID PANEL

Test	Conventional units	SI units
Total cholesterol	< 200 mg/dl	< 5.18 mmol/L
HDL cholesterol	$\geq$ 60 mg/dl	$\geq$ 1.55 mmol/L
LDL cholesterol	< 130 mg/dl	< 3.36 mmol/L
Triglycerides	< 150 mg/dl	< 1.7 mmol/L

THERAPEUTIC DRUG MONITORING

Drug	Laboratory test	Therapeutic range
Digoxin	Digoxin	0.8 to 2 mg/ml (SI, 1 to 2.6 mmol/L)
Phenytoin	Phenytoin	10 to 20 mcg/ml (SI, 40 to 79 μmol/L)
Procainamide	Procainamide	4 to 10 mcg/ml (SI, 17 to 42 μmol/L)
	N-acetylprocainamide (NAPA)	5 to 30 mcg/ml (combined procainamide and NAPA)
Theophylline	Theophylline	10 to 20 mcg/ml (SI, 44 to 111 μmol/L)

THYROID PANEL

Test	Conventional units	SI units
T_3	80 to 200 ng/dl	1.2 to 3 nmol/L
T_4, free	0.7 to 2 ng/dl	10 to 26 pmol/L
T_4, total	5.4 to 11.5 mcg/dl	57 to 148 nmol/L
TSH	0.4 to 4.2 mIU/L	0.4 to 4.2 mIU/L

TUMOR MARKERS

Test	Conventional units	SI units
Alpha-fetoprotein	< 40 ng/ml	< 40 mcg/L
CA 15-3	< 30 units/ml	< 30 kU/L
CA 19-9	< 37 units/ml	< 37 kU/L
CA 27-29	≤ 38 units/ml	≤ 38 kU/L
CA 125	< 35 units/ml	< 35 kU/L
Carcinoembryonic antigen	< 2.5 to 5 ng/ml	< 2.5 to 5 mcg/L
Human chorionic gonadotropin	< 2 ng/ml	< 2 mcg/L
Neuron-specific enolase	< 12.5 mcg/ml	—
Prostate-specific antigen	Age 40 to 49: ≤ 2.5 ng/ml Age 50 to 59: ≤ 3.5 ng/ml Age 60 to 69: ≤ 4.5 ng/ml Age 70+: ≤ 6.5 ng/ml	≤ 2.5 mcg/L ≤ 3.5 mcg/L ≤ 4.5 mcg/L ≤ 6.5 mcg/L

URINE TESTS

Test	Conventional units	SI units
Urinalysis		
Appearance	Clear to slightly hazy	—
Color	Straw to dark yellow	—
pH	4.5 to 8	—
Specific gravity	1.005 to 1.035	—
Glucose	None	—
Protein	None	—
RBCs	None or rare	—
WBCs	None or rare	—
Osmolality	50 to 1,400 mOsm/kg	—

Latex allergy screening

To determine if your patient has a latex sensitivity or allergy, ask the following screening questions:

■ What is your occupation?
■ Have you experienced an allergic reaction, local sensitivity, or itching after exposure to any latex products, such as balloons or condoms?
■ Do you have shortness of breath or wheezing after blowing up balloons or after a dental visit? Do you have itching in or around your mouth after eating a banana?

If your patient answers "yes" to any of these questions, proceed with the following questions:

■ Do you have a history of allergies, dermatitis, or asthma? If so, what type of reaction do you have?
■ Do you have any congenital abnormalities? If yes, explain.
■ Do you have any food allergies? If so, what specific allergies do you have? Describe your reaction.
■ If you experience shortness of breath or wheezing when blowing up latex balloons, describe your reaction.
■ Have you had any previous surgical procedures? Did you experience associated complications? If so, describe them.
■ Have you had previous dental procedures? Did you have any complications? If so, describe them.
■ Are you exposed to latex in your occupation? Do you experience a reaction to latex products at work? If so, describe your reaction.

Magnesium disorders

CLINICAL EFFECTS OF HYPERMAGNESEMIA

Body system	Effects
Cardiovascular	■ Bradycardia, weak pulse, hypotension, heart block, cardiac arrest
Neurologic	■ Drowsiness, flushing, lethargy, confusion, diminished sensorium
Neuromuscular	■ Diminished reflexes, muscle weakness, flaccid paralysis, respiratory muscle paralysis that may cause respiratory embarrassment

CLINICAL EFFECTS OF HYPOMAGNESEMIA

Body system	Effects
Cardiovascular	■ Arrhythmias, vasomotor changes (vasodilation and hypotension) and, occasionally, hypertension
Neurologic	■ Confusion, delusions, hallucinations, seizures
Neuromuscular	■ Hyperirritability, tetany, leg and foot cramps, Chvostek's sign (facial muscle spasms induced by tapping the branches of the facial nerve)

Metric system equivalents and weight conversions

Metric system equivalents

Metric weight

1 kilogram (kg or Kg)	= 1,000 grams (g or gm)
1 gram	= 1,000 milligrams (mg)
1 milligram	= 1,000 micrograms (mcg)
0.6 g	= 600 mg
0.3 g	= 300 mg
0.1 g	= 100 mg
0.06 g	= 60 mg
0.03 g	= 30 mg
0.015 g	= 15 mg
0.001g	= 1 mg

Metric volume

1 liter (l or L)	= 1,000 milliliters (ml)*
1 milliliter	= 1,000 microliters (µl)

Household metric

1 teaspoon (tsp)	= 5 ml
1 tablespoon (T or tbs)	= 15 ml
2 tablespoons	= 30 ml
8 ounces	= 236.6 ml
1 pint (pt)	= 473 ml
1 quart (qt)	= 946 ml
1 gallon (gal)	= 3,785 ml

Weight conversions

1 oz = 30 g
1 lb = 453.6 g
2.2 lb = 1 kg

* 1 ml = 1 cubic centimeter (cc); however, ml is the preferred measurement term used today.

Musculoskeletal system assessment

NORMAL FINDINGS

Inspection
- No gross deformities
- Symmetrical body parts
- Good body alignment
- No involuntary movements
- Smooth gait
- Active range of motion (ROM) and no pain in muscles and joints
- No swelling or inflammation visible in muscles or joints
- Equal bilateral limb length and symmetrical muscle mass

Palpation
- Normal shape, with no swelling or tenderness
- Equal bilateral muscle tone, texture, and strength
- No involuntary contractions or twitching
- Equally strong bilateral pulses

GRADING MUSCLE STRENGTH

5/5: Normal: patient moves joint through full ROM and against gravity with full resistance
4/5: Good: patient completes ROM against gravity with moderate resistance
3/5: Fair: patient completes ROM against gravity only
2/5: Poor: patient completes full ROM with gravity eliminated (passive motion)
1/5: Trace: patient's attempt at muscle contraction is palpable but without joint movement
0/5: Zero: no evidence of muscle contraction

THE 5 P's OF MUSCULOSKELETAL INJURY

To assess a musculoskeletal injury, remember the 5 P's.

Pain
Ask the patient if he feels pain.

Paresthesia
Assess for loss of sensation.

Paralysis
Assess whether the patient can move the affected area.

Pallor
Paleness, discoloration, and coolness on the injured side may indicate neurovascular compromise.

Pulse
Check all pulses distal to the injury site.

Neurologic system assessment

LEVEL OF CONSCIOUSNESS ASSESSMENT

Classification	Description
Alert	■ Follows commands and responds completely and appropriately to stimuli ■ Oriented to time, place, and person
Lethargy	■ Limited spontaneous movement or speech ■ Easy to arouse by normal speech or touch ■ Possible disorientation to time, place, or person
Obtundation	■ Limited responsiveness to environment ■ Mild to moderate reduction in arousal ■ Able to fall asleep easily ■ Answers questions with minimum response
Stupor	■ State of deep sleep or unresponsiveness ■ Arousable (motor or verbal response) only to vigorous and repeated stimulation ■ Withdrawal or grabbing response to stimulation
Coma	■ No motor or verbal response to any stimuli ■ No response to noxious stimuli such as deep pain ■ Unarousable

PUPIL MEASUREMENT

1 MM	2 MM	3 MM
4 MM	5 MM	6 MM
7 MM	8 MM	9 MM

SIGNS OF INCREASED ICP

	Early signs	Late signs
Level of consciousness	■ Requires increased stimulation ■ Subtle orientation loss ■ Restlessness and anxiety ■ Sudden quietness	■ Unarousable
Pupils	■ One pupil constricts but then dilates (unilateral hippus) ■ Both pupils sluggish ■ Unequal pupils	■ Pupils fixed and dilated or "blown"
Motor response	■ Sudden weakness ■ Motor changes ■ Positive pronator drift (with palms up, one hand pronates)	■ Profound weakness
Vital signs	■ Increased blood pressure	■ Increased systolic blood pressure, profound bradycardia, abnormal respirations

Oxygen therapy

Oxygen delivery equipment	Oxygen concentration administered
Nasal cannula	1 to 6 L/min (24% to 40% fraction of inspired oxygen [Fio_2])
Simple mask	5 to 8 L/min (40% to 60% Fio_2)
Partial rebreather mask	6 to 15 L/min (55% to 90% Fio_2)
Nonrebreather mask	6 to 15 L/min (55% to 90% Fio_2)
Venturi mask	4 to 10 L/min (24% to 55% Fio_2, depending on manufacturer)
Continuous positive airway pressure mask	Variable
Transtracheal oxygen	Variable
Aerosol mask	10 to 15 L/min
Handheld resuscitation bag (Ambu bag)	15 L/min

Pacemakers: Transcutaneous placement, malfunctions, and codes

TRANSCUTANEOUS PACEMAKER

Transcutaneous pacing involves the delivery of electrical impulses through externally applied cutaneous electrodes. The impulses are conducted through an intact chest wall using skin electrodes placed in either anterior-posterior (shown below) or sternal-apex positions.

Transcutaneous pacing is the pacing method of choice in emergency situations because it's the least invasive technique and it can be instituted quickly.

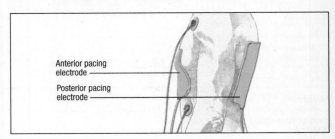

Anterior pacing electrode ——

Posterior pacing electrode ——

UNDERSTANDING PERMANENT PACEMAKER CODES

A permanent pacemaker's three-letter (or sometimes five-letter) code simply refers to how it's programmed.

First letter (chamber that's paced)	Second letter (chamber that's sensed)	Third letter (pulse generator's response)	Fourth letter (pacemaker's programmability)	Fifth letter (pacemaker's response to tachycardia)
A atrium	**A** atrium	**I** inhibited	**P** basic functions programmable	**P** pacing ability
V ventricle	**V** ventricle	**T** triggered	**M** multiple programmable parameters	**S** shock
D dual (both chambers)	**D** dual (both chambers)	**D** dual (inhibited and triggered)	**C** communicating functions such as telemetry	**D** dual ability to shock and pace
O not applicable	**O** not applicable	**O** not applicable	**R** rate responsiveness	**O** none
			N none	

TEMPORARY PACEMAKER MALFUNCTIONS

Occasionally, a temporary pacemaker may fail to function appropriately. When this occurs, you'll need to take immediate action to correct the problem. Take the steps described below when your patient's pacemaker fails to pace, capture, or sense intrinsic beats.

Failure to pace

This happens when the pacemaker either doesn't fire or fires too often. The pulse generator may not be working properly, or it may not be conducting the impulse to the patient.

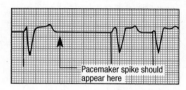
Pacemaker spike should appear here

Nursing interventions

- If the pacing or sensing indicator flashes, check the connections to the cable and the position of the pacing electrode in the patient (by X-ray). The cable may have come loose, or the electrode may have been dislodged, pulled out, or broken.
- If the pulse generator is turned on but the indicators still aren't flashing, change the battery. If that doesn't help, use a different pulse generator.
- Check the settings if the pacemaker is firing too rapidly. If they're correct, or if altering them (according to facility policy or physician's order) doesn't help, change the pulse generator.

Failure to capture

In failure to capture, you see the pacemaker spikes but the heart isn't responding. This may be caused by changes in the pacing threshold from ischemia, an electrolyte imbalance (high or low potassium or magnesium levels), acidosis, an adverse reaction to

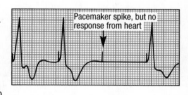
Pacemaker spike, but no response from heart

a medication, a perforated ventricle, fibrosis, or the position of the electrode.

Nursing interventions

- If the patient's condition has changed, notify the physician and ask him for new settings.
- If the pacemaker settings have been altered by the patient (or his family members), return them to their correct positions. Then make sure the face of the pacemaker is covered with a plastic shield. Tell the patient and his family members not to touch the dials.
- If the heart isn't responding, try these suggestions: Carefully check all connections, making sure they're placed properly and securely; increase the milliamperes slowly (according to facility policy or physician's order); turn the patient on his left side, then on his right (if turning him to the left didn't help); schedule an anteroposterior or lateral chest X-ray to determine the position of the electrode.

Failure to sense intrinsic beats

This could cause ventricular tachycardia or ventricular fibrillation if the pacemaker fires on the vulnerable T wave. This could be caused by the pacemaker sensing an external stimu-

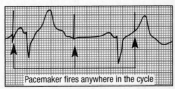

Pacemaker fires anywhere in the cycle

lus as a QRS complex, which could lead to asystole, or by the pacemaker not being sensitive enough, which means it could fire anywhere within the cardiac cycle.

Nursing interventions

- If the pacing is undersensing, turn the sensitivity control completely to the right. If it's oversensing, turn it slightly to the left.
- If the pacemaker isn't functioning correctly, change the battery or the pulse generator.
- Remove items in the room that may be causing electromechanical interference (such as razors, radios, and cautery devices). Check the ground wires on the bed and other equipment for obvious damage. Unplug each piece and see if the interference stops. When you locate the cause, notify the staff engineer and ask him to check it.
- If the pacemaker is still firing on the T wave and all else has failed, turn off the pacemaker. Make sure atropine is available in case the patient's heart rate drops. Be prepared to call a code and institute cardiopulmonary resuscitation if necessary.

Pain medications for adults

OPIOIDS

Drug	Oral dosage	Parenteral dosage
codeine	15 to 60 mg q 4 to 6 hr	15 to 60 mg q 4 to 6 hr
hydromorphone	2 to 4 mg q 4 to 6 hr	2 to 4 mg subQ, I.M., or I.V. (over 2 to 5 min) q 4 to 6 hr
meperidine	50 to 150 mg q 3 to 4 hr	50 to 150 mg subQ or I.M. q 3 to 4 hr
methadone	2.5 to 10 mg q 3 to 4 hr	2.5 to 4 mg subQ or I.M. q 3 to 4 hr
morphine	5 to 30 mg q 4 hr	5 to 20 mg subQ or I.M. q 4 hr or 2.5 to 15 mg I.V. q 4 hr
oxycodone	5 mg q 6 hr	N/A
oxymorphone	N/A	0.5 mg I.V., or 1 to 1.5 mg subQ or I.M. q 4 to 6 hr
propoxyphene	HCl: 65 mg q 4 hr napsylate: 100 mg q 4 hr	N/A
tramadol	50 to 100 mg P.O. q 4 to 6 hr	N/A

Pain rating scales

NUMERIC PAIN RATING SCALE

A numeric rating scale can help the patient quantify his pain. Have him choose a number from 0 (indicating no pain) to 10 (indicating the worst pain imaginable) to reflect his current pain level. He can either circle the number on the scale itself or verbally state the number that best describes his pain.

NO
PAIN   0   1   2   3   4   5   6   7   8   9   10   PAIN AS BAD
                                                      AS IT CAN BE

VISUAL ANALOG SCALE

To use the visual analog scale, ask the patient to place a mark on the scale to indicate his current level of pain.

NO   PAIN AS BAD
PAIN |--| AS IT CAN BE

WONG-BAKER FACES PAIN RATING SCALE

A pediatric patient or an adult patient with language difficulties may not be able to express the pain he's feeling. In such cases, use the pain intensity scale below. Ask the patient to choose the face that best represents the severity of his pain on a scale from 0 to 10.

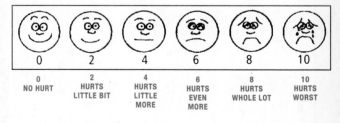

0	2	4	6	8	10
0 NO HURT	2 HURTS LITTLE BIT	4 HURTS LITTLE MORE	6 HURTS EVEN MORE	8 HURTS WHOLE LOT	10 HURTS WORST

From Wong, D.L., et al. *Wong's Essentials of Pediatric Nursing*, 6th ed. St. Louis: Mosby–Year Book, Inc., 2001. Reprinted with permission.

Peripheral vascular assessment

PULSE POINTS

Shown below are anatomic locations where an artery crosses bone or firm tissue and can be palpated for a pulse.

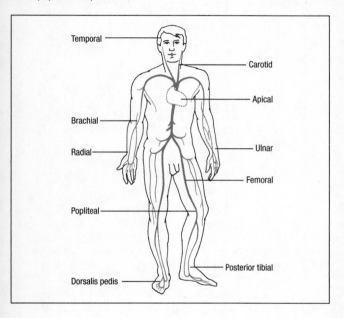

GRADING PULSES

Pulses should be regular in rhythm and strength. Check carotid, brachial, radial, femoral, popliteal, posterior tibial, and dorsalis pedis pulses. Grade them using the numerical scale below.

$$4+ = \text{bounding}$$
$$3+ = \text{increased}$$
$$2+ = \text{normal}$$
$$1 = \text{weak}$$
$$0 = \text{absent}$$

PITTING EDEMA SCALE

0	None observed
+1	Minimal (< 2 mm)
+2	Depression 2 to 4 mm
+3	Depression 4 to 6 mm
+4	Depression > 7 mm

CAPILLARY REFILL

Normal: < 3 sec
Abnormal: > 3 sec

Peritoneal dialysis setup

This illustration shows the proper setup for peritoneal dialysis.

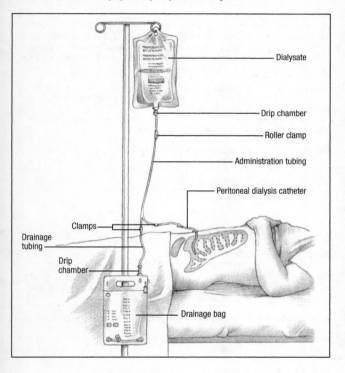

Potassium disorders

CLINICAL EFFECTS OF HYPERKALEMIA

Body system	Effects
Cardiovascular	■ Tachycardia and later bradycardia, ECG changes (tented and elevated T waves, widened QRS complex, prolonged PR interval, flattened or absent P waves, depressed ST segment), cardiac arrest (with levels > 7 mEq/L)
Gastrointestinal	■ Nausea, diarrhea, abdominal cramps
Genitourinary	■ Oliguria, anuria
Musculoskeletal	■ Muscle weakness, flaccid paralysis
Neurologic	■ Hyperreflexia progressing to weakness, numbness, tingling, flaccid paralysis
Other	■ Metabolic acidosis

CLINICAL EFFECTS OF HYPOKALEMIA

Body system	Effects
Cardiovascular	■ Dizziness, hypotension, arrhythmias, ECG changes (flattened T waves, elevated U waves, decreased ST segments), cardiac arrest (with levels < 2.5 mEq/L)
Gastrointestinal	■ Nausea, vomiting, anorexia, diarrhea, abdominal distention, paralytic ileus or decreased peristalsis
Genitourinary	■ Polyuria
Musculoskeletal	■ Muscle weakness and fatigue, leg cramps
Neurologic	■ Malaise, irritability, confusion, mental depression, speech changes, decreased reflexes, respiratory paralysis
Other	■ Metabolic alkalosis

Respiratory assessment:
Breath sounds and breathing patterns

ABNORMAL BREATH SOUNDS

Sound	Description
Crackles	Light crackling, popping, intermittent nonmusical sounds — like hairs being rubbed together — heard on inspiration or expiration
Pleural friction rub	Low-pitched, continual, superficial, squeaking or grating sound — like pieces of sandpaper being rubbed together — heard on inspiration and expiration
Rhonchi	Low-pitched, monophonic snoring sounds heard primarily on expiration but also throughout the respiratory cycle
Stridor	High-pitched, monophonic crowing sound heard on inspiration; louder in the neck than in the chest wall
Wheezes	High-pitched, continual musical or whistling sound heard primarily on expiration but sometimes also on inspiration

ABNORMAL BREATHING PATTERNS

This chart shows several common types of irregular respiratory patterns and their possible causes. It's important to assess the patient for the underlying cause and the effect on the patient.

Type	Characteristics	Possible causes
Apnea	Periodic absence of breathing	■ Mechanical airway obstruction ■ Conditions affecting the brain's respiratory center in the lateral medulla oblongata
Apneustic breathing	Prolonged, gasping inspiration followed by extremely short, inefficient expiration	■ Lesions of the respiratory center
Bradypnea	Slow, regular respirations of equal depth	■ Normal pattern during sleep ■ Conditions affecting the respiratory center: tumors, metabolic disorders, respiratory decompensation, and use of opiates or alcohol
Cheyne-Stokes respirations	Fast, deep respirations of 30 to 170 seconds punctuated by periods of apnea lasting 20 to 60 seconds	■ Increased intracranial pressure, severe heart failure, renal failure, meningitis, drug overdose, and cerebral anoxia
Kussmaul's respirations	Fast (over 20 breaths/minute), deep (resembling sighs), labored respirations without pause	■ Renal failure and metabolic acidosis, particularly diabetic ketoacidosis
Tachypnea	Rapid respirations; rate rises with body temperature—about 4 breaths/minute for every degree Fahrenheit above normal	■ Pneumonia, compensatory respiratory alkalosis, respiratory insufficiency, lesions of the respiratory center, and salicylate poisoning

Respiratory system: Assessment landmarks

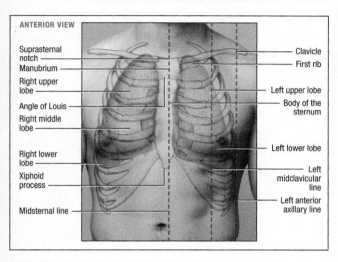

ANTERIOR VIEW

- Suprasternal notch
- Manubrium
- Right upper lobe
- Angle of Louis
- Right middle lobe
- Right lower lobe
- Xiphoid process
- Midsternal line

- Clavicle
- First rib
- Left upper lobe
- Body of the sternum
- Left lower lobe
- Left midclavicular line
- Left anterior axillary line

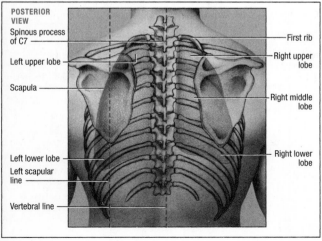

POSTERIOR VIEW

- Spinous process of C7
- Left upper lobe
- Scapula
- Left lower lobe
- Left scapular line
- Vertebral line

- First rib
- Right upper lobe
- Right middle lobe
- Right lower lobe

Sodium disorders

CLINICAL EFFECTS OF HYPERNATREMIA

Body system	Effects
Cardiovascular	■ Hypertension, tachycardia, pitting edema, excessive weight gain
Gastrointestinal	■ Rough, dry tongue; intense thirst
Genitourinary	■ Oliguria
Integumentary	■ Flushed skin; dry, sticky membranes
Neurologic	■ Fever, agitation, restlessness, seizures
Respiratory	■ Dyspnea, respiratory arrest, death (from dramatic rise in osmotic pressure)

CLINICAL EFFECTS OF HYPONATREMIA

Body system	Effects
Cardiovascular	■ Hypotension; tachycardia; with severe deficit, vasomotor collapse, thready pulse
Gastrointestinal	■ Nausea, vomiting, abdominal cramps
Genitourinary	■ Oliguria or anuria
Integumentary	■ Cold, clammy skin; decreasing skin turgor
Neurologic	■ Anxiety, headaches, muscle twitching and weakness, seizures
Respiratory	■ Cyanosis with severe deficiency

Temperature conversions

Fahrenheit degrees	Celsius degrees	Fahrenheit degrees	Celsius degrees	Fahrenheit degrees	Celsius degrees
106.0	41.1	100.6	38.1	95.2	35.1
105.8	41.0	100.4	38.0	95.0	35.0
105.6	40.9	100.2	37.9	94.8	34.9
105.4	40.8	100.0	37.8	94.6	34.8
105.2	40.7	99.8	37.7	94.4	34.7
105.0	40.6	99.6	37.6	94.2	34.6
104.8	40.4	99.4	37.4	94.0	34.4
104.6	40.3	99.2	37.3	93.8	34.3
104.4	40.2	99.0	37.2	93.6	34.2
104.2	40.1	98.8	37.1	93.4	34.1
104.0	40.0	98.6	37.0	93.2	34.0
103.8	39.9	98.4	36.9	93.0	33.9
103.6	39.8	98.2	36.8	92.8	33.8
103.4	39.7	98.0	36.7	92.6	33.7
103.2	39.6	97.8	36.6	92.4	33.6
103.0	39.4	97.6	36.4	92.2	33.4
102.8	39.3	97.4	36.3	92.0	33.3
102.6	39.2	97.2	36.2	91.8	33.2
102.4	39.1	97.0	36.1	91.6	33.1
102.2	39.0	96.8	36.0	91.4	33.0
102.0	38.9	96.6	35.9	91.2	32.9
101.8	38.8	96.4	35.8	91.0	32.8
101.6	38.7	96.2	35.7	90.8	32.7
101.4	38.6	96.0	35.6	90.6	32.6
101.2	38.4	95.8	35.4	90.4	32.4
101.0	38.3	95.6	35.3	90.2	32.3
100.8	38.2	95.4	35.2	90.0	32.2

Selected references
Index

Selected references

Bell, D. "Heart Failure: A Serious and Common Comorbidity of Diabetes," *Clinical Diabetes* 22(2):61-65, Spring 2004.

Broyles, B. *Medical-Surgical Nursing Clinical Companion.* Durham: Carolina Academic Press, 2004.

Heitkemper, M.M., et al. *Medical Surgical Nursing: Assessment and Management of Clinical Problems,* 6th ed. St. Louis: Mosby–Year Book, Inc., 2003.

Huether, S.E., and McCance, K.L. *Understanding Pathophysiology,* 3rd ed. St. Louis: Mosby–Year Book, Inc., 2004.

Ignatavicius, D.D., and Workman, M.L. *Medical-Surgical Nursing: Critical Thinking for Collaborative Care,* 5th ed. Philadelphia: W.B. Saunders Co., 2005.

Koennecke, H.C. "Secondary Prevention of Stroke: A Practical Guide to Drug Treatment," *CNS Drugs* 18(4):221-41, March 2004.

Kuwabara, S. "Guillain-Barré Syndrome: Epidemiology, Pathophysiology and Management," *Drugs* 64(6):597-610, 2004.

Lemone, P., and Burke, K. *Medical-Surgical Nursing: Critical Thinking in Client Care,* 3rd ed. Upper Saddle River, N.J.: Prentice Hall Health, 2003.

Medical-Surgical Nursing Made Incredibly Easy. Philadelphia: Lippincott Williams & Wilkins, 2004.

Nettina, S. M. *Lippincott Manual of Nursing Practice,* 8th ed. Philadelphia: Lippincott Williams & Wilkins, 2006.

Smeltzer, S.C., and Bare, B.G. *Brunner & Suddarth's Textbook of Medical-Surgical Nursing,* 10th ed. Philadelphia: Lippincott Williams & Wilkins, 2004.

Whitman, M.M. "Professional Development: Return and Report: Establishing Accountability in Delegation," *American Journal of Nursing* 105(3):97, March 2005.

Index

A

Abdominal aortic aneurysm, 31-34
  assessment findings in, 31-32
  nursing interventions for, 33-34
  treatment of, 32, 33i
Abdominal quadrants, 476i
Acceleration-deceleration injuries, 2-4
  assessment findings in, 2
  nursing interventions for, 3-4
  treatment of, 2-3, 3i
Acute infective tubulointerstitial
     nephritis. *See* Pyelonephritis,
     acute.
Acute leukemia. *See* Leukemia, acute.
Acute poststreptococcal glomerulo-
     nephritis. *See* Glomerulo-
     nephritis.
Acute tubulointerstitial nephritis. *See*
     Tubular necrosis, acute.
Addisonian crisis, 8
Addison's disease. *See* Adrenal
     hypofunction.
Adrenal crisis, 8
Adrenalectomy, 286-287
  postprocedure care for, 287
  procedure for, 286
  purpose of, 286
Adrenal hypofunction, 8-12
  assessment findings in, 10
  nursing interventions for, 11-12
  treatment of, 10
Alzheimer's disease, 12-14
  assessment findings in, 12-13
  nursing interventions for, 14

Alzheimer's disease *(continued)*
  treatment of, 13-14
Ambulatory electrocardiogram. *See*
     Holter monitoring.
Amputation, 287-289
  postprocedure care for, 288-289
  procedure for, 288
  purpose of, 287-288
  traumatic, caring for body part in,
     394i
  types of, 287
Amyotrophic lateral sclerosis, 15-17
  assessment findings in, 15
  modifying home for patient
     with, 17
  nursing interventions for, 16-17
  treatment of, 16
Anaphylaxis, 17-20
  assessment findings in, 18
  nursing interventions for, 19-20
  treatment of, 18-19
Anemia, aplastic, 20-22
  assessment findings in, 20-21
  nursing interventions for, 22
  treatment of, 21
Angina, 86. *See also* Coronary artery
     disease.
Anthropometric arm measurements,
     205i
Antidotes to drug and toxin overdos-
     es, 477t
Aortic insufficiency, 35-38
  assessment findings in, 35-36, 36i
  nursing interventions for, 37-38

---

i refers to an illustration; t refers to a table.

i refers to an illustration; t refers to a table.

i refers to an illustration; t refers to a table.

i refers to an illustration; t refers to a table.

i refers to an illustration; t refers to a table.

i refers to an illustration; t refers to a table.

i refers to an illustration; t refers to a table.

i refers to an illustration; t refers to a table.

i refers to an illustration; t refers to a table.

i refers to an illustration; t refers to a table.

i refers to an illustration; t refers to a table.

---

i refers to an illustration; t refers to a table.